THE
REALAGE
DIET

Also by Michael F. Roizen, M.D.
RealAge: Are You as Young as You Can Be?

THE

REALAGE

DET MAKE YOURSELF
YOUNGER WITH
WHAT YOU EAT

MICHAEL F. ROIZEN, M.D.
and JOHN LA PUMA, M.D.

Cliff Street Books

An Imprint of HarperCollins*Publishers*

FIRST EDITION

Designed by Stratford Publishing Services

Library of Congress Cataloging-in-Publication Data

Roizen, Michael F.
    The real age diet : make yourself younger with what you eat / by Michael F. Roizen and John La Puma.
        p.   cm.
    Includes bibliographical references and index.
    ISBN 0-06-019679-3
        1. Nutrition.   2. Health.   3. Longevity.   I. La Puma, John.   II. Title.

RA784.R635 2001
613.2—dc21   2001028049

01 02 03 04 05   10 9 8 7 6 5 4 3 2 1

To my family, for their enthusiasm for RealAge and their patience with the project and my endless kitchen and food experiments. They not only help me stay young but are the reason I want to be young.

M. R.

To my patients, for their creativity and spirit, and for allowing me to believe in them and their success. May the pleasures of the table and youthful energy be theirs.

J. L.

Contents

A Note from Michael Roizen, M.D., Author of *RealAge: Are You as Young as You Can Be?*

When I was writing *RealAge,* my colleagues often asked me, "Why are you so excited about writing this book?" The answer was easy. "I've found a way to explain difficult medical concepts so that patients know how much control they have over their health," I told them. "The concept has been so motivating for both my patients and myself that I want to share it. It could very possibly change the health of the nation!"

Those who knew me knew that I set big goals. Those who didn't know me so well just told me I was wasting my time—that it was unlikely a doctor who was so grounded in science and had written only scientific papers and books could write a book that a major publishing house would take. They said it was even less likely that the general public would read it. They often ended the conversation with, "Stick to basic science research." But I couldn't stop.

Well, people bought the book like hotcakes, and they jammed our website, even crashing it twice. *RealAge* became a bestseller in the United States, Canada, Brazil, and Great Britain. The book even temporarily bumped a Harry Potter book from the number one position on the Amazon.com bestseller list.

Why?

RealAge presented a concept that ended the confusion in medicine. Readers could use the concept to make rational decisions about health in the same way they make rational decisions about money. Let's look at the concept of money.

If I gave you a hundred dollars, you could buy a truly great bottle of wine or an incredible new pair of running shoes. You could buy an armful of flowers for someone special. Sure, you could do a lot with a hundred dollars, but you couldn't buy a condominium. Or a new car. You know exactly how far a hundred dollars goes.

Because money has concrete value, we can compare activities as diverse as going to a pro basketball game and paying the phone bill, and then choose between them. We know that a hundred dollars will buy an evening out or a month of phone calls to Mom, but not both. The clearly defined value of money allows us to evaluate our choices.

I did not give readers a hundred dollars. I gave them something better: years of life. *RealAge* taught many people how to add years—vibrant years—to their life. It showed them how to live younger, with a method that makes health decisions as easy to understand as the worth of a hundred dollars.

The biggest problem with understanding health care decisions is that we had no common currency for health matters. We had no way of measuring decisions as diverse as buckling a seat belt, exercising, or taking vitamins regularly. For readers of *RealAge,* all that changed.

As complex as medical science is, there are only two real questions in medicine: How long will you live? How healthy and vigorous will your life be while you're living it? The fundamental motivation for choosing any behaviors, be it eating, taking calcium supplements, or wearing sunscreen, is to have a more enjoyable, longer, healthier life. Unfortunately, medical studies and news reports almost never make it that simple. RealAge determines exactly how an array of health behaviors affect youth and vigor. It correlates these behaviors to a common measurement—years of life.

Remember your school reunion? Although you all were the same age, not everyone looked it. Some people wore the years well, still young and exuberant, despite the passage of time. They had learned how to slow the pace of aging. Others looked as if they had aged ten years more than everyone else—and they probably had. They had probably chosen certain behaviors that had caused their bodies to age much faster than they should.

The RealAge program shows every single one of us *just how simple it is to become one of those people who really are younger than their calendar years.* We really can slow the pace of aging—and even reverse it. Although we've never been able to talk about getting younger before—time moves in only one direction, after all—now we can. Even though you can't change your calendar age, you can make your RealAge younger. That is, you can have the health profile of someone who is chronologically younger and healthy. Best of all, it's not that difficult to do. Slowing the pace of aging can be relatively easy and painless. You can start feeling more invigorated, energetic, and healthful almost as soon as you adopt the RealAge program. You won't just live longer, you'll live younger.

From the hundreds of thousands of people who bought *RealAge,* and the millions who've visited the RealAge website and taken the test online, there's been a recurring question: "What about food?" People write all the time to ask about food. "Is there a diet that will prevent aging?" "What's the healthiest way to lose weight and keep it off?" "Does it matter that I don't like green beans? What can I eat instead?" Questions about food have been far more numerous than any other type of question. Also, of all the tips of the day we e-mail to people from the RealAge website, the most popular have been food tips. People have always liked the food information best. (You can arrange to receive free "Tip of the Day" e-mails at www.RealAge.com.)

Although the four years I worked on the first *RealAge* book had taught me a great deal about nutrition and I had improved my food choices, I felt I still didn't know enough. The unending stream of letters and e-mails about food inspired me to learn more and write this book. In the process, I discovered a great deal. First and foremost, I discovered that eating is a blast and searching out and preparing new foods is an exciting journey. I also learned how to shop for and cook the juiciest, ripest, and tastiest fruits and vegetables available. I discovered how to order healthful food in restaurants and find the age-reducing food at parties, even when the choices seem limited. I learned how to make my eating schedule healthier by adding more small meals and cutting out some large ones, eating breakfast every day, and snacking on fruits and vegetables instead of candy bars.

After a lifetime of eating like many doctors, on the run and poorly, I retrained my palate to enjoy new foods, and I learned how to prepare them so that I relished their taste. I also discovered a lot of helpful, specific information about food—for example, that blueberries have more age-reducing antioxidants than any other fruit and that guavas are a good source of lycopene, an antioxidant associated with a reduced risk of cancer.

To help me write this book, I enlisted the help of Dr. John La Puma, a medical doctor who is also a professionally trained chef. John created and compiled recipes that even I can cook and that will help you bring healthy eating into your life deliciously and easily. He offered valuable insights to the principles of making good food choices—practical advice for incorporating RealAge eating practices into busy lives. *Note:* We've written this book in the first person to make it easier to read, but everywhere you see an "I" you can assume a "we."

I also worked closely with the science and research team at RealAge, Inc., a group of dedicated scientists and health writers and researchers who provide expert health information for the RealAge website. They scoured the literature for the latest research on nutrition and good eating, tracking down studies on such things as the benefits of selecting pink grapefruit over white and corn tortillas over flour ones. The team has translated complicated scientific research into practical advice that you can incorporate into your life and presented it in many of the charts in this book.

To be honest, there's still a lot that scientists don't know about nutrition. For example, we know that people who eat fish at least three times a week are as much as 3.1 years younger in RealAge than people who don't. Studies have consistently shown that people who eat fish have better overall cardiovascular health and are less prone to heart attacks and strokes. Why? No one knows exactly. Scientists *speculate* that the omega-3 fatty acids contained in such cold-water fish as salmon, tuna, and mackerel help protect the arteries from aging. Unfortunately, health magazines and diet books have touted this speculation as fact, urging readers to eat more omega-3s, fish oil supplements, and other sources of the fat. The omega-3 speculations may prove to be right, but at the moment no one can say for sure. It could be a special protein in fish that changes the way your genes function. There is no indisputable scientific evidence. So, what should you do? Eat fish. Eat the fish you enjoy most. We *know* that fish helps prevent cardiovascular aging, whether it's the omega-3s or something else contained in fish. The whys are still to be determined.

As much as RealAge draws on science, you don't eat science. Or nutrients. You eat food. How can you use what we know about science to make good food choices? Can you make healthy foods as tasty and enjoyable as the foods that age you? The answer, I found, is YES! *And,* healthy food can even taste *better* than aging food! The secrets are actually available to all of us. I didn't know them before, and maybe you don't know them now. If you read this book, you will.

Colleagues who now ask why I'm writing *this* book get invited to a delicious, healthy dinner. Not many scoff when I tell them they can learn how to eat to slow their aging processes and can teach their patients to do the same thing, too. They now ask what to eat and how to make those small changes in food choices that make a big difference in the rate of aging. You see, as physicians, most of us received scant training in nutrition, even though for the majority of us, good food choices are absolutely essential for health. In this book I take scientific knowledge about food choices and translate it into practical steps for eating enjoyably and healthfully—for staying younger longer.

M. R.

Preface: Food Can Make You Younger!

Food is celebration. Food nourishes us, sustains us, makes us grow, and gives us energy. It can be a positive force in your life, making you feel good, alive, and growing younger every day.

Eating the RealAge way is eating for good health and a good life, delaying or reversing aging, and having fun while you're doing it. This is *not* another diet book: If there's one thing you'll learn from this book, it's that no matter who you are, if you eat foods that are high in nutrients and low in calories, your body is going to be healthier and younger than you ever dreamed possible. Grow old gracefully? Not you. You'll live life to your youngest!

In this book you'll learn that:

- Nutritious eating can be an easy, fun part of your life.
- Great choices will slow the aging process and even reverse it.
- RealAge eating will help you lose weight and keep it off.
- You can eat sensibly and healthfully, at home or when eating out.
- You can modify the popular weight-loss diets to make them healthier.
- There's no need for yo-yo dieting. You *can* lose weight and keep it off.
- Keeping the RealAge hourglass in mind will help you make smart food choices. Eating foods in the middle of the hourglass widens your middle and speeds up the aging process. Eating foods in the bottom half of the hourglass actually slows or reverses the aging process, slowing the sands of time.
- RealAge foods are nutrient rich, calorie poor, and world-class delicious!
- Eating the RealAge way increases your energy.

It sounds counterintuitive, but you *can* slow aging and even grow younger. Your RealAge, or biological age, can grow younger as your calendar age gets older. RealAge is not only a measurement of how fast your body is aging but also a set of steps for slowing that rate. In my first book, *RealAge: Are You as Young as You Can Be?*, I outlined forty-four factors you can change to affect your rate of aging.

In this book, I examine the food-related factors that multiple studies indicate can cause you to age faster than you should. I also give you strategies for eating tastier, healthier, and more nutritious food—food that will help you stay younger longer. I look at principles of sensible weight loss and weight management and explain how and why certain fad diet plans help you lose weight and whether they cause needless aging. And I provide general principles you can follow to eat younger for the rest of your life, so you'll be healthier and more energetic.

Learning how to eat the RealAge way is the same as learning how to do anything: riding a bike, using a computer, reading. Practice and a little coaching go a long way. Changing your eating habits requires a little time and consistent commitment. If you aren't used to eating foods that make you younger, it isn't second nature. But to make healthy eating an enjoyable, natural part of your life, you just have to take the first step. Making your RealAge younger is easier and more fun than you ever imagined!

Acknowledgments

Mike's Acknowledgments

First and foremost, I thank my patients and the thousands of people who sent questions, notes, cards, and e-mails after the first book and inspired me to write this one. They encouraged me to develop the RealAge concept and motivated me to be passionate, because this approach to thinking about health meant something to them. I hope and believe this book will help them and other readers live younger longer. That would be the best reward any physician could want.

I am also especially indebted to the members of the staff and faculty of the Department of Anesthesia and Critical Care at the University of Chicago who gave me the time to do this project and have the vision to understand that the best medicine happens before a patient ever gets sick.

I am grateful to many, many other people who contributed to this book: Shelly Bowen and Maurina Sherman of the RealAge team, who rewrote and helped develop the early versions of several chapters; Elizabeth Stephenson, who cowrote *RealAge: Are You as Young as You Can Be?* with me and encouraged this book; Tracy Hafen, who taught me an enormous amount about exercise, corrected the errors of my writing, and wrote descriptions of and illustrated the Plan 10 and Plan 60 exercises for the website (she and her partners are the great athletes on the website who demonstrate those exercises); Sukie Miller, who constructively critiqued more than one draft of this book and whose passion proved to be the consistent encouragement I needed; Anita Shreve, for saying the *RealAge* book was possible and that the chapters were just what she wanted to read; Candice Fuhrman, for making it happen; Elsa Dixon Hurley, for making it much, much clearer and never saying no to any request (she made the text flow much better); Pauline Snider (and her stress-buster Timmy), for keeping the English concise and the grammar and style appropriate and consistent; the many gerontologists and internists who read sections of the book for accuracy; Jack Rowe, Jeremiah Stamler, Linda Fried, and the many investigators of the Iowa Women's, the Nurses' Health, and the Physician's Health Studies, for invaluable research and advice that helped make the science better; members of the RealAge team who verified the content and contributed their expertise to the book, including Genina Berger, Jennifer Oliver, Karina Lichtenstein, Lauren Weiss, Elizabeth Karlsberg, Erin Malone, Kevin Kaiser, and Rani Vaughn; the many professional chefs who contributed recipes, including Robin Lenz of Robin's Restaurant in Williamstown, Massachusetts, Rich Tramonte and Gale Gand of Tru in Chicago, and Marisa Curatolo of the Cooking Studio in Winnipeg, and those whose recipes we modified, including the chefs of Canyon Ranch; our amateur chefs, who tested the recipes, especially Donna Szymanski (she has incredible patience—she taught me how to cook and cooked every recipe we tested—more than two hundred—at least three times); our tasters, especially my wife, Nancy, and my children, Jennifer and Jeffrey, and the Wattels of Lettuce Entertain You, the Shermers, the Pelligrinis, and many others who tasted occasionally; the staff of the University of Chicago Program for Executive Health, who understood and encouraged the goals of RealAge; Shivani Chadha and Kate Poneta, the research associates who tirelessly analyzed the nutrients and calculated the RealAge effect of each recipe, not only of this diet but for the other bestseller diets discussed in Chapter 3; Julie Tarr, for her endless patience and good humor in producing the manuscript; Charise Petrovitch, for inspiring and improving the charts and slides; David Ward, for his work on the hourglass; Brisa Kilfoy, who enthusiastically worked late into the night and on weekends to produce corrections to many of the more than thirty drafts of each chapter and the final copies of the manuscript; Anne-Marie Ruthrauff, for doing so much so well and doing it so calmly in the midst of a constant storm; Andy Davis, M.D., who on many days saw my internal medicine patients to allow me to do this project; Susan Muller, Shara Storandt, Mary Lou Trepac, and William Germino, who each made this a better book than it would have been; Arline McDonald, Tate Erlinger, Linda Van Horne, Carol Peck, Mark Rudberg, Mike Parzen, and especially Keith Roach, Axel Goetz, and Harriet Imrey, the scientists who helped evaluate the data and scientific content of RealAge; Sidney Unobskey and Martin Rom, who inspired the process and named it; Charlie Silver, who funded the research and assembled the innovative RealAge team who continually evaluate and update the RealAge program and its website; Jill Siegel-McDermott and Donna Gould, who promoted the concept; the group at HarperCollins and Cliff

Street Books, whose encouragement keeps me going—Richard Rhorer, Pam Pfeifer, Janet Dery, and especially Diane Reverand, whose faith in the work inspired me to make it better and who herself improved it, not just a little, and not just once. She conveyed her excitement to me and infused the book with it. I would not passionately believe that RealAge could change the health of the world without her excitement about the project. And, of course, I am grateful to my co-author John La Puma, who really taught me that nutritious food could and should be world-class delicious.

Finally, I would like to thank my wife, Nancy, for her constant love and support and my children, Jeffrey and Jennifer, for their encouragement and patience. I dedicate this book to them.

John's Acknowledgments

The people to whom I am most grateful, like my friend Mike Roizen, are my patients and clients, especially those from CHEF Clinic. They gave me the courage to reveal the pleasures of healthy eating, too often buried beneath the fears of weight gain and uncertainty about what to eat.

I had many other wonderful teachers and incurred several large debts of gratitude in writing this book. The first is to Gary Hopmayer, of Fox and Obel Market in Chicago, who promotes understanding of others' needs as a way of success in life. Gary is an inspirational mentor who gives generously and from his heart, and has creativity, insight, tact, and perseverance to which I can only aspire. His belief in my abilities allowed me to give myself to this work. The second debt is to Meme, his wife and companion and my friend.

I thank Karen Levin of Highland Park, Illinois, for her terrific recipe development and testing skills. Karen's carefulness and care and our mutual passion for great ingredients and new flavors made every kitchen session a delight. Executive chef Kimberly Schor of Chicago Gourmet Productions and Nordstrom's Michigan Avenue, so filled with enthusiasm and possessed of a terrific palate, also assisted with the development and testing of recipes. Karen and Kimberly bear no responsibility for anything in this book or its website that doesn't taste great.

Lisa Drayer, R.D., now of www.dietwatch.com in New York City, did much of the original research for the chapters on eating out and worked with me to improve drafts of them. And Laura Walsh, R.D., a thoughtful, first-rate clinical dietitian in private practice in Elmhurst, Illinois, did a brilliant job of researching and assembling resources.

John Reyes, remarkably wise and humanistic and grounded, helped me put one foot in front of the other. Bill Raynor did the same—with his ambitious and friendly way of helping me create food that everyone will want to eat.

I am also grateful to Sandy Blumofe, Jennifer Becker, Kathy Zant, Jeanne McMahon, Judy Kolish, Janet Miller, and the staffs of CHEF Skills and CHEF Clinic for caring for our patients and permitting me to devote stolen time to completing the book. They are excellent clinicians to whose care I would trust any member of my family. I am especially grateful to Jeanne for the early care of the puppy, Madeline, so I could concentrate on writing, cooking, and eating (tough job, I know). Kelley Clancy, Dean Grant, and Nancy Hellyer, of Alexian Brothers Medical Center in Elk Grove Village, Illinois, deserve many thanks for providing the space and time to allow me to continue this work. I also thank chef Chris Stoye, whose personal touch with so many of our patients taught me that great professionalism and great knife skills can be melded with great hands-on teaching.

Milo Falcon, Stefanie Lewis, and Brenda Mooney of American Health Consultants deserve special credit for allowing me to test some of the menu plans on two hundred physicians. Working with Gregg Zeringue, executive chef at the Grand Hyatt Atlanta, on a conference menu plan was a pleasure— great chefs like Gregg love making food that is good for you taste good. And Leslie Coplin and Paula Cousins have my deep daily gratitude for their faultless work on Alternative Medicine Alert.

I also owe special thanks to the chefs Rick Bayless, Tracey Vowell, Kevin Karales, and Geno Bahena and the staff of Frontera Grill and Topolobampo for opening their hearts and generously sharing what they knew. All four chefs took me by the hand, sometimes literally and often after having worked ten or more hours straight in the hot kitchen, to make sure I knew how to make a new sauce, to let me taste a new special, or to show me how to grill something new. Their commitment to local farmers when possible, to flavor, and to organic seasonal foods forms the foundation for the RealAge Diet. Manny Valdes of Frontera Foods offered regular, welcome sparks of entrepreneurial encouragement to seek a specialty food path. David and Kim Schiedermayer offered their kindness, kitchen, and editorial support many times (and in season, David's eye for morels and wild asparagus) during the two years in which I worked on this book and for fifteen years before that.

Pamela Sheldon Johns, a Tuscan cooking school teacher, encouraged me to try my hand at this complementary partnership. Santa Barbara's Juliana Middleton inspired me with her love of plants grown with care and then prepared with her magic hands. Dun Gifford and Sara Baer-Sinnott of Oldways in Cambridge, Massachusetts, are champions who know the synergy of traditional diets and great health, and who allowed me to hear the ancient wisdom and sample the traditional foods of the Mediterranean. Also, I am grateful to writer Peter Jaret, for believing so deeply in a hands-on approach to food and medicine. His brilliance on paper is matched only by his modesty in person.

Finally, I thank Mike Roizen for the exceptional opportunity to work with, learn from, and most of all become part of the RealAge team. His absolute focus and visionary leadership move and excite me. Mike's passion for science is now joined by the pleasures of the table—and of a healthy, younger RealAge.

Introduction

The RealAge Diet: A Giant Menu of Possibilities

Good food choices help you not only live healthier and lose weight, but also grow younger and stay young. How can you make *informed* choices about food?

The RealAge Diet is not a diet prescription and not a fad diet. It's not a stringent routine you follow morning, noon, and night. It's also not about restricting yourself or measuring calories day after day. Instead, the RealAge Diet is a giant menu of possibilities: a menu of choices for growing younger and staying young. A menu for a lifetime—a long and healthy lifetime—of good eating.

Every single day, you make hundreds of choices that affect your health and rate of aging. Choosing to exercise or not to exercise is such a choice. If you aren't physically active, you age more rapidly, because your heart, arteries, and immune system grow old prematurely. If you exercise regularly, you age more slowly, postponing the decline of your arteries and immune system. Choosing your bedtime is another health choice. Everything from brushing your teeth to buckling your seat belt to spending time with friends is a health choice that speeds up or slows down your rate of aging.

One choice that you make several times a day is whether or not to eat, and what to eat. Over and over, each and every day, you decide, "I'm hungry. I want to eat." How can you learn to make better decisions about food? How can you make food part of your plan to stay young longer?

For starters, you have to learn to love food. You may already love food, and that's great. Eating should be fun—a main course of the good life. Your diet shouldn't be a prison sentence. When we think "diet," we think restriction, deprivation, and endless calorie counting. It doesn't have to be that way.

Unfortunately, too many of us have been raised to think about food the wrong way. Instead of celebrating food, we feel ambivalent about it. As a result, we get caught in a cycle of overindulgence and deprivation. Although we're obsessed with staying thin, as a nation our waistlines are widening. More than 55 percent of the U.S. population considers itself overweight. And for the most part, we eat uninteresting, unhealthful food that makes us gain weight. We eat food out of habit and convenience, instead of making our meals a focal point in our lives.

I spent many years eating food I didn't much think about—pizza, vending machine snacks, carbonated sodas—only to go on semi-annual diets to lose the pounds that accumulated from this diet. I felt sluggish, and I was harming my body. My eat-now, diet-later approach was causing me to age faster than necessary. Worst of all, it wasn't much fun. I wasn't enjoying eating, and a lot of my food choices made me feel guilty.

Any activity you do every day of your life shouldn't be a burden. It should be a pleasure and a joy. The more you know about food and the more you make new foods a part of your life, the better you will eat and the more likely you will be to lose weight and feel good about yourself. Good eating should be an adventure for a lifetime. Don't worry about diet plans and punishing yourself when you fall off the wagon. Instead, set out on a new beginning: food for life.

Eating the RealAge Way

The response to *RealAge: Are You as Young as You Can Be?* was overwhelming. I received thousands of e-mails and letters of thanks. People told me they loved having a way to measure their rate of aging and, even better, had found some simple steps for slowing that process. Most of all, they said, they liked knowing they were in the driver's seat, able to make choices that would affect their health. Indeed, genetics plays a far smaller role in aging than we thought. Almost 70 percent of premature aging is caused by choices we make. By making better choices, you can slow—or even reverse—aging, regardless of your genetics.

 What Is RealAge?

RealAge gauges how fast you're aging biologically. Some people age faster than average. Others age more slowly. What can you do to slow the sands of time and stay younger longer? If you have not yet calculated your RealAge, please take the full test online at www.RealAge.com, or complete the test in *RealAge: Are You as Young as You Can Be?*, now available in paperback.

Science-Based Research

I'm a medical doctor and a scientist. My co-author, John La Puma, is a medical doctor, too. We are committed to the highest scientific standards. Indeed, the guiding principle of the RealAge concept is that only factors that have been scientifically proven to affect longevity and/or the quality of life are used to calculate a person's RealAge. Each factor must have been proven to affect longevity and/or the quality of life in no fewer than four peer-reviewed studies involving people, not animals.

When the RealAge team applied those criteria to more than *twenty-five thousand* scientific studies, we identified 127 factors that affect a person's RealAge, or rate of aging. These factors, which we discuss in detail on our website and in *RealAge: Are You as Young as You Can Be?*, include everything from cessation of smoking to flossing your teeth. Twenty-five of the factors concern exercise, food choices, and factors that affect food choices. In the four years since *RealAge* was written, we continued to study advances in scientific research for new factors that help you stay young. Even more factors—like eating an ounce of nuts five days a week—have been repeatedly shown to make your RealAge younger. In this book we discuss old and new nutritional factors and choices that make you younger relatively easily.

Every recommendation in this book is based on scientific evidence. Whenever a recommendation is not a purely scientific fact, it is always a suggestion about practical ways to achieve something that has been shown likely to be correct. When little is known on a subject, I tell you so and suggest how you might want to proceed, on the basis of what is known. I always point out that this information is an opinion, hypothesis, or educated guess.

As an accompaniment to this book, the RealAge team has built the RealAge Diet Nutrition Center on our website. There we offer many online tools and assessments that help you evaluate your own diet and eating needs. The assessments are personalized to you, so you get answers that fit your individual needs and profile.

Finding the Balance of Nutrients, Calories, and Fats

If there's one thing to remember about eating, it's this: Eat nutrient rich, calorie poor, and delicious.

Almost all of what is known about nutrition and eating healthfully can be reduced to that one thought. And, lucky for us, nature makes it even easier.

The foods with the most nutrients—fruits, vegetables, whole grains, lean meats, and fish—are also the foods that tend to have the fewest calories. By focusing on nutrients, you go a long way toward cutting out excess calories.

I won't tell you to forget about calories, but I do want to emphasize that although calories are an important consideration when you're trying to develop a healthy eating plan, they are not the most important consideration. This attitude is in stark contrast to the way most of us have been conditioned to think about our diets. However, by switching your focus from calories to nutrition, you are more likely to find the right caloric balance without giving it much thought.

The first step in any diet plan is to boost nutrients. By focusing on nutrients first, you will already have done much of the initial work to cut calories. Then you can begin to figure out how to cut out more calories. Finally, you must strike a balance with that tricky third factor, fats. Good eating is a balance of nutrients, calories, and fats.

The Consumption of Nutrients and Fiber

Remember the adage, "You are what you eat"? Well, in RealAge terms, you are as old or young as what you choose to eat. Eating a nutrient-rich diet is the best way to stay younger longer. Since foods with the most nutrients tend to have the fewest calories, increasing your nutrient intake simultaneously decreases your calorie intake.

Learn to choose the foods that give you the most bang for your buck, that is, the most nutrients and flavor for the calories. Choose lots of fruits and vegetables, of course. Whole grain carbohydrates—whole grain breads and pastas, for example—provide fiber and important minerals. Low-fat and no-fat dairy and soy products are valuable sources of protein and calcium. Every time you eat a red pepper or a blueberry, you're also getting fabulous antioxidants that help lower your risk of cardiovascular disease and cancer.

The Consumption of Calories

How important are calories? Important, but more important is getting the right amount. Your aim should be, "Not too many, not too few." This will help you keep your weight in balance and avoid on-again, off-again dieting. When you start messing drastically with your caloric intake, you start altering your basic metabolic rate—and that generally causes you to gain weight more easily and makes it more difficult to keep weight off (the specifics are explained later).

The key to eating for youth is not to starve yourself but rather to find your caloric balance. Your goal should be to find a comfortable body weight for your frame and profile and adopt an eating plan that keeps you more or less at that weight. Most women's ideal weight is what they weighed at age eighteen, and most men's ideal weight is their weight at age twenty-one. A comfortable body weight for you is as individual as you are and may be measured better with a favorite pair of jeans than with a scale.

The Consumption of Fats

Fats are the trickiest part of eating. When we hear the word "fat," we think "bad," because we equate eating fat with becoming fat. That's not so. Fats are a specific type of molecule. Their purpose is to store and harness energy. All of us have fat, and all of us need fat. If you understand fats, you will learn how to use them to help you stay healthy and trim. There are three rules for eating fats:

1 **Do eat fats.** Going fat free is not the best way to lose weight or keep the weight off for good. You need *some* fat. Fats help you feel full faster. People who eat moderate amounts of fats actually eat fewer calories if they eat the right fats and eat them at the right time.
2 **Eat the right fats.** There are several kinds of fats. The best fats for you are monounsaturated and polyunsaturated fats, which are found in olive oil, avocados, and other plant and fish sources. The worst fats are saturated and trans fats, the fats found in animal products and in many processed foods.
3 **Eat fats early.** By eating your fats early in the meal, you will eat less throughout the meal—and will eat less throughout the day. Fats make you feel full faster and keep you feeling full longer.

Throughout the book, I keep coming back to the following formulation. These core principles will help you identify an eating path that will keep you young:

**Eat nutrient rich and calorie poor. Eat the right fats at the right time.
And make sure that eating is fun!**

The Non-Diet Diet

I started out by saying that this is not a diet book. Why not? Because this is a book about eating healthfully and youthfully for the rest of your life. The RealAge Diet is not a plan you go on, lose ten pounds with, and go off in eight weeks, only to start over grimly in six months when the ten pounds creep back on. It's not a plan with strict rules or criticism for slip-ups. It's a philosophy to guide you through eating for the long term, helping you make better food choices every day. Diet books focus on what *not* to do and what to avoid. Here I suggest what *to do*.

A key drawback of many diet plans is that they are moralistic. People who don't stick to a diet plan because they lack willpower are made to feel like a failure. Thin people aren't thin because they have more willpower. It isn't self-control that makes you thin. Many thin people don't really think about how much they eat. A complex relationship between eating habits, exercise, body metabolism, and genetics determines your weight.

The main thing is to understand your body and what's healthiest for it. Losing twenty pounds may or may not be good for you. If you do decide it's time to lose twenty pounds, why not lose them slowly, sensibly, and just once? Why lose a total of 140 pounds as your weight cycles up and down? Who wants to be on a never-ending diet, when you can do just a few simple things and lose the original twenty pounds just once? Losing twenty pounds in two weeks, or even eight weeks, is definitely not a good long-term move for you. It's the best prescription for gaining back that weight—and more. Weight loss that occurs too fast can also do long-term damage to your bones, arteries, kidneys, and more.

Unlike conventional diet books, *The RealAge Diet* does not list foods that you can or can't have. Rather than forbidding a specific nutrient group—carbohydrates, proteins, or desserts—our book aims to give you the information you need to make good decisions about when and how to eat to make and keep your RealAge younger.

I'm glad there will be times you'll choose the chocolate cake—and that there are times it will be the right choice. Knowing the implications of your choices will help you make better choices more often. The RealAge Diet is not a food regimen set in stone, but a group of strategies that will have you eating more of the food that keeps you young and less of the food that makes you old.

1

The Enjoyable Miracle

Using Food to Regain the Energy of Your Youth

Good nutrition can be confusing. Even without all the tempting wonder diets, newest nutritional fads, and prepackaged refined food, it's difficult to know which foods have enough (or too many) calories, fats, proteins, carbohydrates, or nutrients. The good news is that behind all the hoopla, there's a simple method you can adopt to become younger and healthier:

Choose food that's nutrient rich, calorie poor, and *delicious!*

I call this the RealAge Diet. You can start getting younger right now, simply by making small nutrient-rich and calorie-poor substitutions in your meals. Time and again, my patients have expressed amazement at how a very small change made a big difference in their rate of aging. For example, if you have a choice between potato chips and walnuts or almonds, the nuts win hands down. The nuts not only have great protein, but, most important, contain a healthy fat that makes your RealAge younger. Nuts have the same or fewer calories as potato chips but are much better for you. Over the long haul, small, easy substitutions like this make a *big* difference. Whenever you eat, make every calorie delicious and nutrient rich. I call that world-class eating. Every item you choose to eat should be world-class in taste and nutrients. If you choose great-tasting foods that are full of vitamins, minerals, nutrients, and fiber rather than empty calories—nuts rather than chips, brown rice rather than white rice, onion soup rather than cream of mushroom soup—you're on the RealAge Plan.

Your Health and the RealAge Diet Plan

Your Arteries

Simply put, you're as young as your arteries.

> Keeping your arteries young and healthy is the single
> most important thing you can do for your health.

Aging of the Arteries

More Americans die from cardiovascular disease than from any other cause. Current statistics predict that 50 percent of us will be affected by cardiovascular disease, and 40 percent of us, both women and men, will die from it. Cardiovascular disease, which is brought on by aging of the arteries, is the major cause of heart attacks, strokes, many types of kidney disease, and memory loss. Even mild forms of vascular disease, which won't actually kill you, can sap your energy and make you feel old and tired. Aging of the arteries also causes impotence, diminished quality of orgasm, and even wrinkling of the skin.

Food choices and small, easy-to-make changes can profoundly affect your arterial health and can reverse a great deal of the aging that has already taken place. Simply eating certain foods outlined in the RealAge Diet can reduce the fatty buildup on arterial walls that can lead to vascular disease. This serious health problem can make your RealAge as much as twenty years older.

REALAGE CAFÉ TIP 1.1
Start Early to Stay Young

You're never too young to begin adopting good habits that make your RealAge younger. A recent study reported in the *Journal of the American Medical Association* evaluated the arterial health of a randomly selected group of people between the ages of fifteen and thirty-four. The researchers found that even the teenagers were beginning to show fatty streaks and atherosclerotic plaques in the walls of their arteries. This fat and plaque buildup is a primary cause of arterial aging and ultimately leads to cardiovascular disease, memory loss, impotence, and even wrinkles in the skin. One way to reduce fatty buildup is to avoid saturated and trans fats—that is, fats that are liquid when heated and solid at room temperature.

The Latest on Cholesterol

As it turns out, the cholesterol story is more complex than we thought. Sure, it's good to have a low total cholesterol level, but we now know that many other factors are even more important to aging than cholesterol. These factors include

- high blood pressure,
- smoking,
- lack of exercise,
- high levels of an amino acid called homocysteine,
- diabetes,
- chronic inflammation (such as gum disease or sinus infections), and
- a diet that is heavy in saturated fats and trans fats and poor in nutrients.

Choosing olive oil rather than stick margarine can importantly influence your cholesterol levels and your health. That's what I mean by making a small change in choice of foods that will have a big impact on aging.

JUST WHAT IS CHOLESTEROL? Cholesterol is a type of lipid (fat) combined with alcohol (not the alcohol in a drink but a type of chemical molecule) that's found in three places: in our cells, in our food ("dietary cholesterol"), and in our blood ("blood cholesterol"). Cholesterol is a vital nutrient that our body needs to manufacture hormones, build cell walls, and produce bile acids, which are essential for the breakdown and digestion of fats. In some areas of the body, cholesterol levels are high, and that's a very good thing. For example, skin cells contain a lot of cholesterol, which makes the cells highly water resistant and protects them from dehydration. The brain also contains high levels of cholesterol.

HOW IS CHOLESTEROL MEASURED? When doctors measure cholesterol, we measure the amount of cholesterol circulating in the blood. More specifically, we measure the three kinds of cholesterol in the body: low-density lipoproteins (LDL), high-density lipoproteins (HDL), and very-low-density lipoproteins (VLDL). The last kind—VLDL cholesterol—is rarely measured directly. So cholesterol tests usually give three values: the total amount of cholesterol, the amount of LDL cholesterol, and the amount of HDL cholesterol. Often, the value for LDL is obtained by subtracting the amount of HDL cholesterol from the total amount of cholesterol.

WHEN DOES CHOLESTEROL BECOME A PROBLEM? Problems arise when we have too much cholesterol *and* too much of the wrong type of cholesterol in our blood, where it can damage our arteries. In general, having a high total cholesterol level is bad because it promotes arterial aging. For example, for each 1 percent increase—say, from 200 to 202 milligrams/deciliter (mg/dl)—in overall cholesterol level in middle-aged men, the risk of cardiovascular disease increases by 2 percent. Even among such high-risk populations as middle-aged men, only 9 to 12 percent of those who have high total cholesterol levels (over 200 mg/dl) will actually have symptomatic cardiovascular disease as a direct result of cholesterol. So, with regard to health of the heart and arteries, other important things are going on besides just high total cholesterol levels.

THE DIFFERENCE BETWEEN GOOD AND BAD CHOLESTEROL. Far more important than a person's total cholesterol reading is the ratio of his or her LDL cholesterol to HDL cholesterol. Most people who have high total cholesterol also have a high level of LDL cholesterol. LDL cholesterol is called the "bad cholesterol" because it ages the arteries (remember "L" for "lousy"). LDL molecules *deliver* cholesterol to cells throughout your body. When cholesterol rises, excess LDL molecules in the bloodstream can attach to small ruptures or lesions in the lining of the artery wall. This triggers a process that can lead to arterial plaques and aging of the arteries.

In contrast, HDL cholesterol is called the "good cholesterol" because it *removes* excess cholesterol from the arteries (remember "H" for "healthy"). The more HDL cholesterol you have, the less excess LDL cholesterol you'll have in your blood and the less your arteries will age. Unfortunately, people with high HDL (over 56 mg/dl) are the exception, not the rule.

WHAT ARE THE IMPORTANT NUMBERS? The following levels correlate with a high rate of arterial aging. If any of these levels applies to you, have a serious talk with your doctor about how you can control your cholesterol:

- A total cholesterol level of over 200 mg/dl
- A bad (LDL) cholesterol level of over 120 mg/dl
- A healthy (HDL) cholesterol level of less than 35 mg/dl

THE REALAGE EFFECT? Having either a high level of bad cholesterol or a low level of good cholesterol can make your RealAge 3 to 6 years older. Having both a high level of bad cholesterol and a high ratio of bad to good cholesterol can make your RealAge 6 to 18 years older, depending on the ratio.

It's Easy to Keep Your Arteries Young

Believe it or not, you can make easy substitutions that keep your arteries from getting old by lowering your lousy (LDL) cholesterol and raising your healthy (HDL) cholesterol. How does having some healthy fat first in each meal sound? Starting every meal—breakfast, lunch, and dinner—with nuts, olive oil, or a little avocado can really be healthy. You can also make your arteries younger with other food choices that reduce blood pressure, decrease homocysteine levels, raise potassium or fish intake, or contain lycopene. And, as you probably can tell by now, I think it's pretty easy and tastes terrific once you know which nutrient-rich foods to adopt.

Your Immune System

Cancer is the second leading killer in the United States and may soon overtake cardiovascular disease as number one. More than a half million Americans die from cancer every year. Despite decades of research by scientists, no cure has been found for most cancers. The best way to fight cancer is not to get it in the first place.

Your immune system protects your body from disease by finding and destroying potentially harmful bacteria, viruses, and cells that have gone bad. Allowing your immune system to age increases the risk that it will fail, which could mean letting an abnormal cell, such as a cancer cell, grow unchecked.

Very fortunately, cancer is not just a matter of fate. Simply eating the foods that are part of the RealAge Diet can profoundly strengthen the health of your immune system and thereby substantially enhance your body's ability to fight off cancer. And it's easy: Try orange juice fortified with vitamin D and calcium rather than plain orange juice, or grilled onions (grilled in olive oil or without fat) or tomato sauce rather than mayonnaise to moisten a sandwich. Those choices will strengthen your immune system functions.

A healthy immune system is a powerful weapon in your fight to stay young and healthy. Nutrient-rich and calorie-poor foods can help you stave off arthritis, connective tissue diseases, allergies, cancer, and even heart disease. Protecting your immune system can make your RealAge more than 6 years younger.

Energy

Eating nutrient-rich and calorie-poor foods has an immediate big payoff: energy. Good nutrition generates more usable energy—energy to jog an extra mile, to keep pace with the kids, to tackle that long-delayed home-improvement project, and to have better sex more often. Researchers know that such foods as tomatoes and fish make us more energetic. Our genes respond as if they were years younger. Relatively calorie-poor, nutrient-rich foods seem to tell our genes to produce beneficial proteins—and more of them.

The amount of energy you feel at any given time depends on several factors. Mental attitude affects your energy level; most other factors are influenced by nutrition. When you walk up two flights of stairs or chase a soccer ball, your arteries must be able to dilate (widen) to allow more oxygen (in the blood) to reach those now-activated muscle cells. Too much fat in the bloodstream has two effects, one immediate and one chronic. Both decrease your energy.

The immediate effect is that the arteries don't dilate properly. It's almost as if someone suddenly poured concrete along the inside of your arteries. A meal rich in fats or simple sugars inhibits dilation of the arteries for at least two hours. When that happens, muscles don't get enough oxygen, you're less energetic, and you tire faster.

The chronic (long-term) effect of too much fat is that the artery walls thicken with fat and become permanently less able to dilate. The effect is chronic because it takes years to layer (or unlayer) the fat in the arteries.

Of course, if you tire easily, you're not likely to be physically active, which is why an unhealthy diet and a sedentary lifestyle often go hand in hand. Regular physical activity is crucial for the health of your vascular and immune systems. It can lower your blood pressure, raise your level of healthy (HDL) cholesterol, prevent blood clots, and put you at a far lower risk of heart attack. If you're not getting enough exercise, you're allowing your arteries and immune system to age unnecessarily.

Eating the RealAge way will help you have plenty of energy. More energy means more physical activity, which keeps you healthy and makes your RealAge younger.

The Fundamentals of the RealAge Diet

Calories

It takes at least twenty minutes to work off the calories you can consume in about thirty seconds, even if those calories came from healthy foods. When you realize how long it takes to burn off calories, you see how important it is to make every calorie count, to make every calorie nutrient rich.

Unfortunately, a lot of the foods we use to "reward" ourselves—cookies, chips, and candy—have empty calories. You already know this. Empty calories lurk in other places you wouldn't expect. For example, such foods as white bread and white rice have been stripped of many of their nutrients. Even though you may not be getting a lot of fat from these foods, you're getting empty calories. Darker breads, like rye bread, and darker rice, like brown, contain many natural nutrients and are more flavorful. Better tasting *can* be more healthful. Even when a food is fat free, it still could be fattening, meaning high in empty calories—calories you could be spending on something even more delicious.

Calories themselves aren't bad—they are simply a way of measuring how much energy a food contains that your body is capable of absorbing. You use this energy for everything you do—breathing, walking, and talking, as well as more vigorous activities. When you are low on calories, you might feel faint, sluggish, or sleepy. Above all, you'll probably feel hungry. If you don't use them right away, calories get stored as fat that, ironically, can sap your energy and make you feel more tired. Once that fat is stored, it takes a lot of effort to burn off.

Lucky for us, the most nutrient-rich foods are relatively calorie poor. So when you choose fruits and vegetables that are full of nutrients, vitamins, and fiber, you're also choosing fewer calories—whether you realize it or not. **Healthy food choices are usually good calorie choices.**

What are some other healthy foods that are nutrient rich and relatively calorie poor?

Whole grain breads and whole grain pastas are relatively calorie poor (compared with equal servings of refined pastries or snacks) and provide important minerals and fiber, the cornerstones of good nutrition. Low-fat and nonfat dairy products, including skim milk, nonfat yogurt, and cottage cheese, are relatively calorie poor and contain protein and calcium. The bottom line is this: Think nutrients first, calories second, and world-class taste always.

Eating too many calories for your needs will do more than make you gain weight. Overeating can hasten the aging of your arteries and immune system and increase your risk of such chronic problems as diabetes, low back pain, arthritis, high blood pressure, and certain cancers.

How many calories should you consume to keep your weight at an ideal level? Chart 1.1, the Calorie Chart, will give you a starting point for figuring this out. However, you must determine your own best value, based on your activity level, eating patterns, and metabolic rate. Ideally, your present weight should be what it was at age eighteen if you're a woman or what it was at age twenty-one if you're a man. You should try to get enough calories and exercise (see Chapter 9) to allow you to keep that weight or a weight that's comfortable and healthy for you. The ideal quantity of calories varies, depending on your weight, height, level of activity, how muscular you are, and your body's ratio of muscle to fat. This ratio matters, because in general a pound of muscle burns about 150 calories a day, whereas a pound of fat burns only 3 calories a day.

As you get older, the number of calories you need to maintain your ideal weight usually decreases. One reason: Starting at age twenty, you lose approximately 5 percent of your muscle mass and you gain about an equal amount of fat every ten years. This does not have to happen. You do not have to lose muscle mass as you age. With just thirty minutes of muscle building a week, you can maintain your muscle mass. These resistance exercises help you build and maintain muscle and bone, and are extremely important for maintaining your ideal weight and health.

And, yes, your activity level and even pattern of eating affect your metabolic rate. If you don't eat for just sixteen hours, your metabolic rate tends to drop to a protective "starvation" level. Your body thinks it may not get food for a long time and tries to preserve every calorie it has by decreasing the metabolic rate.

 REALAGE CAFÉ TIP 1.2
Calories and Color

The key to making your RealAge younger is to find foods that have a lot of nutrients and few calories.

What's a calorie? A calorie is the amount of energy that a food provides that will raise the temperature of 1,000 grams of water 1° Celsius. A food calorie is the same amount of energy as an exercise kilocalorie. In any case, when it comes to food value, nature did it right: Generally, the more brightly colored and appealing to the eye a food is—such as brightly colored fruits and vegetables—the more nutrients you get per calorie. Brightly colored tomatoes, strawberries, blueberries, squash, pumpkins, mangoes, bananas, broccoli, green beans, soybeans, and red, green, and yellow peppers are all nutrient-rich and beautiful RealAge choices.

Nutrients

Nutrients are substances you use to build, maintain, or repair your body. If you were going to lay a new floor, you would recycle wood from an old house or use brand-new wood, or both. In the same way, to perform its functions,

CHART 1.1

The Calorie Chart: The Number of Calories You Should Consume Daily, Depending on Your Muscle Mass and Physical Activity

Your Weight in Pounds at Age 18	You Are Not Very Muscular or Active	You Are Average in Muscle Mass and Activity	You Are Very Muscular and Active
MEN			
110	1,460–1,780	1,680–2,220	1,920–2,520
120	1,510–1,845	1,745–2,300	1,990–2,615
130	1,560–1,910	1,810–2,380	2,060–2,710
140	1,620–1,975	1,875–2,460	2,130–2,805
150	1,670–2,040	1,940–2,540	2,200–2,900
160	1,715–2,105	2,000–2,625	2,265–3,000
170	1,760–2,170	2,060–2,710	2,330–3,100
180	1,805–2,240	2,120–2,795	2,390–3,200
190	1,860–2,310	2,180–2,880	2,450–3,300
200	1,905–2,380	2,240–2,965	2,510–3,400
210	1,950–2,450	2,300–3,050	2,570–3,405
220	1,995–2,520	2,360–3,135	2,630–3,505
WOMEN			
90	1,200–1,450	1,400–1,680	1,510–1,900
100	1,240–1,500	1,445–1,725	1,560–1,960
110	1,280–1,550	1,490–1,770	1,610–2,020
120	1,320–1,600	1,535–1,815	1,660–2,080
130	1,360–1,650	1,580–1,860	1,710–2,140
140	1,390–1,700	1,625–1,905	1,760–2,220
150	1,420–1,750	1,665–1,955	1,805–2,265
160	1,450–1,800	1,705–2,005	1,850–2,330
170	1,480–1,850	1,745–2,055	1,895–2,395
180	1,510–1,900	1,785–2,105	1,940–2,450

Some readers may think the ranges in this table are too wide to be helpful, but friends and users of the RealAge website have told me they wanted a guideline, even if the ranges were large.

your body breaks down existing tissues to obtain nutrients, uses brand-new nutrients in their raw form, or both. Some nutrients it converts from one form to another. For example, the body easily converts sugar to fat. Some nutrients cannot be produced by such conversions: Calcium can be obtained only from calcium-containing substances or calcium in tissues. Nutrients that are called "essential" nutrients are those that the body cannot manufacture or convert from another substance—we must get them from food. Since our bodies do not produce the essential nutrients, we must provide ourselves with them to keep our bodies energetic and healthy. In the scientific sense, nutrients are all of the proteins, carbohydrates, fats, minerals, vitamins, and water. In the RealAge sense, nutrients are the substances that make your RealAge younger—the substances that provide more than calories. Examples of nutrients that make you younger include vitamin D, the flavonoids in onions, and the lycopene found in tomatoes, which I discuss in more detail in the following chapters.

Antioxidants and Free Radicals

Although no one food can prevent or cure cancer, much research has shown that a combination of many nutrients, most notably antioxidants, may keep the immune system healthy. Antioxidants protect your cells from the damage caused by free radicals. Free radicals are by-products formed by cells when the body converts oxygen into fuel. Sometimes the free radicals can be beneficial, but most often they're harmful. These free radicals cause cell damage (oxidation) that can lead to such illnesses as cancer.

Fortunately, some antioxidants occur naturally in the body, and these natural antioxidants can be increased by certain foods or exercise. Other antioxidants can be obtained from certain foods. Both types of antioxidants—natural and those obtained from food—help block most of the damage. If you don't get enough antioxidants in your diet, damaged cells can accumulate over time and make you very sick. Think of your body as an exclusive club. Free radicals are the nonmembers who crash the club; the body can't get rid of them without some help. Antioxidants are the "bouncers." They find the roving oxygen radicals and bind to them—a chemical handcuff. Bound together, the free radical and the antioxidant form an entity that the body can then flush out. As long as you have enough "bouncer" antioxidants, free radicals won't build up in your body. Without antioxidants, you can hasten the aging of your arteries and immune system, and its consequences: cancer, heart disease, strokes, memory loss, impotence, cataracts, and a much older RealAge.

Vitamins

Fruits, vegetables, and whole grains are the food groups that contain the highest amounts of vitamins, minerals, fiber, and other nutrients that have been linked to the health of the immune system and the prevention of cancer. Some vitamins, thus, have two effects. At low doses, they are essential for life functions. At high doses, they appear to retard aging by an antioxidant action. The vitamins that are themselves antioxidants or facilitate antioxidant effects are vitamins C, E, and D, folate, and several other B vitamins.

It's fairly easy to incorporate antioxidants into your diet. For example, eating fruits and vegetables that are rich in vitamin C (such as mangoes and sweet potatoes) and in lycopene (another antioxidant that is found in tomatoes, watermelon, guava, and pink grapefruit) may reduce your risk of aging and illness and make your RealAge more than 3 years younger.

Flavonoids

Flavonoids are like vitamins: They make biological processes work faster, and they act as antioxidants. Also, some flavonoids increase the ability of certain enzymes to metabolize potential cancer-causing compounds into harmless compounds. On the other hand, vitamins are essential to life, and flavonoids are not. Eating four servings of foods that contain flavonoids each day will reduce your risk of illness and make your RealAge as much as 6 years younger.

Which foods contain flavonoids? The best sources are onions, green tea, cranberries (and cranberry juice), broccoli, celery, apples, grapes, raisins, and leafy green vegetables—the darker green, the better. Other good sources are strawberries, tomatoes and tomato products, and red peppers.

Although all alcohol in moderation has benefits, red wine may have even greater benefits. Red wine is full of flavonoids, and one of these is resveratrol, a substance that early (but consistent) research data indicates makes the immune system younger and thus provides anticancer effects. All grapes—red, green, and blue-black—have resveratrol in their skin. However, only red wine is made with the grape skin in significant contact with the wine. When red wine is made, the grape juice is fermented in contact with the skin—that is what makes the wine red. Thus, all grapes and red wine have resveratrol. Although definite data are lacking, resveratrol may be responsible for some of the anti-aging effects that come from drinking one glass of red wine a day.

REALAGE CAFÉ TIP 1.3

Fill Your White Wine with Flavonoids and Serve It at the Right Temperature

Red wine is loaded with the flavonoids obtained from the skin of grapes during fermentation. So when you drink red wine, you obtain both the benefit to the arteries from the alcohol and the benefits to your arteries and RealAge from the flavonoids.

In contrast, white wine offers only the benefit of alcohol. But you can change that and also make your wine more beautiful and even more flavorful. Wash a few grapes of any color, and then freeze them. The next time you have a glass of white wine, put one or two of the frozen grapes in the glass with the wine. It looks beautiful, makes the wine RealAge smarter by adding the flavonoids, and even brings out the flavor of the white wine. (A toast to Sydney and Nancy Unobskey for the tip!)

All wine is best if stored at 55° F. Some red wine is said to be most flavorful when consumed at that temperature, but the flavor of white wine is best at 40–45° F. Adding a frozen grape or 2 to 4 ounces of white wine not only makes your RealAge younger, it also lowers the wine's temperature, bringing out its flavor.

Carotenoids

Carotenoids are vitamin-like substances found in many fruits and vegetables. Carotenoids, unlike vitamins, are not required for survival. Of the many types of carotenoids, the best known is beta-carotene, a substance the body turns into vitamin A. The most important carotenoid for life may be lycopene. Other carotenoids include alpha-carotene, cryptoxanthin, lutein, and zeaxanthin.

For a long time, scientists didn't know whether most carotenoids had any nutritional benefit. It's become increasingly clear that many of them have antioxidant—and hence anti-aging—properties. A key function of carotenoids is to attach to free radicals, "handcuffing" to them so they can be washed out of the body, preventing them from damaging our cells.

Since carotenoids are pigments, they make foods colorful. You can be fairly sure your fruit or vegetable contains carotenoids if it is red, orange, or yellow. Tomatoes, carrots, and apricots all contain carotenoids, as do other fruits and vegetables of the same hues. Lycopene, which may be the most important carotenoid, is found in tomatoes, guava, watermelon, and pink grapefruit.

Carotenoids can also be found in such dark green vegetables as spinach, broccoli, and kale. Carotenoids are one of the big reasons that eating a diet rich in fruits and vegetables can help keep you young.

REALAGE CAFÉ TIP 1.4
Attack Arthritis with Antioxidants

How do you help keep your joints ache free and arthritis free? Antioxidant-rich fruits and vegetables may be the answer.

Since arthritis can be the result of an immune system problem, keeping the pain of arthritis at bay is another reason for keeping your immune system young and healthy with the foods you eat. Studies have shown that the antioxidants found in fruits and vegetables may protect joints—especially the knee joint—from the ravages of osteoarthritis. In particular, the antioxidants lutein and lycopene—both found in tomatoes—have been linked to a lower risk of osteoarthritis. Other studies have demonstrated that people with high intakes of vitamin C and beta-carotene (which can be found in red peppers, broccoli, and sweet potatoes) and vitamin D and calcium also have a substantially lower risk of knee pain and arthritis.

Carbohydrates

Carbohydrates are the body's first choice when it needs energy. Maybe that's why you crave carbohydrates when you're hungry. Most people get about half their daily caloric intake from carbohydrates.

Simple or Complex Carbohydrates?

Simple carbohydrates are the sugars—refined sugars and sugars found in honey, corn syrup, and many fruits. These simple carbohydrates, also called "simple sugars," make up much junk food and are not a component of good RealAge nutrition.

Complex carbohydrates—starches that the body breaks down into simple sugars—are RealAge wise and are part of good nutrition. Complex carbohydrates are found in cereals, whole grain breads, whole grain pasta, vegetables, beans, legumes, and some fruits.

You might ask, if complex carbohydrates break down into simple sugars, why are they any better than the simple sugars? Don't both types provide the same amount of energy?

Yes and no. The biggest difference is that most complex carbohydrates are found in foods that are rich in vitamins, nutrients, and fiber. Even though complex carbohydrates do provide the same amount of calories and energy per sugar molecule that simple carbohydrates provide, the body treats the two differently. Complex carbohydrates break down more slowly and consume more metabolic energy in digestion. Since the breakdown from complex carbohydrate to simple sugar occurs more slowly, blood sugar levels are more stable and stay lower when you consume complex carbohydrates. This lower blood sugar level is important, because high blood sugar causes your body to age faster. Extra sugar causes the proteins in your body to be less functional and, as a result, directly ages your immune and arterial systems and even your joints (knees, neck, and elbows).

Unfortunately, most of us eat fewer complex carbohydrates than simple sugars. Why? Because we've reinforced our natural palate preference to like sweet substances. Humans have a natural liking for the taste of simple sugars, as demonstrated by the love of even newborns for sugar. We make that preference even stronger by consuming too much sugar. Our taste buds get used to the higher level of sugars.

But it's easy to retrain your palate! Just start substituting complex carbohydrates for simple carbohydrates. Have an apple instead of a candy bar or a roasted sweet potato instead of French fries. In eight weeks, you'll find your former food favorites too sweet, and you'll be on your way to really preferring complex carbohydrates.

Once you've retrained your taste preferences, eating a diet high in complex carbohydrates—fruits, vegetables, and whole grains—is easy good nutrition, is enjoyable, and helps you grow younger. Forget those old myths that breads and pastas are fattening. They aren't, *if* you eat the same amount of whole grain breads and pastas, and do not overload them with fats, such as butter and stick margarine, that age your arteries. Carbohydrates contain far fewer calories per gram than fats do: 4 calories per gram of carbohydrates versus 9 calories per gram of fat. Complex carbohydrates such as nutty or rye breads, brown rice, whole grain bread, corn, and cereal products are all healthy foods and are an important part of your RealAge diet.

Although it's much less aging to eat complex carbohydrates than to eat simple carbohydrates, there's simply no data available to say how much or how little consumption of carbohydrates is necessary to reduce aging. We do know that avoiding simple sugars does make your RealAge younger.

The Glycemic Index

The glycemic index of a food is a measurement of how that food affects your blood sugar level in the hours after you eat it. Foods that have a high glycemic index—a baked potato, white bread, or pure sugar—are converted into energy quickly. Foods that have a low glycemic index—plums, peaches, skim milk, and yogurt—are converted more slowly, which means that your blood sugar level stays lower.

REALAGE CAFÉ TIP 1.5
Spotting Simple Sugars on Food Labels

How can you tell if a food contains a lot of simple sugars? Check the label: A food is likely to be high in simple sugars if one of the following substances is first or second in the list of ingredients, or if the list contains several of these substances:

Brown sugar	Glucose	Malt syrup
Corn sweetener	High-fructose corn syrup	Molasses
Corn syrup	Honey	Raw sugar
Dextrose	Invert sugar	Sucrose
Fructose	Lactose	Syrup
Fruit juice concentrate	Maltose	Table sugar

Source: Dietary Guidelines for America, 2000.

WHAT'S WRONG WITH HIGH BLOOD SUGAR? Glucose is a simple sugar. A high blood glucose (sugar) level causes your body to put an extra glucose molecule on proteins. The extra glucose make the proteins less functional, which produces aging. For example, the addition of a glucose molecule on hemoglobin (a protein) inhibits the ability of the hemoglobin to deliver oxygen to your tissues. As a result, you're less energetic. An extra glucose molecule on collagen (another protein) causes arthritis that ages your joints and makes you feel older.

High blood sugar levels cause undue aging of the arteries. Just as we have peaks and dips in our blood sugar levels during the day whenever we eat, we also have changes in blood pressure as we perform our activities. During regular activities, a process protects our arteries from possible damage from variations in blood pressure. A high glucose level disables this protective process. Whenever blood sugar levels are high, blood pressure is conveyed to the arterial wall more intensely. This pressure can cause breaks or nicks in the arterioles (very small arteries) and cause your arteries to age faster.

HOW TO HAVE A HIGH-GLYCEMIC FOOD AND EAT IT, TOO! Some nutritionists and diet book authors recommend that you eat only foods that have a low glycemic index. That's a little like asking you to drive under twenty miles an hour for the rest of your life. That wouldn't be a safe thing to do. Avoiding nutrient-rich foods that have a high glycemic index—such as carrots, cantaloupe, or watermelon—is not healthy. What can you do about healthy foods that have a high glycemic index?

Here's a trick that diet books won't tell you:

Many foods that have a high glycemic index can be made to act like low-glycemic foods. How? By eating a little healthy fat first.

For example, eating a carbohydrate, like French bread, with a little olive oil, or wheat bread with peanut butter, decreases the bread's ability to increase blood sugar. Why? Because glucose is absorbed in the intestine, not the stomach. By slowing the emptying of your stomach into your intestine, you slow the rise of sugar in your blood, and thus decrease the glycemic index of the food.

Another thing to consider is how nutritionists obtain the glycemic index. They calculate the value by tracking the blood glucose level of a person who has consumed 50 grams (g) of carbohydrate from a particular food. For most of us, 50 g is more than one serving. For instance, you'd have to eat about thirty carrots to get the 50 g of carbohydrate needed for the determination of the glycemic index of carrots. If you consumed fewer carrots—which is the normal case—your blood sugar levels would rise more slowly. Also, you don't usually eat carrots all by themselves, and the other foods can make a difference. If you eat a food that contains fat, such as a tiny bit of olive oil (one-third of a teaspoon) or six or seven nuts beforehand, or dip the carrots in some guacamole, you will greatly slow the emptying of your stomach, decrease the rise of sugar in your blood, and protect your arteries. That's RealAge-smart nutrition.

Fiber

A key reason that fruits, vegetables, and whole grains help you grow younger is that they contain a lot of fiber. Fiber is a substance found mainly in plants. Because it is largely indigestible, it passes through the digestive tract intact and has no calories. However, it does make you feel full sooner, which can help control overeating. Fiber helps regulate metabolism and digestion, helps stabilize blood glucose levels, and helps slow the absorption of nutrients. Fiber reduces the risk of diverticulitis and inflammatory bowel disease, two conditions that cause inflammation of the gastrointestinal tract. A high-fiber diet also helps reduce the incidence of hemorrhoids. Eating 25 grams or more of fiber a day can make you more than 2.5 years younger in RealAge than the person who eats only 12 g a day, the national average.

Several studies have shown that people who eat a breakfast that contains fiber are not as hungry in the late afternoon (for most of us, around 4:00 p.m.) as those who don't get fiber in the morning. Soluble fiber, found in foods like

Cheerios, oatmeal, barley, beans, and rye, slows the emptying of your stomach and your intestine. So, four to eight hours after you eat these foods, you might find yourself skipping your usual afternoon snack and reducing your total calorie intake for the day.

The RealAge goal is to get 6 g of fiber for breakfast. Here are some of my favorite breakfasts.

- Rye or some other whole grain bread, toasted for flavor and crunch, topped with a little almond butter or whole apricot preserve, followed by an oat and/or barley breakfast cereal with both raisins and grapes.
- A veggie burger on a toasted whole grain English muffin with a squirt of ketchup or a slice of tomato and onion.
- A bowl of oatmeal (use rolled oats for extra youth, not the instant kind) with a swirl of apple butter, plus chopped dates or fresh plums, or a teaspoon of your favorite nut butter.

Fiber also appears to be necessary for the health of the digestive tract. High-fiber diets speed up digestive processes, adding bulk to stool and helping the body rid itself of waste products more quickly. This means that possible carcinogens spend significantly less time in the bowel. This nutritional advantage appears to reduce aging by decreasing your chance of intestinal disorders and diseases that age your arteries.

 REALAGE CAFÉ TIP 1.6
Foil Fat with Fiber

Getting your fill of fiber may be an even smarter way to keep pounds off than cutting fat. Researchers in Boston report that men and women who ate a diet high in fiber gained the least weight over a ten-year period, regardless of how much fat they had consumed. The people who gained the most weight had diets low in both fiber and fat. Of course, you still don't want to fill up on fats, and, when you do eat fats, opt for the healthful, monounsaturated variety (olive oil and canola oil).

You can get your fiber in several forms. Some high-fiber cereals contain almost double the amount of fiber found in vegetables such as broccoli and cauliflower. Grapes, grapefruit, oranges, and apples are also great sources of fiber.

RealAge Benefit: Eating a high-fiber diet can make your RealAge up to 3.5 years younger.

For example, one study found a connection between low-fat, high-fiber diets and reduced blood estrogen levels in women. This relationship may help explain why women on high-fiber diets have a lower incidence of breast cancer. Also, a study at Northwestern University showed that a 10-g increase in the daily intake of cereal fiber decreased the risk of heart attack by 29 percent. Eating oatmeal or bran cereal for breakfast every day would make the RealAge of a fifty-five-year-old person 1.9 years younger.

As you may already know, whole grains are a great source of fiber. Numerous studies indicate that whole grains slow your rate of aging. The Nurses' Health Study on stroke showed that whole grain intake is associated with more youthful arteries. Similar youth-giving effects were found for whole grains in the Iowa Women's Health Study, which indicated that the soluble fiber from whole grains makes your RealAge younger. Other studies have confirmed the importance of whole grains, including the Scottish Heart Study; the Cancer Prevention Study II; and the study of eleven thousand vegetarians and health-conscious people, reported by Keyes and colleagues. Be sure to check the labels on processed food, which are now required to indicate the overall fiber content.

Don't go on a high-fiber diet all at once. Do it gradually. Go one-fourth of the way to 25 g of fiber a day the first week, halfway there the second week, etc. Some people who rapidly increase the amount of fiber consumed may notice an increase in flatulence (gas). This is less likely with a slow increase in dietary fiber and will resolve for others with some dietary changes. Make sure to drink lots of water, because fiber tends to absorb water. That is RealAge-smart nutrition.

Protein

Protein is an essential part of our diet. We just can't live without it. The building blocks of proteins are amino acids. Amino acids that the body cannot manufacture on its own are called "essential" amino acids, meaning they are essential to eat, since our body can't manufacture them. When you eat a food that contains protein, your body rearranges the amino acids (the building blocks of that protein), to build the protein it wants. It uses the new protein to rebuild and grow such tissues as muscles.

Although protein can be a source of energy, the body burns fat and carbohydrates first and uses protein as its last resort. One recent discovery is that the protein you eat may turn some of your genes on or off, making you younger or older.

The specific proteins you eat may be very important to your rate of aging.

There are two kinds of protein: the protein in your food (dietary protein) and the protein in your body. When you think of sources of protein in food, your first thought is probably meat. It's true that meat, poultry, eggs, and milk are similar to our own body proteins, so they can easily be incorporated into our bodies. You may not realize that protein is also available in other foods that *don't* contain much saturated fat, such as fish, nuts, beans, soy, and vegetables. These nutrient-rich proteins are RealAge-smart.

Soy is a popular source of vegetable protein. It's available in a variety of forms, including fresh or frozen bean pods (called "edamame"), soy milk, cereal, nuts, and tofu, which is the curd produced from soaked, pressed, and briefly cooked soybeans. Other sources of protein are nuts, legumes and beans, and seeds. By themselves, these selections contain a narrower variety of proteins than do meats. However, when you combine these healthy proteins with such whole grains as brown rice, barley, and wheat, all your protein needs will be met.

In fact, recent studies suggest that diets high in these healthy kinds of protein can help you live longer and younger. Although it has not yet been determined scientifically what ratio of protein to carbohydrates is the least aging, many experts say that getting 15 to 25 percent of calories from protein, 50 to 60 percent from carbohydrates, and 25 percent from fat is about right. Is more protein better? This, too, hasn't been determined scientifically. We do know that too much protein from red meat ages you, since red meat contains saturated fat. We do *not* know if getting more than 20 percent of calories from protein causes aging.

You don't have to deny yourself the steak or poultry dishes you enjoy. Just choose your meats wisely—extra lean beef and lean pork—and broil or bake them without added butter and oil. Also, keep the portions small.

> Think of red meat as an occasional side dish and try to limit your consumption of it to one serving a week. For the rest of the week, a diet rich in fish, the skinless white meat of poultry, beans, rice, soy, and almonds and other nuts can fill your plate and please your heart. And that's good nutrition—nutrient rich, calorie poor, delicious, and making your RealAge younger.

How do you know which foods have the most protein, and the most beneficial protein? See Chart 1.2 for a selection of foods ranked by protein content. You will see that meats have more protein and fat than vegetables do. In each case, the portion size is 100 g, or a little less than one-fourth of a pound. (Much of the remaining weight of the food is water.)

CHART 1.2
Protein by the Numbers

Protein Source (100 g or about ¼ of a Pound)	Protein (g)	Fat (g)	Eating This Food Usually Makes Your RealAge:
Chicken: Broiler or fryer, white meat, no skin, roasted	30.9	4.5	Younger
Pork: Fresh, loin or sirloin (chops), bone in, lean only, cooked or broiled	28.5	10.1	Older
Luncheon meat: Beef, sliced thin	28.1	3.8	Older
Beef: Top sirloin, lean, fat trimmed to ¼ inch, choice, cooked or broiled	27.6	16.7	Older
Chicken: Broiler or fryer, dark meat, meat only, cooked or roasted	27.4	9.7	Younger
Fin fish: Salmon (Coho), prepared without oil	27.4	7.5	Younger
Fin fish: Tuna, light, canned in water without salt, drained	25.5	0.8	Younger
Turkey breast	22.5	1.6	Younger
Chicken: Broiler or fryer, meat and skin, cooked, battered, and fried	22.5	17.4	Older
Nuts: Mixed, dry roasted, with peanuts, no salt	17.3	51.5	Younger
Hamburger: Single meat patty, plain	16.5	16.7	Older
Nuts: Cashews, dry roasted, no salt	15.3	46.4	Younger
Tofu: Extra firm, prepared with nigari (a substance made from sea water that makes tofu firm)	10.4	6.2	Younger
Bread: Whole wheat, commercially prepared	9.7	4.2	Younger
Beans: Kidney, California red, mature seeds, cooked or boiled, no salt	9.1	0.1	Younger
Soybeans: Mature seeds, sprouted, cooked or steamed	8.5	4.5	Younger
Bread: White, commercially prepared	8.2	3.6	Older
Rice: White, long-grain, regular, cooked	2.7	0.3	Older
Rice: Brown, long-grain, cooked	2.6	0.9	Younger

Protein Source (100 g or about ¼ of a Pound)	Protein (g)	Fat (g)	Eating This Food Usually Makes Your RealAge:
Brussels sprouts: Cooked or boiled, drained, no salt	2.6	0.5	Younger
Asparagus: Cooked or boiled, drained	2.6	0.3	Younger

Source: U.S. Department of Agriculture and calculations by RealAge, Inc.

Fat

There are two kinds of fat: food fat and body fat. The fat found in food—from plant and animal alike—is called "dietary fat." This is the fat you eat and the fat that's listed on food labels. Dietary fat is different from body fat: If you eat 10 g of fat, that doesn't mean you're going to gain 10 g of body fat. The fat you eat is digested and processed. You can use the processed fat for energy right away; it can be transformed into other substances, such as hormones and portions of cell walls; or it can be stored. Stored fat is called "body fat." Body fat results when you have excess calories, no matter what the food source—proteins, fats, or carbohydrates.

There are four major types of dietary fat: saturated, polyunsaturated, monounsaturated, and trans fat. The first three occur naturally. The fourth, trans fat, is an artificially created product that mimics saturated fat. Although trans fats do occur naturally (there's a little in cows), they're usually produced by applying an artificial process to vegetable oil. The first popular trans fat product was margarine.

All four kinds of dietary fat have the same amount of calories—120 per tablespoon or 9 per gram—but they affect your body differently. Saturated and trans fats age your arteries and immune system. In contrast, polyunsaturated fat seems to decrease aging. Of all the fats, monounsaturated is the best. It helps boost the level of healthy cholesterol in your blood and in this way makes you younger. However, polyunsaturated and monounsaturated fats are beneficial only if they're consumed in moderation.

No matter what kind of fat you eat, it is "fattening." Fats, whether in our bodies or in the plants and animals we eat, are energy stores that are loaded with calories. Remember: Fat contains more than twice as many calories per gram as protein and carbohydrates do.

The average American consumes about 95 g of fat per day, which is about 33 percent of his or her total calorie intake.

> Your RealAge will be more than 3.5 years younger if you limit
> your total fat intake to around 25 percent of your daily calories
> and make sure that less than 30 percent of that fat (less than
> 8 percent of your total calories) is saturated and trans fats.

This is even more important if you're at special risk for aging of the arteries. See Chapters 2 and 4 to find out more about reducing your risk of accelerated arterial aging.

Saturated Fats ("Four-Legged Fats")

Saturated fat has long been thought to be the worst of the fats. It is found in red meats, full-fat dairy products, palm and coconut oils, and, to a lesser extent, poultry and other animal products. What's the difference between a saturated fat and an unsaturated fat? What is a "saturated fat" saturated *with*? In a word, hydrogen. All fats are mixtures of carbon, hydrogen, and a little oxygen. These mixtures, called fatty acids, are classified according to the amount of hydrogen they contain. If a fatty acid contains all the hydrogen it can, it's said to be saturated. If it does not, it's said to be unsaturated. We do not know *why* having all of the hydrogens possible is unhealthy, but repeated studies show that it is. And, we do know *how* more hydrogens make a fat unhealthy.

In fact, no foods have been more closely linked to substantial aging of the arteries and immune system than saturated fat and its cousin, trans fat. This relationship was confirmed by a twenty-five-year study that evaluated coronary heart disease and the long-term risk of death. This study and many others have found the same result: Saturated fat ages you.

Here's how it happens: First, saturated fats promote the first stage of arterial aging and cardiovascular disease—the buildup of fatty tissue on the inner lining of arteries.

Specifically, saturated fats make it easier for the level of bad cholesterol to rise in the bloodstream. In fact, consuming saturated fat, *not cholesterol,* is the biggest dietary contributor to an elevated level of cholesterol in the blood. Excess consumption of saturated fats is also linked to an elevated level of triglycerides. Triglycerides are another form of fat that occurs in the body. These fats can be made when sugar hits the bloodstream. Triglycerides are used to store fat. Elevated triglyceride levels have been linked to aging of the arteries.

Excess saturated fat in your diet can also increase your risk of cancer. Although the link between fat consumption and cancer remains unclear, several studies show a strong correlation. Some experts estimate that as many as one-third of cancers may be provoked by the dietary choices we make, and saturated fat appears to be a leading culprit. The Iowa Women's Health Study indicates that postmenopausal women who have been diagnosed with breast cancer have a better survival rate if they manage their weight and consume a diet low in saturated fats. Other studies have noted a connection between greater fat intake and a higher incidence of lymphomas and lung, ovarian, and prostate cancers.

It's easy to find out whether the food you're eating has a lot of saturated fat in it. The Food and Drug Administration (FDA) requires that every food label list the percentage of saturated fats in the food. In response to consumer concern, companies announce on the front of their packages whenever their products are low in saturated fat. However, many companies are finding a way around the saturated-fat dilemma by using something even more dangerous: trans fat.

Trans Fat

Trans fat—also called "trans fatty acid"—is created when unsaturated fats are hydrogenated (combined with hydrogen). The purpose of this chemical process is to create fats that are solid at room temperature rather than liquid, their normal state at room temperature. For example, most solid margarine is produced by transforming (through partial hydrogenation) good vegetable oils into bad vegetable oils. Even though a food label doesn't use the exact words "trans fat," if you see "partially hydrogenated vegetable oils" as ingredients, you can be sure the product contains trans fat.

Any fat that is liquid when heated but hardens when cooled to room temperature is probably made of either saturated or trans fat. If the fat is solid when cool, it likely will age you. For example, most stick margarine is a trans fat, as is the glaze on most doughnuts.

WHY IS TRANS FAT HARMFUL? Trans fats, like saturated fats, alter metabolic processes and increase the hardening (and thus aging) of your arteries. Studies show that the more trans fat a person eats, the faster the cardiovascular system ages. In one study of more than eighty-five thousand people, women who ate more than 4 teaspoons of margarine a day had a 70 percent higher risk of cardiovascular disease than those who rarely ate margarine. So, if a fifty-five-year-old woman consistently cooked with stick margarine, her body would be 2.7 years older than if she used olive oil instead. Some researchers have attributed as many as thirty thousand deaths a year to the consumption of trans fat. Other researchers believe the figure is several times higher.

The full effects of trans fats are still not understood. Most scientists believe that the artificial molecular structure of trans fat actually causes more harm than naturally occurring molecules of saturated fat. For example, it seems to

be healthier to use small amounts of butter than most stick margarines. However, this hypothesis has not been proven.

**What we do know is that avoiding all partially hydrogenated
vegetable oil will make your RealAge as much as 2.7 years younger.**

THE HIDDEN FAT. Since food producers are not required to list trans fats on
their nutrition labels, trans fat is called the "hidden fat." The FDA has proposed
that the trans fat content of food be listed on labels by mid-2002, but some food
manufacturers are fighting this requirement. Many packaged foods—cookies,
crackers, and chips—contain these oils, because they give food a longer shelf
life. Many companies advertise their cookies and crackers as "baked, not fried,"
or as having "no saturated fat" or "no cholesterol." This implies they're low in
fat, when in fact they're often full of trans fat. It doesn't matter if the product is
cholesterol free; if it contains trans fat, it will age your arteries.

Be aware, too, that many restaurants, especially fast-food restaurants, cook
their food in trans fat. Why? Before trans fat was available, some restaurants
used lard, a saturated animal fat, or palm or coconut oils, also saturated fats.
Then came the revelations about saturated fats. In order to keep the flavor of
food cooked in lard without, technically, using saturated fats, many restaurants turned to such trans fat products as solid shortening.

How can you know what kind of fat a restaurant is using? You have to ask. If
the restaurant used a solid shortening or hydrogenated or partially hydrogenated vegetable oils to fry the potatoes or cook your food, you're getting trans
fatty acids, which may increase your bad cholesterol levels.

Avoiding Unhealthy Fats

One basic step in good nutrition is avoiding unhealthy, aging fats. How can you
avoid hidden trans fat? Your best bet is to say no to most fast food—especially
the fried kind. When you're grocery shopping, check all your nutrition information labels for total fat content and saturated fat content. Subtract the saturated fat and unsaturated fat from the total fat. This number will tell you how
much trans fat is in the product. For example, the label on the Oreos cookie
package says that three Oreos have 7 g of total fat, 1.5 g of saturated fat, 0.5 g of
polyunsaturated fat, and 3 g of monounsaturated fat. How many grams of trans
fat do those three Oreos have? Seven minus the rest (1.5 + 0.5 + 3) leaves 2 g of
trans fat. So three Oreos have 3.5 g of aging fat (1.5 g of saturated and 2 g of
trans). Not bad as cookies go, but almost all store-bought, processed cookies
are nutrient poor and calorie rich, the opposite of RealAge-smart nutrition.

Another trick is to look at the ingredients label. If you see hydrogenated or partially hydrogenated oils listed before polyunsaturated or monounsaturated oils, the product contains lots of trans fat. The ingredients label (listed right below the nutrient table) must list the ingredients in order of quantity, from most to least. If the label lists unsaturated or monounsaturated oils, olive oil, or canola oil first, the fats are probably okay. Some experts say that 25 to 60 percent of all the fat in processed food is trans fat and that 15 to 30 percent of all the fat in most people's diets is trans fat. See Chapter 7 to learn how to avoid this aging fat when you eat out.

Polyunsaturated and Monounsaturated Fats

The other two types of fats are the naturally unsaturated fats: the monounsaturated and polyunsaturated fats, found in vegetable and nut oils. These fats remain liquid at room temperature. (The prefixes "poly" and "mono" refer to the chemical structure of the fats.) Unsaturated fats are found mostly in plants, and we consume them largely as vegetable oils.

Polyunsaturated fats appear to prevent premature aging. Some very preliminary studies question whether these fats might be linked to the onset of certain cancers, yet other studies link these oils to *reduced* aging of the immune system. Corn oil, soybean oils, and most vegetable oils contain mostly polyunsaturated fats.

Monounsaturated fats are actually good for you. Unlike saturated fats, monounsaturated fats help reduce bad cholesterol and boost healthy cholesterol in the blood. Olives, olive oil, and cold-pressed canola oil are key sources of monounsaturated fats. Flaxseed and nuts are also great sources of this type of fat.

Avocados are a good source of monounsaturated fat and are also high in fiber, beta-carotene, potassium, and vitamin E. Remember that a small avocado contains almost 20 g of fat, about one-third of your daily fat allowance. If you have a choice, consider "Florida" avocados, which are not as creamy tasting as "California" avocados but contain significantly less fat. In either case, it's best to consume only small amounts.

When you buy oil, canola and olive oils are your best choices. Still, use them sparingly, because, like all fats, they're fattening.

How do you know if what you're eating is aging you? How do you determine which foods will help you grow younger right now? The next chapters tell you more about how you can answer these questions and how you can use great-tasting food to regain and keep the energy of your youth.

2

What Is the Effect of Your Food Choices on Your RealAge Now, and How Much Younger Do You Want to Be?

Now that you know a little more about the general principles of nutrition, you can begin to see how they might apply to you. To know what first steps to take, you need to know where you stand.

What Is Your RealAge Now?

The best way to find out where you stand is to calculate the differences that your current nutritional choices have made in your RealAge. By answering easy questions about your health factors and food choices, you can determine whether you are aging more quickly or more slowly than your contemporaries. You can do this in two ways:

1 Fill out Chart 2.1, which gives you an *approximation* of how your nutritional choices affect your RealAge. Or
2 Complete the questionnaire on the RealAge website (www.RealAge. com).* This produces a more accurate calculation, and the RealAge computer database does all the work for you.

*Use of the RealAge website is currently free. The company hopes to continue that (but makes no guarantee). At the site, follow the instructions for opening a personal account and answering the survey from which we calculate your RealAge. Your account stores information about you that you can access as often as you like. All information is completely confidential and accessible only to you. As you adopt new age reduction strategies, you can chart your progress and literally "watch the years disappear."

If you've already taken the online test or filled out the chart in the first book, *RealAge: Are You as Young as You Can Be?*, you have a head start on setting your goals. At the end of the test were suggestions that would make your RealAge younger. Those recommendations are the perfect launch pad for your journey to improved health and fitness. The suggestions might have been to do strength-building exercises, enjoy fish more often, or use a helmet when you ride your bike. Whatever your individual results, knowing exactly what changes you can make right away is extremely helpful.

Note: The RealAge effect specified for each factor mentioned in the charts and chapters in this book, other than Chart 2.1, is the effect of the factor being considered—for example, eating vegetables—*individually*. It does not take into consideration the interaction between factors. This is important, because many factors contribute to the effect of eating vegetables—for example, cholesterol levels, fiber and sodium intake, and potassium levels. Therefore, some of the effects attributed to eating vegetables are attributable to other things as well. For example, eating vegetables lowers your lousy (LDL) cholesterol level: 0.4 years of the 6 years' difference in RealAge between a fifty-year-old man who enjoys five vegetables a day on average and one who consumes no vegetables is attributable to the change in LDL cholesterol levels.

How We Calculate Your RealAge

You may be wondering how the RealAge team can calculate a number that's supposed to be your true physiologic age. How can we say with confidence that some people are physiologically younger and others physiologically older, even though they have the same calendar age? Especially since people are so different from one another? For every person who has a heart attack from eating a lot saturated fat, there's always someone who's had steak and eggs every day since age twelve and is going strong at ninety. So how can we say that eating an ounce of nuts a day will make you 3.3 years younger? Or that taking a folate supplement every day can make your RealAge not 55 but 52.5?

This chapter gives you a short course in the calculation of RealAge. It shows how much care the RealAge team put into the calculation of the values. Even though the mathematics for quantifying the effects of overall health factors (the focus of the first book) are considerably different from the mathematics for quantifying the effects of nutritional factors (the aim of this book), the basic principles are the same:

People age at different rates because of their choices and genetics, and you can make your genetics less important than your choices.

Everyone Ages at a Different Rate

If you examine the human population as a whole and track any one biological function, say, kidney function or mental ability, you see that it declines with age. In general, each biological function decreases 3 to 6 percent per decade after age thirty-five. This decrease is a measure of the *average* for the population as a whole. Although this sort of measurement has been the standard used by scientists to calculate the rate of aging, it doesn't take into account the variation *among* individuals.

For older populations, the variation *among individuals* is so great that it's often meaningless to calculate an average at all. An average is meaningful only if it represents what's truly happening for most people. With aging, averages don't tell the true story. You see this at high school reunions. When you graduated, everyone looked pretty much the same, but by your twentieth reunion, some look much younger and some look much older than others.

In fact, if you really look at the numbers, there is so much variation among individuals that the "average" obscures more than it shows. In every age group, there are people who represent every degree of function, from dramatic decline to virtually no decline. For every seventy-year-old who's debilitated from cardiovascular disease, there's another one who's running road races or traveling the globe.

In fact, for certain functions—mental acuity and IQ, for example—some people show almost no decline and even improve as they progress from age thirty-five to seventy-five. The question is how can *you* be one of them? Living not just longer, but more healthfully. You can start by knowing your RealAge now.

Using Age to Compare Your Health with That of Others

RealAge is a calculation of *your* relative risk of dying compared with that of the population as a whole, based on the law of averages. If your relative risk matches that of the average person who is ten years younger (because you make smart food and behavior choices), that is the same thing as saying that your RealAge is ten years younger. You are at the same risk of suffering severe aging or a major health problem as someone that much younger. Physiologically, you are equal.

This calculation of risk is the clearest measure we have for determining the rate at which you are aging. We take data from clinical studies that have calculated the risk of dying for a variety of factors and integrate these factors into your likelihood of surviving, creating Kaplan-Meier survival curves. With these curves we can evaluate the effects that individual habits and food choices have on physiologic age. Our computer-based equations use the most recent and reliable medical information available, which is then modeled by statisticians.

In our calculations, we start with the most general statistic: the average life expectancies for American males and females at specific ages. For example, the average life expectancy of a twenty-five-year-old man might be 77.2, that of a twenty-eight-year-old woman might be 80.2, and that of a fifty-one-year-old woman might be 81.5 years. That is where we start—life expectancy individualized to the age and gender of the person. We then break each category into smaller and smaller categories. For example, we consider weight-to-height ratios. The fifty-one-year-old woman who is 5′4″ tall and weighs 126 pounds might have a life expectancy of 81.7 years, while a 5′4″ fifty-one-year-old woman who weighs 185 pounds might have a life expectancy of 77.9 years.

Further examples: We calculate the long-term effects of eating fruit, eating nuts, or lifting weights. The 126-pound, 5′4″ fifty-one-year-old woman who eats 6 ounces of nuts a week and an average of four servings of fruit a day and lifts weights 30 minutes a week might have a life expectancy of 84.8 years, compared with the same woman who does not eat nuts or lift weights and averages one serving of fruit a day and has a life expectancy of 78.9 years.

Astounding differences, as you can see. Yes. That's what science tells us. And each breakdown allows us to refine our measurement and consider how much impact each action has on the aging process.

Finally, we consider all the categories together. The resulting equation allows us to evaluate all these diverse factors together and calculate a unique RealAge value tailored to each person's health profile. For RealAge in general—that is, all health factors considered—we found that 129 factors significantly affect aging. For RealAge as it relates to nutrition, we found that 71 factors affect aging.

Sound complicated? It is. But don't worry. To participate, all you have to do is answer a set of questions that allows us to calculate your RealAge. We do the rest.

Where Do the Numbers Come From? The Studies That Provide the Data

RealAge is an information system. Instead of providing new scientific data, it is a way of reinterpreting already published results. We use data from the most recent studies done by the leaders in each field of medical research, so that you are getting the best information the medical community has to offer. We tell you of the concepts and health choices that have been repeatedly and reproducibly shown in published studies to affect the quality or length of your life. What we do is unify all that information: We integrate specific recommendations from hundreds of studies into a general framework, so you can understand how all of this information relates to *you*. Whereas most medical researchers calculate their statistics in relation to the "risk of disease," we recalculate their data to determine what the risk of aging is for *you*. RealAge translates currently available research into information you can use—something you can integrate into your own life.

Seven medical experts make up the RealAge scientific advisory team for nutrition-related factors. We now have pored over more than *twenty-eight thousand* medical studies, evaluating what those studies have told us about aging and, more important, about the *prevention* of aging. Our calculations are based on data from more than 950 of those twenty-eight thousand studies and have been checked against a huge proprietary database (a database owned by a company and not generally available to the public). As new research data becomes available and statistics change, we recalculate our equations to accommodate the changes. Our online computerized RealAge program is updated whenever new and important research appears. For example, because Americans are becoming progressively heavier, we have modified our weight-to-height ratios to reflect expanding waistlines.

Although my colleagues and I rely on all kinds of scientific information for our calculations, our major sources of data are clinical studies of two types: large-scale studies on risk factors and smaller-scale randomized trials.

How Do We Decide Which Factors Affect Aging?

What are our criteria for deciding what factors do or do not affect aging?

> **We select only factors that have been shown to make a quantifiable difference in risk (that is, *aging*) or quality of life in at least four peer-reviewed studies.**

How do we come up with a RealAge value? We integrate and compare the various studies that have pertained to a certain factor—for example, heart attacks—calculate what each study tells us about choices that affect that factor—for example, the effect of eating nuts on risk of a heart attack—and then tell you in one easy-to-understand number—years—the impact of each behavior on *your* rate of aging.

Using Chart 2.1 to Get an Approximation

Chart 2.1 provides a way to quantify how nutritional factors affect your RealAge. For each factor, simply choose the description that fits you and fill in the corresponding "Tally" column. Because of the complexity of the mathematics involved in calculating your RealAge, Chart 2.1 provides a less accurate reading than the computer program we use at our website, www.RealAge.com. In fact, the RealAge program is possible only because of the tremendous calculating power of computers of the twenty-first century. Our computer programs can make subtle statistical differentiations rapidly. This allows us to draw on a huge database to account for the subtle effects that these factors have on one another. The charts you fill in by hand provide a relatively accurate reflection of your present RealAge due to nutritional choices. These values have been modified to account for many interactions and have been tested on many individuals and on countless hypothetical cases, so they represent the best possible approximation.

Filling Out Chart 2.1

The far left column in Chart 2.1 is a list of health factors, including food choices. To the right of each factor are descriptors about it. Check the one that best describes you. For example, one factor is "Portions of fish (excluding shellfish) you eat per week," and the answers range from "3 or more portions" to "none." Mark the one that best describes your consumption of fish. Then look at the top of the column. Depending on your answer, it will read something like "years younger –3" or "years older +3."

Write the number that corresponds to your answer in the "Tally" column at the far right, making sure to write the positive or negative sign. (My publisher says copy this chart, don't write in the book.) When you are done with the questionnaire, add up all the numbers. Remember that a negative number should be subtracted. For example, (+2) + (–3) = (–1). When you have added all your answers, you will get a total tally. Multiply that by the "multiplier," an age-conversion factor that is provided at the bottom of the chart, to get your "net RealAge change from nutritional and related habits and choices." If that number is a positive number, your RealAge is that much older than your calendar age. If you get a negative number, your RealAge is that much younger than your calendar age. For example, if you are now fifty and get a final number of +4, then your RealAge due to nutritional choices is 54. Likewise, if the final number is –5, your RealAge is 45. The calculation is simple and easy, and taking the quiz and tabulating the numbers should not take more than forty-five minutes.

Interpreting the Results

After you have finished computing how nutritional and related choices affect your RealAge, look back over your answers. Wherever you marked a plus number, you marked a food or related choice that is causing you to age prematurely. Write those choices down and read the rest of this book to learn how and why they are causing you to age.

CHART 2.1

How Old Are You, Really? Your Current RealAge
due to Food and Health Choices

This chart gives you an approximation of your RealAge based on your food choices and health behaviors if you are between twenty-five and one hundred years of age and don't have an acute or chronic disease.

Go down the chart, factor by factor. For each one, find the description that best fits *your* situation. Then look at the column heading to find out whether your action is making you younger or older. Write the number in the "Tally" box at

Health Factor	Years Younger –3.0	Years Younger –2.5	Years Younger –2.0	Years Younger –1.5	Years Younger –1.0	Years Younger –0.5
<u>YOU KNOW THESE:</u>						
Compared with the health of others your age, your health is					Excellent	
Ounces of nuts you eat per week				5 or more		
Portions of fish (excluding shellfish) you eat per week (a portion is the size of a pack of cards)				3 or more portions	2 portions	
Number of times you eat meat per week					None	
Water, adequate amounts						
Number of colorful vegetables you eat per day			5 or more	4		2 or 3

the end of each row. Remember, if your response made you younger, the number should have a negative sign (for example, –1.5). If none of the descriptions for a factor exactly fit your situation, choose the closest one or skip that factor.

At the end of the chart, multiply the number at the bottom of the Tally column by the multiplier that's right for your age. (There's a box that shows you what that multiplier is.) The result is the change in your physiologic age that your food choices and health behaviors have made.

Then calculate your RealAge by adding or subtracting this number from your calendar age.

No Change	Years Older +0.5	Years Older +1.0	Years Older +1.5	Years Older +2.0	Years Older +2.5	Years Older +3.0	TALLY
Very good or fair						Poor or bad	
	1–4		Less than 1				
Fewer than 2 portions			None				
Once	More than once						
No known effect on RealAge							
		1		Less than 1 a day, or 1 or 2 and I don't pay attention to color			

Health Factor	Years Younger –3.0	Years Younger –2.5	Years Younger –2.0	Years Younger –1.5	Years Younger –1.0	Years Younger –0.5
Number of times you eat breakfast per week						More than 5
Number of times you eat whole grain cereal fiber per week					5 or more	
When it's whole grain *vs.* processed grains, how often do you choose whole?				Always		Usually
Have you learned how to cook? Are you continuing your education?			Yes			
Number of servings of tomato paste, tomato sauce, or tomatoes you eat per week (see also Chart 4.7)					More than 10	7–10
Taking multivitamins						
Number of days you snack between meals per week						Rarely, or only fruit

No Change	Years Older +0.5	Years Older +1.0	Years Older +1.5	Years Older +2.0	Years Older +2.5	Years Older +3.0	TALLY
4 or 5	2 or 3	Less than 2					
3 or 4	1 or 2		Less than once a week				
	Rarely	Never					
				No			
	Fewer than 2						
Provided you eat a diverse diet, there is no known effect of multivitamins on RealAge							
Occasionally, and not usually fruit	3–5 days, and not usually fruit	Almost every day, and not usually fruit					

Health Factor	Years Younger –3.0	Years Younger –2.5	Years Younger –2.0	Years Younger –1.5	Years Younger –1.0	Years Younger –0.5
Have you been in a mutually monogamous relationship with a partner of the opposite sex for more than 10 years?						
Males: How many orgasms do you have per year? Females: How satisfied sexually are you?	Male: 300 or more		Male: 200–300	Female: Satisfied with quantity and quality	Male: 100–200	Female: Satisfied with quantity or quality
If you have not been in a mutually monogamous relationship for over 10 years, do you use condoms regularly?						
How often do you floss and brush your teeth, and do you have dental disease?			Every day, and no dental disease			
Percentage of food you eat that is prepared without fatty sauces and is not fried						

No Change	Years Older +0.5	Years Older +1.0	Years Older +1.5	Years Older +2.0	Years Older +2.5	Years Older +3.0	TALLY
Yes				No			
Male 40–100	Female: Unsatisfied with quality and/or quantity	Male: 25–40		Male: 5–25	Male: Fewer than 5		
Yes	No						
	Not every day, and/or I have gingivitis			Rarely or never, and I have periodontitis			
No known effect on RealAge, other than that from saturated fat or fat in the diet							

Health Factor	Years Younger –3.0	Years Younger –2.5	Years Younger –2.0	Years Younger –1.5	Years Younger –1.0	Years Younger –0.5
Do you consume fat-soluble vitamins with a little fat?					Yes	
Taking iron *in* *supplements*						
Minutes of total physical activity of any kind (e.g., walking) per day in the last 3 years (give yourself the most positive rating)				More than 90	More than 60	More than 20
Minutes per week of physical activity that gets your heart rate to over 70% of its maximal (220 – chronological age)					More than 60	40–60
Minutes per week of strength-building activities (weights, resistance exercises, treadmill on incline) in which you exercise at least 8 of the 12 major muscle groups*					More than 30	20–30
Hours of exposure to secondhand smoke per day						

*The major muscle groups are the rotator cuff; upper back; lower back; biceps; abdominals; chest; triceps; shoulders; gluteals, hamstrings; gastrocnemius; quadriceps; and foot, ankle, and calves.

No Change	Years Older +0.5	Years Older +1.0	Years Older +1.5	Years Older +2.0	Years Older +2.5	Years Older +3.0	TALLY
					No		
	Any iron supplement, if you are not iron deficient						
More than 10	More than 5	Less than 5	None				
20–40	10–20	Less than 10					
10–20	5–10	Less than 5					
None		0–1		1–3		More than 3	

Health Factor	Years Younger −3.0	Years Younger −2.5	Years Younger −2.0	Years Younger −1.5	Years Younger −1.0	Years Younger −0.5
Maximum number of alcoholic drinks you've consumed in 1 day in the last year (one drink is 5 oz of wine, 12 oz of beer, or 1.5 oz of spirits)						
Number of alcoholic drinks you have in an average day					Males over age 40: 1–2	Males over age 40 and females over age 50: one-half to 1
How often do you drive after drinking?						
Do you eat regularly?					3 meals a day and rarely skip	
THESE MAY TAKE A LITTLE INQUIRY:						
Do you consume monounsaturated fat first at every meal?					Most meals	
Do you make smart food choices in uncontrollable situations?				Most meals		Occasion-ally

No Change	Years Older +0.5	Years Older +1.0	Years Older +1.5	Years Older +2.0	Years Older +2.5	Years Older +3.0	TALLY
3 or fewer	4 or fewer	5 or fewer	More than 5				
Males over age 40 and females over age 50: more than 2 but fewer than 3	More than 3 or none						
Never		Less than once a month		More than once a month	More than twice a month		
2 or 3 meals a day and frequently skip		Don't eat regularly					
Occasion-ally		Rarely	Never				
	Rarely		Never				

Health Factor	Years Younger −3.0	Years Younger −2.5	Years Younger −2.0	Years Younger −1.5	Years Younger −1.0	Years Younger −0.5
Diversity in your diet: How many of the following do you eat at least one of per day on average: fruit, vegetables, whole grains, protein (meat, fish, nuts, beans), low-fat milk or milk substitute?						
Minutes of sun you get per day						
Your average green tea consumption per week in the last 3 years						
Number of pills and tablets you take per day (excluding vitamins and minerals)						0–4
Do you take all necessary (and only necessary) medications?						

No Change	Years Older +0.5	Years Older +1.0	Years Older +1.5	Years Older +2.0	Years Older +2.5	Years Older +3.0	TALLY
More than 2		2 or fewer					
Less than 20 and had no blisters before age 20		More than 20 and/or had blisters before 20					
No known effect on RealAge in women; may retard aging from prostate cancer in men							
5–7	More than 7						
Perfect or near-perfect adherence	Not perfect or near-perfect adherence			Poor adherence; I often stop or start medications without talking to doctor			

Health Factor	Years Younger −3.0	Years Younger −2.5	Years Younger −2.0	Years Younger −1.5	Years Younger −1.0	Years Younger −0.5
Do you take medicines correctly with food?					Yes. I asked the doctor or pharma-cist how to take the medica-tion and I follow the instruc-tions	
How many of the healthy recipe substitutions in Chart 6.1 do you make?					6	3–5
How many servings of fruit do you eat per day?					4 or more	
Have you trained your palate to enjoy "peasant foods"?					Yes	
Do you read food labels and avoid unhealthy fats?				Yes, and I avoid saturated and trans fats and simple carbohy-drates		
Do you avoid conta-minated or unsafe foods?					I shop for food at a variety of places	

No Change	Years Older +0.5	Years Older +1.0	Years Older +1.5	Years Older +2.0	Years Older +2.5	Years Older +3.0	TALLY
	No. I don't know how to take my medication or follow instructions for it						
	1 or 2	None					
		No					
Occasionally, and I avoid saturated and trans fats and simple carbohydrates		Rarely		Never			
		I always buy or eat food from the same place					

Health Factor	Years Younger –3.0	Years Younger –2.5	Years Younger –2.0	Years Younger –1.5	Years Younger –1.0	Years Younger –0.5
Weight changes in any 5 years						
Body mass index (see Chart 9.1)†						19 or less without acute or chronic diseases
Weight gain since age 18 for females, since age 21 for males						
Number of social groups, friends, or relatives you see more than once a month‡				6	3–5	2
Do you make healthy eating fun?	Yes					
Do you frame things positively?					Yes	
Can you laugh in stressful situations?						Yes
Do you use relaxation or other stress-relieving therapies?					Yes	

†Body mass index (BMI) is the ratio of your weight to your height. It's expressed in the unit of kilograms per meter squared. To determine your BMI, divide your weight in kilograms by your height in meters. Take the resulting number and divide again by your height in meters. The resulting number, your BMI, should be somewhere between 13 and 60; if not, you've done the math incorrectly. See Chart 9.1 for already calculated BMIs based on height and weight.

‡People who offer support during disruptive events (applicable only in case of two or more such events).

No Change	Years Older +0.5	Years Older +1.0	Years Older +1.5	Years Older +2.0	Years Older +2.5	Years Older +3.0	TALLY
At most 5%		At most 10%		Over 10%			
19.1–26.9				27–31.9		32 or higher	
Less than 20 lb		20–40 lb			More than 40 lb		
1				None			
	No						
No							
	No						
	No						

Health Factor	Years Younger −3.0	Years Younger −2.5	Years Younger −2.0	Years Younger −1.5	Years Younger −1.0	Years Younger −0.5
THESE ARE A BIT HARDER TO KNOW:						
How much vitamin C do you get in food and supplements per day?					Males over age 40 and females over age 50: more than 1,000 mg	Males over age 40 and females over age 50: 160–1,000 mg; Males age 40 or younger and females age 50 or younger: more than 1,000 mg
How much vitamin E *in supplements* do you take daily?					Females over age 50 and males over age 40: more than 400 IU	Females under age 50 and males under age 40: more than 400 IU
How much potassium *in food* do you get daily?						More than 3,000 mg
How much vitamin B$_6$ in food and supplements do you get daily?						More than 6 mg
How much vitamin A in food or supplements do you get daily?						

No Change	Years Older +0.5	Years Older +1.0	Years Older +1.5	Years Older +2.0	Years Older +2.5	Years Older +3.0	TALLY
Males age 40 or younger and females age 50 or younger: 160–1,000 mg	Less than 160 mg						
	None						
	2,500–3,000 mg	Less than 2,500 mg					
1.5–6 mg	Less than 1 mg						
Less than 15,000 IU	More than 15,000 IU	More than 25,000 IU					

Health Factor	Years Younger −3.0	Years Younger −2.5	Years Younger −2.0	Years Younger −1.5	Years Younger −1.0	Years Younger −0.5
How much calcium in food and supplements do you get daily?						More than 1,200 mg
How much vitamin B_{12} in food and supplements do you get per week?						
How much folate (folic acid, a B vitamin) in food and supplements do you get daily?						More than 700 mcg
Do you eat a balanced diet that is low in calories and high in nutrients?	Yes					
How much of your diet is fat?					20–30%	31–40% or less than 20%
How many grams of fiber do you get per day?					More than 21.1	15.2–21.1
Number of these foods with flavonoids you eat daily: onions, strawberries, apples, broccoli, tomatoes, tea, or oranges (see Chart 4.5)					At least 3	
How many days a week do you eat legumes (peas, beans, lentils)?						More than 5

No Change	Years Older +0.5	Years Older +1.0	Years Older +1.5	Years Older +2.0	Years Older +2.5	Years Older +3.0	TALLY
800–1,200 mg	500–800 mg	Less than 500 mg					
	If you don't eat meat, or get less than 15 mg per week as a supplement						
224–700 mcg	Less than 224 mcg						
					No		
			More than 40%				
9.2–15.1		3.2–9.1		Less than 3.2			
			Rarely eat 3				
2–5	Fewer than 2						

Health Factor	Years Younger –3.0	Years Younger –2.5	Years Younger –2.0	Years Younger –1.5	Years Younger –1.0	Years Younger –0.5
Do you cut out excess simple sugars?			Yes			
THESE REQUIRE SOME WORK TO FIND OUT:						
Your blood pressure (systolic/diastolic, mmHg)?	90/65–120/81		Lower than 90/65, no heart disease		121/82–129/85	
Your total cholesterol level?					You're under age 70, level is lower than 160 mg%, and you have no chronic disease	You're age 70 or older and level is lower than 160 mg%
Your HDL (healthy) cholesterol level?					Male or female age 50 or older, and level is higher than 55 mg/dl	Female under age 50, and level is higher than 55 mg/dl
What is your fasting triglyceride level?						Lower than 89.3 mg/dl

No Change	Years Older +0.5	Years Older +1.0	Years Older +1.5	Years Older +2.0	Years Older +2.5	Years Older +3.0	TALLY
				No			
130/86	Females: 131/87–140/90	Males: 131/87–140/90	Females: 141/91–150/95	Males: 141/91–150/95	Females: 151/96 or higher	Males: 151/96 or higher	
You're under age 70 and level is 161–200 mg% OR you're age 70 or older and level is 161–240 mg%	You're age 70 or older and level is 241–280 mg%	You're under age 70 and level is 201–240 mg%	You're over age 70 and level is higher than 280 mg%	You're under age 70 and level is 241–280 mg%		You're under age 70 and level is higher than 280 mg%	
Male or female and level is 45–54 mg/dl	Female under age 50 and level is 40–44 mg/dl	Male, or female age 50 or older, and level is 40–44 mg/dl	Female under age 50 and level is 30–40 mg/dl	Male, or female age 50 or older, and level is 30–40 mg/dl	Female under age 50 and lower than 30 mg/dl	Male, or female over age 50, and level is lower than 30 mg/dl	
89.3–208.8 mg/dl	Higher than 208.8 mg/dl						

Health Factor	Years Younger -3.0	Years Younger -2.5	Years Younger -2.0	Years Younger -1.5	Years Younger -1.0	Years Younger -0.5
What percentage of your calories is from saturated fat?				Less than 6.7%		6.7–10%
What percentage of your calories is from trans fat?					Less than 1.5%	
What percentage of your calories is from polyunsaturated fat?					More than 5.8%	
Do you get selenium in food and supplements?						

Total Tally from Chart

Multiplier (see Chart at Right to Find the Correct Multiplier)

Net RealAge Change from Nutritional and Related Habits and Choices

Chronologic Age

Your RealAge

☐ × ☐ = ☐ + ☐ = ☐

No Change	Years Older +0.5	Years Older +1.0	Years Older +1.5	Years Older +2.0	Years Older +2.5	Years Older +3.0	TALLY
10.1–13.3%			More than 13.3%				
1.5–2.6%		More than 2.6%					
4.26–5.8%		Less than 4.2%					
Effect is not known yet; more data are expected within 3 years							

TOTAL: ☐

Age	Multiplier
<40	0.1
40–50	0.15
50–60	0.2
60–70	0.3
70–80	0.3
80–90	0.2
90–100	0.1

Developing an Age Reduction Plan: Go from Knowing Your RealAge to Making Yourself Younger

Now that you have calculated your RealAge based on your current food choices in Chart 2.1 or online, it's time to develop your own nutritional age reduction plan. Reread Chart 2.1 to see what you can do to become younger. If you used our website to calculate your RealAge, look back over the age-reducing suggestions given to you by the computer program. Evaluate your options. What changes are you willing to make? Which ones aren't you willing to make, at least, right now?

Some choices may already be part of your life. Perhaps you already eat a few nuts at the start of dinner every evening, or maybe you've never had any problems with weight gain. That's great. Those factors are helping to keep you young. What else could you be doing? The information in this book is appropriate for you in either case: It can help you become younger if you are already at your proper weight, and it can help if you want to adopt a nutrition plan to get to the weight that is right for you.

Look over the list of age reduction strategies in Chart 2.2 and determine which ones could help you to get younger. Begin with the Quick Fixes, such as taking the right vitamins in proper doses, eating an ounce of nuts every day, and enjoying fish. There's no reason not to adopt them—they can take 3 to 6 years off your RealAge with almost no effort. Then, work your way down the list, through Moderately Easy Changes to the Most Difficult Changes, adding age reduction behaviors as you see fit. Always check with your physician before initiating or stopping any age reduction strategy. But *do* make some choices. Food choices can make your RealAge as much as 13 years older than the average person of your calendar age. But easy substitutions can reduce your RealAge by 2 to 14 years. And you can do this easily and with world-class taste.

CHART 2.2
51 Food and Behavior Choices That You Can Enjoy to Make Your RealAge Younger
QUICK FIXES

These age-busters are simple things that anyone can do. You can become 3 to 6 years younger with hardly any effort at all.

1 Eat an ounce of nuts five days a week.

❑ I do it
❑ I will do it
❑ I might do it later

• Eating an ounce of nuts (and we do not mean doughnuts) before dinner is a great way to start the meal with a little healthy fat. Although this tasty habit reduces your chances of arterial aging and its consequences, be careful to limit yourself to an ounce or so, since nuts pack a lot of calories.

RealAge benefit:
Women: 1.1 years younger in ninety days
      3.4 years younger in three years
Men: 1.5 years younger in ninety days
      4.4 years younger in three years

2 Take vitamins C and E daily for their antioxidant and antiaging power.

❑ I do it
❑ I will do it
❑ I might do it later

• Consume food that contains vitamin C three times a day. Get more than 1,200 milligrams (mg) a day of vitamin C through your diet or supplements, spread out so that you get at least 400 mg in any twelve-hour period.
• Consume 400 international units (IU) of vitamin E a day. To be optimally absorbed, fat-soluble vitamins need to be consumed with a little fat, so take your vitamins when you're eating a little monounsaturated fat.

RealAge benefit: Up to 3 years younger

3 Take calcium and vitamin D daily to keep your bones young.

❑ I do it
❑ I will do it
❑ I might do it later

• Consume 1,200 mg of calcium a day in food or supplements if you're a woman or 1,000 mg a day if you're a man. Add another 200 mg for each hour you are physically active and for each six cans of diet soda you drink.

- Consume 400 IU of vitamin D in food or supplements, or get ten to twenty minutes of sun a day.

RealAge benefit: 1.3 years younger

4 Consume the fat-soluble vitamins, such as D and E, with some fat.

❏ I do it
❏ I will do it
❏ I might do it later

- So that your body absorbs the fat-soluble vitamins and nutrients, take them with a little fat (one-half ounce or so).

RealAge loss: If you don't take the fat-soluble nutrients and vitamins with a little fat, you'll lose the extra years those substances can give you: Up to 1.3 years for vitamin D, 2 years for vitamin E, and 3.1 years for the flavonoids and carotenoids, such as lycopene.

5 Take folate daily to reduce your level of homocysteine, an artery ager.

❏ I do it
❏ I will do it
❏ I might do it later

- Consume 700 micrograms (mcg) of folate (folic acid) a day through your diet or supplements to reduce arterial aging and probably decrease immune aging. The usual supplement requirement is 400 mcg.

RealAge benefit: 1.4 years younger

6 Take vitamin B_6 daily.

❏ I do it
❏ I will do it
❏ I might do it later

- Consume 4 mg of vitamin B_6 daily in food or supplements to make and keep your arteries younger.

RealAge benefit: As much as 1 year younger

7 Don't take needless vitamins and supplements.

❏ I do it
❏ I will do it
❏ I might do it later

- Every day, take a multivitamin that contains all the necessary vitamins and minerals—especially vitamins C, D, and E, folate, and calcium—in the correct amounts, but contains no iron and not more than 8,000 IU of vitamin A. Do not take vitamin A as a supplement, and do not take iron as a supplement, except under the supervision of a physician.

RealAge loss: For taking needless vitamins or supplements, 1.7 years older

8 *Floss and brush your teeth daily; see a dental professional regularly.*

❏ I do it
❏ I will do it
❏ I might do it later

- Dental problems such as gingivitis (inflammation of the gums) and periodontal disease (disease of the bone and tissue that support the teeth) can ruin the pleasure of eating. Even worse, gingivitis and periodontitis can work through your immune system to damage arteries. We don't know why gum disease and chronic infections cause aging, but they do. For example, in terms of RealAge, a fifty-five-year-old man who is free of periodontal disease is 2 years younger than a peer who has gingivitis and 4 years younger than a peer who has full-blown periodontal disease.

RealAge benefit: If you're free of gingivitis and periodontitis, up to 6.4 years younger

RealAge loss: If you have full-blown periodontal disease, up to 3.4 years older

9 *Eat fish.*

❏ I do it
❏ I will do it
❏ I might do it later

- Eat fish—*any kind that's not fried*—three times a week. A total of 13 ounces is all it takes to gain substantial benefit. Since we don't really know if fish oil supplements give you the same benefit, eat and enjoy fish.

RealAge benefit: 1.6 to 3.4 years younger, depending on your age and gender

10 *Develop an age reduction program.*

❏ I do it
❏ I will do it
❏ I might do it later

- Developing an age reduction program is the quickest, easiest, and most important step in keeping you young. It can make the RealAge of a seventy-year-old as much as 29 years younger. It's relatively easy to make yourself the first 3 to 6 years younger from nutritional changes alone. Getting younger than that requires some work.

  Some people find it difficult to control their blood pressure through food choices, to take charge of their nutrition every time they pay for food, to retrain their palate to enjoy the healthy fats, and to go for the colorful foods. But isn't it worth some work to have a RealAge of 56 just from nutritional choices alone or of 42 to 45 from adopting all of the health choices when your calendar age is seventy? In this book I give you strategies to accomplish these and other goals.

RealAge benefit: As much as 29 years younger

MODERATELY EASY CHANGES

These choices will make you younger fast, and they require only a little more effort than the Quick Fixes. Some, like eating a little monounsaturated fat before each meal, are as easy as the Quick Fixes but require a little more thought to implement. These changes can help your RealAge become 5 to 8 years younger.

11 Eat a little monounsaturated fat before each meal.

❑ I do it
❑ I will do it
❑ I might do it later

- The only thing that makes this change moderately easy rather than a quick fix is that it takes a little effort to remember it at every meal. It may be easy to start dinner off with a few nuts (see Chapter 4 for how many nuts of each variety), but what about breakfast? Be inventive. Try nut butter, freshly ground flaxseeds on your cereal, a granola cereal made with olive oil, or an egg white omelet made in a little olive oil. Sharing your inventive taste delights with the rest of us at the www.RealAge.com website probably gives you even more youth than just this food choice alone.

RealAge benefit: 1.8 years younger in three years

12 Don't let situations you can't control stop you from making smart food choices. Take charge of your nutrition every time you pay for food.

❑ I do it
❑ I will do it
❑ I might do it later

- If you eat out frequently, the most powerful anti-aging strategy you can have is to ask servers about the ingredients in each food choice and whether they can be modified to make the dish more age reducing. ("Can you ask the chef if that onion soup can be made without the cheese and white bread?") By the way, consider tipping the server extra if he or she helps you stay younger.

RealAge benefit: At age seventy, 6 to 14 years younger, depending on how frequently you eat out

13 Diversify your diet.

❏ I do it ❏ I will do it ❏ I might   do it later

• Eating a diverse diet that daily includes four servings of fruit, five servings of vegetables, some whole grains, protein (meat, fish, nuts, or soybeans), and low-fat milk or milk substitute (rice or soy milk) will help keep you feeling young.

RealAge benefit: Up to 4 years younger

14 Get enough sun, but not too much.

❏ I do it ❏ I will do it ❏ I might   do it later

• Getting some sun—ten to twenty minutes every day—makes your RealAge 0.9 years younger by producing active vitamin D. Wearing sunscreen when you're in the sun for longer than this, avoiding tanning salons, and avoiding excessive sun exposure will help prevent aging.

RealAge benefit: 1.7 years younger

15 Now for women as well as men: Eat tomato paste and sauce.

❏ I do it ❏ I will do it ❏ I might   do it later

• Eating ten servings of tomato paste and tomato products a week helps prevent prostate cancer. When eaten with a little oil, lycopene, the carotenoid found in tomatoes, provides an immune-strengthening antioxidant that seems to inhibit prostate cancers. Lycopene, which is also found in watermelon, guava, and pink grapefruit, may also decrease the risk and growth of other cancers and may make your arteries younger. The evidence for a benefit from lycopene has increased since publication of the first RealAge book, and so has the RealAge benefit of this tasty, colorful choice.

RealAge benefit:
For men, as much as 1.8 years younger
For women, as much as 1.1 years younger

16   Avoid exposure to passive smoke, especially while eating.

❏ I do it ❏ I will do it ❏ I might   do it later

• Don't tolerate working, living, or eating in a smoke-filled environment. Passive smokers experience almost as much aging as real smokers.

RealAge loss: For those exposed to four hours a day or more of passive smoking, 6.4 years older

17   Get your flavonoids.

❏ I do it ❏ I will do it ❏ I might   do it later

• Flavonoids are antioxidants—substances that help protect the body from damage by free radicals—found in plants. One reason red wine has an anti-aging effect is that it is rich in flavonoids. For age reduction, the optimal amount of flavonoids is 31 mg a day. The richest sources are onions, (about 4 mg from one small onion), green tea, cranberries, broccoli (1 cup, about 4.2 mg), celery, tomatoes (1 medium, about 2.6 mg), apples (1 medium, 4.2 mg), garlic, strawberries (1 cup, 4.2 mg), and grapes (see Chart 4.5).

RealAge benefit: 3.2 years younger

18   Drink alcohol in moderation.

❏ I do it ❏ I will do it ❏ I might   do it later

• Women who have one alcoholic drink a day and men who have one or two drinks a day have a younger RealAge. However, people who are at potential risk or have a family history of alcohol abuse or addiction should not drink alcohol at all.

RealAge benefit: 1.9 years younger

19   Take all necessary (and only necessary) medicines, and take them correctly in relation to food.

❏ I do it ❏ I will do it ❏ I might   do it later

• Taking medications as prescribed by your doctor makes your RealAge 0.9 years younger. Avoiding drug interactions makes your RealAge 0.7 years younger.

   Many medicines interact with food. For example, grapefruit and grapefruit juice radically change the concentration of many drugs in the blood. The grapefruit or grapefruit juice doesn't have to be consumed near the time of the pills—just tell your doctor if you wish to add grapefruit to your diet or that you already eat it regularly, and he or she can adjust your dosage.

Some fat-soluble drugs require fat for absorption, and some drugs have decreased absorption in the presence of foods. For example, tetracycline binds calcium into a compound that is not easy to absorb, so neither is absorbed well in the presence of the other. Fosamax (alendronate), a drug used to prevent bone loss, similarly is bound by coffee and should be taken only with water.

These interactions can be reviewed by your doctor or pharmacist, but they are least problematic when you take each medicine at the same time each day and in the same relationship to meals. Discuss your medication with your doctor and pharmacist and always disclose all prescriptions, over-the-counter drugs, vitamins, and herbal or other supplements that you take both regularly and occasionally.

RealAge loss: If you take medicines incorrectly, 1.6 years older

20 Eat breakfast daily.

| ❏ I do it
❏ I will do it
❏ I might
   do it later | • No one is sure why, but eating breakfast makes you younger.

RealAge benefit: 1.4 years younger |

21 Have cereal or soluble fiber every day.

| ❏ I do it
❏ I will do it
❏ I might
   do it later | • A 10-gram (g) increase in the daily intake of cereal fiber decreases the risk of heart attack and arterial aging by 29 percent. Soluble fiber helps regulate metabolism and digestion and stabilizes blood glucose levels by moderating the rate of nutrient absorption. Soluble fiber is found in grains such as oats, oatmeal, barley, and rye; legumes such as beans, peas, and lentils; and cereals such as Cheerios and Kashi. |

RealAge benefit:
For men, 2.4 years younger
For women, 4.5 years younger

22 Eat fiber, and eat it early in the day.

❑ I do it
❑ I will do it
❑ I might do it later

• Fiber helps reduce the risk of diverticulitis and inflammatory bowel disease and helps prevent peaks in glucose levels that accelerate aging. Insoluble fiber can be found in many foods: grapefruit, oranges, grapes, raisins and dried fruit, okra, sweet potatoes, peas, zucchini, whole wheat bread, granola, papaya, and peaches. Whether it's soluble or insoluble, fiber slows the emptying of the stomach and first part of the intestine, making you feel fuller and less hungry four to eight hours later. If you have foods with fiber in your breakfast, you will have less desire for a large afternoon snack.

RealAge benefit: For eating insoluble fiber, 0.6 years younger

MODERATE CHANGES

These age reduction strategies require a little more work and commitment than the Moderately Easy Changes, but once you put your mind to it, you'll watch those needless years fade away.

23 Eat like a peasant. Eat a balanced diet that's low in calories, high in nutrients, and delicious.

❑ I do it
❑ I will do it
❑ I might do it later

• This is a good way to remember what food choices are the healthiest. Peasants had to eat whole grain foods, rather than refined or processed flours and foods (remember "Let them eat cake"?). Everyone in the working class had to eat less fancy forms of fats and proteins—fish and olive oil rather than steak and butter. Fish and olive oil are far less aging than steak and butter. Also, coarse bread is much better for your genes than croissants and makes you feel full faster. Peasant-style food can help you lose weight slowly and stay young longer.

RealAge benefit: 6 to 8 years younger

24 Eat a diet low in "four-legged" (animal) saturated and trans fats.

❏ I do it
❏ I will do it
❏ I might do it later

• Aim to keep your fat intake to no more than 25 percent of your daily calories—about 60 g of fat a day. Of this, no more than 20 g should be saturated or trans fat.

Trans fat—"the hidden fat"—is not listed on food labels. If you see "partially hydrogenated vegetable oil" on the label, or more fat than can be accounted for by adding up all the saturated, polyunsaturated, and monounsaturated fats, you can assume that the rest is artery-aging trans fat.

RealAge benefit: Up to 6.4 years younger

25 Make sure your diet contains monounsaturated and polyunsaturated fats, and eat them at the right time.

❏ I do it
❏ I will do it
❏ I might do it later

• Even though you should avoid saturated and trans fat, to make your RealAge as young as possible you need to consume about 25 percent of your calories as fat and to eat them early in each meal. Most of this fat should be healthy monounsaturated and polyunsaturated fats such as those found in olive oil, avocados, flaxseeds, canola oil, fish, and nuts.

RealAge benefit: 3 years younger

26 Make substitutions you enjoy.

❏ I do it
❏ I will do it
❏ I might do it later

• A few substitutions can make a big difference in your rate of aging. They also make food taste great! Try olive oil instead of butter or margarine on bread, or canola or olive oil instead of 1 to 3 tablespoons of butter in smaller recipes. Substitute fruit for cookies; orange slices for orange juice; orange juice fortified with calcium and vitamin D for unfortified orange juice; dark chocolate for milk chocolate; nuts for chips; and cooked garlic salsa or marinara sauce for a cream sauce.

RealAge benefit: Up to 12 years younger

27 Don't forget the fruit.

❑ I do it
❑ I will do it
❑ I might do it later

- The lengthening of the average life span has paralleled the availability of fresh fruit. Fruits are rich in vitamins, fiber, carotenoids, and other nutrients. Remember to wash fruit well, but to keep the peel on. If you peel an apple or pear, you're tossing most of the fiber. Also, processed juices don't have the same fiber content as whole fruit. When you're making your daily choices, reach for two or three pieces of whole fruit.

RealAge benefit: For eating four servings of fruit a day, 0.5 years younger

28 Become a lifelong nutrition learner, and learn how to cook.

❑ I do it
❑ I will do it
❑ I might do it later

- People who have higher levels of education and those who continue to be involved in activities that stimulate their mind undergo less mental aging. In RealAge, the college graduate is 2.5 years younger than the high school dropout.

Of course, you get extra benefits if you learn about nutrition and cooking! You could subscribe to the free e-mail "Tip of the Day" at the RealAge website. You could also subscribe to a favorite nutrition newsletter, like the *Nutrition Action Health Letter,* published by Consumer Science in the Public Interest, 1875 Connecticut Avenue N.W., Suite 300, Washington, DC 20009.

Becoming a lifelong nutrition learner has three benefits: You'll make your food make you younger, your mind will stay young, and it's fun. We credit you with the benefit of a younger mind from this choice.

RealAge benefit: 2.5 years younger

29 Have safe sex.

❑ I do it
❑ I will do it
❑ I might do it later

- In Chapter 10 you'll see my rating scale for food choices (Chart 10.2). You need a scale to compare the quality of food, and a 10 means it's almost as good as great sex. (We snuck this one in since people liked it so much in the first RealAge book.) The more orgasms you have a year, the younger you are. The average fifty-five-year-old American has sex fifty-eight times a year. Increasing the number to 158 through mutually monogamous and safe sex can make your RealAge as much as 8 years younger.

RealAge benefit: 1.6 to 8 years younger

30 Identify your genetic risks from your food choices and use age reduction strategies to reduce those risks.

| ❏ I do it
❏ I will do it
❏ I might
   do it later | • If, for example, cardiovascular disease runs in your family, take extra precautions with enjoyable food substitutions to keep your arteries young. Such choices might include olive oil for butter, an additional piece of fruit a day, eating a few nuts regularly, or drinking a glass of wine each evening. Similarly, you can reduce your risk of cancer, arthritis, and many other chronic conditions that might run in your family. |

Your RealAge will be 4 years younger if both your parents (or grandparents, if your parents aren't that old yet) lived past the age of seventy-five. If no first-degree relative (parent, brother, or sister) had breast, colon, or ovarian cancer diagnosed early, you are an additional 0.2 to 11 years younger than if a first-degree relative had received one of those diagnoses.

RealAge benefit: If both parents lived past seventy-five, 4 years younger

MODERATELY DIFFICULT CHANGES

These age reduction steps require commitment and work, but the payoff is in many "years younger."

31 Retrain your palate to enjoy peasant food.

| ❏ I do it
❏ I will do it
❏ I might
   do it later | • When you were born, your palate didn't automatically love foods with saturated or trans fats—Krispy Kreme doughnuts, Cinnabons, or "Blumin Onions." The saturated and trans fat in one of these is more than three days' worth of the amount of fat that promotes optimal aging. Also, each of these will make you more than three days older. |

If you've gotten to like those items, you'll need to retrain your taste buds (palate) to again enjoy what they originally did—whole grain foods and foods that contain less saturated ("four-legged") fat and trans fats.

Retraining the palate to prefer olive oil or cold-pressed canola oil or fish is just that—retraining. If you drank whole milk and switched to skim, it probably took eight weeks before you preferred the skim milk. For baked goods, for the first four weeks, if a recipe calls for 3 tablespoons of butter, try 2 tablespoons of butter and 1 tablespoon of canola oil. Then, for the next four weeks, try 1 tablespoon of butter and 2 tablespoons of canola oil. After eight weeks, you and your family will love the taste, and all of your RealAges will be significantly younger.

RealAge benefit: Depending on your present choices, 6 to 12 years younger

32 Retrain your intestine.

| ❏ I do it
❏ I will do it
❏ I might
   do it later | • Your food is digested, to a large extent, in the intestine, which is accustomed to your current pattern of eating. Just as you have to retrain your taste buds to prefer less saturated fat and enjoy more healthy fat, fruits, vegetables, and nuts, you need to retrain your intestine. If you don't, the result is often flatulence (gas). |

As you increase your intake of fiber, fruits, vegetables, nuts, and soy protein, your intestine makes the necessary adjustments in metabolism and produces less gas. However, people who are deficient in lactase, an enzyme that breaks down lactose, one of the sugars found in milk, will always produce flatulence when they consume milk. Other people cannot digest beans. In those cases, the person can take the enzyme (for example, lactase) that helps in the digestion of the problem food. Another option is to eat only a small portion of the food.

If you switch from a low-fruit, low-vegetable, low-fiber diet to the RealAge Diet all at once, you may not feel very well. You most likely will have bloating and gas, and perhaps nausea and an upset stomach. Your intestine has become used to unhealthy food, so retrain it gradually. The training period for the intestine, just like that for the palate, is about eight weeks.

RealAge loss: If you do not retrain your intestine, about 8 years older (depending on how many friends you lose)

33 Retrain your eye.

❑ I do it
❑ I will do it
❑ I might do it later

• Think "healthy" at the grocery store, the restaurant, and the coffee shop. Retrain your eye. Think about the control you have over your choices when you go shopping for food. If you buy only nutrient-rich food, you'll eat only health-giving food. Before you put any item in your cart, ask yourself, "Will it help keep me young?" If the answer is no, get it out of your cart. Fast!

Part and parcel of retraining your eye is to read between the lines at all places you pay for food. That means becoming a label reader, a menu reader, and a good observer.

RealAge loss: If you do not retrain your eye, 2 to 13 years older, depending on your present age

34 Be a label reader.

❑ I do it
❑ I will do it
❑ I might do it later

• Be aware of hidden fats, simple sugars, and needless calories. For all prepared foods, learn to read what is first, second, third, fourth, and fifth in the list of ingredients. Notice what the label calls one serving. Most saturated fats, trans fats, and sugars are hidden ingredients in many processed foods, but the package label may provide the clues you need.

For example, many commercial brands of cereal and processed breads contain lots of added fats and sugars. What are some other common foods that may have hidden unhealthy ingredients? Canned soups and vegetables, and even granola, can contain high quantities of sugars and saturated fats or trans fats. By becoming a label reader, you won't consume needless calories that you didn't know were there.

Remember, "fat free" doesn't necessarily mean healthier or age reducing. Many "fat-free" products are good for you and form part of an age reduction diet, but not all are. You have to read the label. Fat-free cookies, muffins, and ice cream may be "fat free," but they are usually full of added simple sugars and calories, and low on nutritional value. Ask to see the label or nutritional value listing; you'll be years younger because you did.

RealAge benefit: 2 to 27 years younger

35 Lower your lousy cholesterol and increase your healthy cholesterol.

❑ I do it
❑ I will do it
❑ I might do it later

• Try to keep your total cholesterol level below 200 milligrams/deciliter (mg/dl) and your healthy (HDL) cholesterol level at or above 46 mg/dl. There are at least four ways to increase HDL cholesterol: Eat healthy fats; get plenty of physical activity; drink a little alcohol every day; take certain statin drugs; and, if you're a woman, take certain estrogens. Statin drugs, such as Lipitor or Pravachol, or Zocor, are commonly used to treat high lousy (LDL) cholesterol levels, and some of them, such as Lipitor, also increase healthy (HDL) cholesterol levels. Niacin is sometimes combined with these. Increasing your good cholesterol is important because, as we age, the amount of good cholesterol in our blood becomes much more significant to our arteries than the amount of lousy cholesterol or the total cholesterol.

RealAge benefit: 3.7 years younger

36 Exercise regularly, expending at least 3,500 kilocalories of energy a week.

❑ I do it
❑ I will do it
❑ I might do it later

• Walking the equivalent of an hour a day, or doing more vigorous exercise for a shorter time, can bring your level of physical activity up to the optimum age reduction range. Walking just a half hour a day gives you half the extra years that general physical activity can provide.

RealAge benefit: 3 to 8 years younger

37 Build stamina.

❏ I do it
❏ I will do it
❏ I might do it later

- Do stamina-building exercises that boost your heart rate and aerobic intake for at least twenty minutes three times a week. You should exercise vigorously enough to raise your heart rate to 70 percent of the maximum for your age group, or to break a sweat in a cool room.

RealAge benefit: Up to 6.4 years younger

38 Make yourself strong.

❏ I do it
❏ I will do it
❏ I might do it later

- Do strength-building exercises, such as weight lifting, three times a week for at least ten minutes. This is particularly important for women, since it helps maintain bone density.

RealAge benefit: 1.7 years younger for men and 2.2 years younger for women

39 To avoid the possible accumulation of unsafe contaminants, eat foods from a variety of sources.

❏ I do it
❏ I will do it
❏ I might do it later

- Eat a variety of foods from a variety of sources. Remember to wash all fruits and vegetables carefully, and to cook all foods that should be cooked. None of us can predict where contamination will occur in the food chain. It isn't only pesticides, either. Some organically grown fish have been contaminated, as have native soy and corn crops. The best protection is to vary your food sources, so you're less likely to accumulate a toxic dose of any contaminant. (I discuss the controversy on genetically engineered food later in the book.)

RealAge loss: If you don't vary your food sources and don't cook appropriately, 1 year older

40 Make your vegetables delicious and eat them often.

❏ I do it
❏ I will do it
❏ I might do it later

- One of the tricks to a diet that is moderate in fat, low in calories, and full of nutrients is to eat lots of vegetables. Since vegetables contain lots of fiber, they help you fill up fast. With only 20 to 50 calories a serving, vegetables help you feel full and keep your weight down. They are also full of vitamins, carotenoids, and flavonoids, many of which have antioxidant properties that will help keep you young. Try to eat five or six servings of vegetables a day.

Just because you hated vegetables as a kid doesn't mean you won't like them now. Try steaming them with a little lemon juice or sautéing them lightly. Cook green vegetables just until they turn bright green. If they go all the way to gray, you've cooked them way too long.

Each day, try to eat some kind of dark, green, leafy vegetable and one serving of a cruciferous vegetable (broccoli, cauliflower, or cabbage). The prettier and brighter your plate, the younger the foods will make you.

Make vegetables your new snack food. Buy bags of pre-cut vegetables and keep them in the fridge. I even keep veggie burgers (largely soy and vegetables) in the freezer in a lunchroom at work and microwave them for snacks. Cucumbers, celery, peppers, radishes, and even mushrooms all make great snacks. Eaten raw, vegetables keep all of the nutrients and fiber that cooking can deplete.

RealAge benefit: As much as 6 years younger

41 Use food choices to help manage chronic disease.

❑ I do it
❑ I will do it
❑ I might do it later

• Learning how to manage such diseases as diabetes, cardiovascular disease, arthritis, and many other chronic conditions can dramatically decrease the impact they can have on aging. Arterial aging can be largely prevented and even treated by eating in the enjoyable RealAge way. Nutrient choices like vitamins C, D, and calcium for preventing arthritis, and such foods as fruits, nuts, and whole grains for diabetes, can make aging less a part of these chronic conditions.

RealAge benefit: Depending on the disease, how much it ages you can be diminished considerably, sometimes to an almost indiscernible effect

42 Find out what a legume is and how to make it enjoyable for you.

❏ I do it
❏ I will do it
❏ I might
   do it later

- What are legumes? Green beans, red beans, black beans, lima beans, lentils, peanuts, peas, chickpeas—almost any pea or bean that comes in a closed pod. Four studies have shown that eating legumes decreases blood pressure and arterial aging and their consequences—heart disease, stroke, memory loss, impotence, decay in the quality of orgasm, and even wrinkling of the skin. Consumption of legumes also reduces autoimmune diseases, many forms of arthritis, and cancer.

RealAge benefit: The same 0.6 years younger you get for eating fiber, plus the benefit produced by the other nutrients in the legumes you choose

43 Get enough water.

❏ I do it
❏ I will do it
❏ I might
   do it later

- Your body is about 60 percent water, and it works hard to make sure it stays that way, through the opposing mechanisms of stimulating your thirst and reducing the amount of urine you produce. If you have not taken vitamins in the last four hours and your urine tends to be darker, you need more water. And all of us need lots of fluid (at least eight glasses a day). Although water is best, juices, soups, and skim milk can also provide fluid. Make sure you drink extra water to keep yourself properly hydrated, especially if you are exercising, the weather is hot, or you drink dehydrating drinks such as caffeinated coffee or alcohol. What's the best kind of water? We don't know. But most experts agree that as long as your town treats its water and the water is free of excess minerals and bacteria, tap water is usually okay.

RealAge benefit: We cannot put an age value on adequate hydration because the necessary period of dehydration would not be ethically acceptable for studies on humans.

44 Find out which foods contain selenium and enjoy them.

❑ I do it
❑ I will do it
❑ I might do it later

- Selenium is one of the minerals that is clearly needed in small amounts but causes harm in excess. We should know soon if aiming for the high end of the safe range—up to 1,000 mcg a day—is age reducing. There are just not enough studies yet, but selenium appears to strengthen the immune system and reduce the rate of many cancers.

  Don't supplement with more than 200 mcg a day, and do use organic as opposed to inorganic selenium. Even better, get your selenium from food. Foods high in selenium are Brazil nuts, garlic, whole grains, cereals, meats, and some seafood.

RealAge benefit: Perhaps as much as 6.8 years younger, although there's not enough data yet to say this with confidence

THE MOST DIFFICULT CHANGES

Choices 45 to 51 refer to the things that age you the most and are the hardest to fix. Working to overcome these obstacles is one of the most important things you can do to keep your RealAge young.

45 Make nutritional choices to keep your blood pressure low: Increase your calcium, potassium, vegetable, and fruit intake; perhaps reduce your weight gradually; and cut back on salt.

❑ I do it
❑ I will do it
❑ I might do it later

- Keeping your blood pressure at the ideally low level—115/76 mmHg or lower—makes your RealAge 9 years younger than if your blood pressure were at 130/86 mmHg, the national average for middle-aged Americans. It also makes your RealAge more than 25 years younger than someone who has a blood pressure of 160/90 mmHg or higher (moderately high blood pressure).

  Reducing your blood pressure from the national average to the ideally low level makes you 4.5 years younger in six months and 9 years younger in three years, provided you do so before any permanent structural damage occurs in the arteries.

Blood pressure of 120–130/80–85 mmHg is considered normal but not ideal.

Increased intake of fruit, potassium, calcium, olive oil, fish, and garlic; increased physical activity; and decreased weight, saturated fats, trans fats, and perhaps salt can all help lower blood pressure.

RealAge benefit: For a blood pressure of 115/76 mmHg or lower, 10 to 15 years younger

RealAge loss: For a blood pressure of 140/90 mmHg or higher, 10 to 15 years older

46 Eat regularly throughout the day.

❑ I do it
❑ I will do it
❑ I might
   do it later

• Many people believe they will lose weight if they starve themselves all day, waiting until dinner to eat, at which time they gorge. If you starve yourself for long periods of time, your body may switch to a starvation mode in which your metabolism may act as though you need to conserve energy and may cause weight gain even when your calorie intake is normal. Moreover, most people feel so hungry they sneak an aging snack—a saturated fat-laden cookie or a bag of aging trans-fat chips—sometime in the mid-afternoon. Make sure to eat regular meals, and don't skip breakfast.

RealAge loss: For keeping a stable weight, up to 6 years younger. This is the same benefit provided by Choice 47.

47 Maintain a steady weight.

❑ I do it
❑ I will do it
❑ I might
   do it later

• Reduce your weight gradually to what it was at age eighteen, if you're a woman, or twenty-one, if you're a man. Your goal should be to reduce your body mass index to less than 23 (see Chapter 9). Even if you can't achieve these ideal weights, reducing your weight to a lower level, one that is comfortable for you, and keeping it there still produces a RealAge benefit. Lose weight slowly and consistently and avoid yo-yo dieting, since rapid weight gains and losses cause aging.

RealAge benefit: 6 years younger

48 Cut back on excessive consumption of alcohol.

❏ I do it
❏ I will do it
❏ I might do it later

• Alcohol addiction and abuse can cause severe aging, bringing about liver failure and triggering cancers. Drinking more than three drinks a day causes you to age needlessly.

RealAge loss: 3 years older

49 Cut out excess sugars.

❏ I do it
❏ I will do it
❏ I might do it later

• Remember, carbohydrates were meant to be complex. Even though simple sugars in your food add empty calories, that's not the worst effect. Simple sugars in food are absorbed quickly in the intestine and increase the amount of sugar in the blood for at least one to two hours. A high concentration of sugar in the blood eradicates the natural protective control your body has over the usual, everyday variations in blood pressure. High blood sugar levels also increase triglyceride levels in the blood.

RealAge benefit: For eliminating added and simple sugars, 5 years younger

50 Not so difficult, but perhaps most important: Make healthy eating an enjoyable and aesthetic social event.

❏ I do it
❏ I will do it
❏ I might do it later

• Having three or more stressful major life events in one year can create more than 30 years of aging. Having lots of friends, strong support networks, and strategies for coping with stress can minimize the effect.

• Use the time and situation of eating to reduce stress. Connect with friends, and laugh a lot. Laughter is a whole-body stress reducer. It helps open lines of communication with others and reduces anxiety, tension, and stress. Laughter makes your immune system younger. Having a network of close friends and/or family can help prevent aging from excessive stress.

• Make the place you eat special. Always sit down when you're eating, and decorate that special place with colors and furniture that are particularly pleasing to you and yours.

RealAge benefit: For people who use times (but not quantities) of eating as a great stress reducer, 8 to 16 years younger

RealAge loss: For people who don't have strategies for stress reduction, 30 to 32 years older during high-stress times. For people who do have effective strategies for stress reduction, as little as 2 years older during high-stress times

---

51 Not so difficult, but also very important: Stay on your RealAge Diet steps!

| ❏ I do it
❏ I will do it
❏ I might
    do it later | *RealAge benefit:* For making the best food choices versus the worst food choices, up to 27 years younger |

Keeping Yourself on Track: Easy Does It!

Once you have identified strategies that could make your RealAge younger, you'll want to read the rest of this book to understand why and how the different choices will make you younger and learn strategies that other people have come up with to make these substitutions enjoyable and easier. You might also reconsider your decision *not* to adopt an age reduction strategy, once you see the kind of impact it can have. For example, many of my patients are at first hesitant to ask a lot of questions and make requests at restaurants, a practice I discuss later in the book, especially in the presence of friends who aren't familiar with RealAge ideas. Once they learn how easy and important this is, many decide to be more assertive when eating out.

Use Chart 2.3 to develop a step-by-step plan for age reduction. Don't try to do everything at once.

Begin by adopting just two or three steps.

Trying to do too much at once can be overwhelming. A common problem with all health initiatives—whether diet plans or exercise regimens—is that we take on too much at once. After a few days of playing the superhero, we give up on everything, never to return to the plan.

The patients in my clinical practice who have been the most successful at age reduction have begun by choosing only two or three steps. They stayed on those steps for three months and, after successfully incorporating them into their daily routines, added two or three more steps, and so on, climbing an easy staircase to success. Climbing just two or three steps at a time makes it easy. They frequently recalculate their RealAge. They modify and update their age reduction plans. One patient calls me every Monday morning. "Mike," she says, "I've adopted such-and-such. What's my RealAge now?" Although you may modify your plan as often as you like, most people make modifications every three months.

Try the Easier Steps First

By adopting the steps in the Quick Fix category first, you can begin reducing your RealAge in just a few days or months with little effort. Reducing your RealAge further requires a little more resolve. Most of the choices are not that difficult; you just need practice. What better payoff than adding quality years to your life?

The decisions that are going to require the most commitment are maintaining a steady weight, getting regular physical activity, avoiding secondhand smoke, retraining your palate to prefer healthy foods, training your eye to spot aging ingredients on labels, cutting out excess sugars, making healthy eating a happy social event, and controlling your blood pressure through food choices. But the payoff is huge.

The RealAge difference between two people who are the same chronologic age but have made different nutritional choices can be as much as 27 years.

If you decide to retrain your palate, you'll start to feel the difference—and others will start to see the difference—after the first eight weeks. You'll enjoy food more, you'll probably lose weight, and you'll definitely feel more energy.

Prioritize Your Steps

Which steps are easy for you? Which steps are difficult but important? Which are less important? Deciding that you will start every dinner with an ounce of nuts requires only that you buy the nuts and remember to eat them first each evening. Other decisions involve more work. Reducing portion size is more difficult, but it is easier if you've eaten the nuts first. You'll soon agree.

Decide the load you can handle. If you have two age reduction goals that are in the Most Difficult Changes category, you probably won't want to adopt both at the same time. Pick one and stay on it. Once you've got the hang of it, pick another. Don't, for example, try to manage your blood pressure by nutritional choices and retrain your palate at the same time. Choose one, and once you've succeeded with that, adopt the other.

Break a Large Task into Parts

If you're trying to lose weight, begin by eating a diet that is rich in fruits, vegetables, and whole grains. Then work on cutting back the amount of saturated and trans fats you eat. Don't worry about watching pounds right away; start by developing healthy eating steps. You might be surprised to see that the pounds come off on their own. Once you have eating under control, start to cut back on calories or begin to integrate exercise into your life. The most important thing about age reduction steps is not that you start them but that you stay on them. Exercise, for example, gives little benefit three months after you stop.

Put your age reduction plan where you can easily see it. Tape it to the bathroom mirror, near a phone, on the refrigerator, or inside the kitchen cabinet you open most often. Look at it often and remember what you can do to get younger. Recalculate your RealAge every few months, or whenever you adopt a new age reduction step. That way, you'll know just how young you've become.

The Difference between RealAge *Maximums* and RealAge *Interactions:* The Impact on *You*

As you read this book and review the choices that help make you younger, remember that the RealAge numbers presented in all the charts except Chart 2.1 and in all the chapters are the *maximum possible* effects. As I explained at the start of this chapter, they presume only that nutritional choice alone is affecting age reduction and do not account for interactions between factors. The numbers are *not* cumulative. This method has the benefit of allowing you to compare the relative value of food choices, but the drawback of not accounting for multiple interactions.

Let's consider an example. In Chapter 5, I state that taking vitamins C and E in food or supplements can make you 3 years younger. The impact is astounding. Is it true? Yes. Is it true for you? Not necessarily. Although a person who does nothing else to protect him- or herself from aging may well have a RealAge benefit of as much as 3 years simply by taking these two vitamins, most of us make many other health decisions as well. The vitamin benefit is moderated by other choices, including exercising, eating nuts, and eating a vegetable- and fruit-rich diet.

Indeed, none of us has only one factor that affects his or her rate of aging. For all of us, many, many factors affect our rate of aging. You cannot simply add up all the years of benefit that certain behaviors provide and subtract those from your calendar age. Let's say you floss your teeth regularly (6+ years younger), eat monounsaturated fat and little saturated fat (3 years younger), exercise (9 years younger), and have an appropriate stable weight (6 years younger). You cannot simply total these years, subtract them from your calendar year, and say that you are twenty-four years younger than your calendar age. If you did that, you might work your way back into childhood, even into negative years!

Instead, when you calculate your RealAge, the effect of any one step depends on your other health behaviors and choices. Calculating that effect involves complex equations and complex mathematics, which is why modern computer technology is necessary. But we have done this, and can tell you the relative and absolute values of your choices. This is what makes the RealAge program so revolutionary: It calculates the effects of complex and multiple behaviors on aging *all at once.*

RealAge Means Informed Choices

In the rest of the chapters, I go over the scientific research studies and discuss the biological impact of the fifty-one choices, most of them related to nutrition, presented in Chart 2.2. I show you which ones help keep you young longer and suggest strategies for incorporating those changes into your life.

I begin by reviewing factors that make you older: aging of the arteries, aging of the immune system, and aging from environmental causes. In subsequent chapters I explain how specific factors, such as taking the right vitamins in the proper doses, eating monounsaturated and polyunsaturated fats, getting plenty of physical activity, and ordering wisely in a restaurant can all make you younger. I give you the information you need to stay healthy and vitally young and, incidentally, slimmer. You make the choices about how you want to grow old.

And, yes, it's *that* important.

CHART 2.3

Your Personal Age Reduction Plan

My RealAge is: _____

I want my RealAge to be: _____

Now that I have calculated my RealAge, what nutritional and related steps can I adopt to make myself younger?

1 _____

2 _____

3 _____

4 _____

5 _____

6 _____

7 _____

8 _____

Which steps am I willing to change?

1 _____

2 _____

3 _____

4 _____

5 _____

Which three steps are the most important?

1 _____

2 _____

3 _____

Which three steps are the easiest?

1 _____

2 _____

3 _____

(continued)

Dates: _____ to _____

In the next three months, I will adopt these three RealAge Diet age reduction steps:

1 _____

2 _____

3 _____

Dates: _____ to _____

After three months, I will continue the first three steps and also adopt the following three:

1 _____

2 _____

3 _____

In three months, my RealAge will be: _____

In one year, my RealAge will be: _____

In three years, my RealAge will be: _____

3

The Bestseller Diets: Do They Make Your RealAge Younger or Older?

Modifying the Bestseller Diets to Make Them Healthier

Many people are willing to do almost anything to lose a few pounds: eat only cabbage soup, drink only canned diet shakes, or even eat bacon and cheese at every meal, week after week after week. Most people lose weight in the first two weeks when they're on these diets. That's why there are so many bestseller diet books and so many different diets that seem to contradict each other.

If you are one of the millions of people buying these books, you know what I'm talking about. In fact, you may be on a bestseller diet right now, and you may have already lost weight. Do you wonder if it's making you younger? I did, and so did many of my patients. In fact, it was the experience of one of these patients, Dr. Marks, that motivated me to write this chapter.

Dr. Marks was the newly appointed chair of a well-known department of internal medicine on the East Coast. Previously, he had been a section chief who guided the clinical and research activities of about twenty busy physicians. In his new position as department chair for almost two hundred physicians, that task was ten times greater. The previous chair was a tough act to follow. In addition to the normal stressors of his position, the situation of declining reimbursement in the face of rising costs in the health care industry was causing him a great deal of extra stress. These circumstances caused him to acquire habits that were aging his body.

He used to be able to keep his weight stable by strictly controlling how much he ate, but now denial was not working. He had gained 40 pounds in just six months. This put him 110 pounds over a body mass index of 25, the point at which you should consider losing a little weight. He worried about his weight and the possibility that his blood pressure was skyrocketing. He also began to have low back pain and decreased stamina at work. He realized that his obese condition made him a likely candidate for type II diabetes. In desperation, he returned to a method that had worked for him in the past—the Atkins diet. He had lost weight on the Atkins diet in the past, but gained back that weight, and more.

Yes, he knew that a healthy diet would work, but he didn't want to wait that long. So he put himself on the Atkins diet, a regimen of mainly protein and fat and no carbohydrates, and lost 40 pounds. After a few weeks, he started feeling uneasy about taking shortcuts with his health and, knowing I was writing this book, sought my advice: "Is this Atkins diet good for my overall health? Is there any data suggesting that this diet may be bad for me if I continue it indefinitely? Because, I've got to tell you, Mike, it's working well for me."

Although Dr. Marks seemed to have finally found the secret of weight control, he worried that it was too easy. Although many of my patients have tried a variety of diets with varying results, the question he asked was the most important one: "Is this diet good for my overall health?"

Of course, I had to tell him what he already knew: If it seems too good to be true, it probably is. Eating an unbalanced diet is bound to have a not-so-good effect on your health. However, losing weight and keeping it off might be worth the risk if the diet prevents high blood pressure, diabetes, and arthritis and promotes physical activity. These were platitudes. I wanted to know a lot more about the subject. Which diets are people following? What are the costs and benefits of each? Do these diets affect a person's RealAge? After all, Americans spend $33 billion a year on the diet industry. We deserve to know what we are getting for our money.

The RealAge Team Analyzes the Popular Diet Books

Several of the RealAge nutrition experts and I gathered the dozen most popular diet books and analyzed each of them. Some bestseller diets are called "fad diets," because they are not widely accepted by mainstream medicine. The current popularity of these diets—as evidenced by both the number of books bought and the number of people advocating the diets—indicates that they have indeed moved well into the mainstream of American thought about nutrition. Many of these diets have helped their readers achieve some success at accomplishing their goals. Within that framework, we examined these diets and assessed how well they measure up to their stated goals and the ultimate goal—optimizing *your* individual health.

For each of the books, the RealAge team and I analyzed the diet itself, the theories and recommendations, the supporting scientific evidence, and the recipes. We also assessed how well the claims and theories of the books agreed with widely accepted principles of physiology (as presented in two well-known physiology textbooks and the peer-reviewed medical literature from 1966 to the present).

To determine whether each diet affects the rate of aging, the RealAge team and I subjected it to two tests.

The First Test: Does the Diet Fight Aging?

We first looked at each diet in terms of the factors known to make your RealAge younger:

- Is the diet nutrient rich and calorie poor?
- Does it try to provide 25 percent of its calories from fat?
- Does it restrict the consumption of animal fat and promote the consumption of monounsaturated fat?
- Does it provide 25 grams (g) of fiber per day?
- Does it include four servings of fruit per day?
- Does it include five servings of vegetables per day?
- Does it contain ten servings of foods that contain lycopene, for example, tomatoes, watermelon, or guavas, per week?
- Is it a diverse diet that contains low-fat dairy or dairy substitutes (like soy milk), protein, fish, vegetables, and fruit?
- Does it include three or more servings of fish per week?
- Does it encourage you to consume complex carbohydrates and avoid simple sugars?
- Does it encourage consumption of legumes (green beans, red beans, black beans, lima beans, lentils, peanuts, peas, and chickpeas)?
- Does it include 5 ounces of nuts per week?

- Does it limit the dietary intake of salt to 2,400 milligrams (mg) or less per day?
- Does it promote water intake?
- Does it promote regular meals?
- Does it promote adequate intake of potassium (3,000 mg per day)?
- Does it promote adequate intake of calcium (1,200 mg per day) and other minerals?
- Does it promote optimal intake of vitamins?
- Does it promote weight loss by calorie restriction?
- Does it promote long-term weight loss management?
- Is there evidence that people can maintain weight loss and an ideal weight on this diet?
- Is there evidence that the diet promotes health?

We also, of course, had to rate the following:

- Is the diet easy to understand?

Since these criteria are not all equally important to aging, we gave each a "weighting" factor. From analyzing the scientific literature, we know that no diet can make your RealAge more than 14 years younger or 13 years older than average. Therefore, we adjusted our statistical methods to take this range into account.

Three people independently read each diet book and used a scale of 0–5 to rate how well the menus and recommendations in it meet each of the above criteria. Their results were independently rated, compared, and discussed. When there was substantial disagreement, the differences were resolved by a fourth independent reader. We subjected the resulting data to standard statistical methods to calculate the RealAge effect of each diet.

The Second Test: How Much Nutrition Does the Diet Provide?

We also analyzed each diet for its nutritional contents. That is, we randomly sampled menus representing ten days of meals. We then used three well-known nutritional programs to analyze the nutritional content of each of the recipes. By using three programs we tried to avoid errors that using only one program might introduce. Any major discrepancies between nutrient analyses were reviewed. We regret if we accidentally let any errors slip in, but we think these analyses are fair and accurate representations of the diets. For the flavonoid content of salads, we did uniform estimates among all the diets for each nutrient. Since the type of lettuce was not specified in many diets (endive and romaine and lettuces that are dark green have many more flavonoids than iceberg), we assumed all lettuce was endive or romaine when not specified. Also, our analyses excluded beverages other than milk (cow, rice, or soy, when specified) and tea but included recommended snacks. Supplements were not included in these analyses.

The resulting values were averaged, and the nutritional content determined.

How the Diets Stack Up

The results of both tests are presented in Chart 3.1. As you can see, the two tests yielded consistent results. Guess what? As it turns out, many of the diet books we examined offer relatively healthy programs. Here are the astonishing results.

CHART 3.1
How the Bestseller Diets Affect Your RealAge, as Determined by Two Tests

Diet Book	Test 1: Analysis of the Book's Recommendations Versus Our Aging Factors	Test 2: Nutritional Analysis of the Book's Recipes (without Modification)	Average of the Two Tests
The RealAge Diet: Make Yourself Younger with What You Eat	Could make your RealAge 14 years younger	Makes your RealAge 11.8 years younger	12.9 years younger
Eating Well for Optimum Health, by Andrew Weil, M.D.	Could make your RealAge 9 years younger	Makes your RealAge 3.3 years younger	6.2 years younger
Eat More, Weigh Less, by Dean Ornish, M.D.	Could make your RealAge 5.8 years younger	Makes your RealAge 4.3 years younger	5.1 years younger
The Anti-Aging Zone, by Barry Sears, Ph.D.	Could make your RealAge 1.8 years younger	Makes your RealAge 6.7 years younger	4.3 years younger

(continued)

Diet Book	Test 1: Analysis of the Book's Recommendations Versus Our Aging Factors	Test 2: Nutritional Analysis of the Book's Recipes (without Modification)	Average of the Two Tests
Everyday Cooking with Dr. Dean Ornish, by Dean Ornish, M.D.	Could make your RealAge 5.8 years younger	Makes your RealAge 0.7 years younger	3.3 years younger
The Carbohydrate Addict's Diet, by Rachael F. Heller, Ph.D., and Richard F. Heller, Ph.D.	Could make your RealAge 3.4 years younger	Makes your RealAge 3.1 years younger	3.3 years younger
The New Pritikin Program, by Robert Pritikin	Could make your RealAge 2.3 years younger	Makes your RealAge 3.4 years younger	2.9 years younger
The Omega Diet, by Artemis Simopolos, M.D., and Jo Robinson	Could make your RealAge 6.7 years younger	Makes your RealAge 2.6 years older	2.1 years younger
Sugar Busters! Cut Sugar to Trim Fat, by H. Leighton Steward, M.D., and others	Could make your RealAge 0.8 years older	Makes your RealAge 0.9 years younger	0.1 years younger
Eat Right for Your Type, by Peter J. D'Adamo, N.D. (average of all four diets)	Could make your RealAge 2.8 years older	Makes your RealAge 1.2 years younger	0.8 years older
Protein Power, by Michael Eades, M.D., and Mary Dan Eades, M.D.	Could make your RealAge 3.8 years older	Makes your RealAge 0.9 years younger	1.5 years older
Suzanne Somers' Get Skinny on Fabulous Food, by Suzanne Somers	Could make your RealAge 0.6 years older	Makes your RealAge 2.9 years older	1.8 years older
Total Health Makeover, by Marilu Henner	Could make your RealAge 3.5 years older	Makes your RealAge 1.0 years older	2.3 years older

Diet Book	Test 1: Analysis of the Book's Recommendations Versus Our Aging Factors	Test 2: Nutritional Analysis of the Book's Recipes (without Modification)	Average of the Two Tests
Dr. Atkins' New Diet Revolution, by Robert Atkins, M.D.	Could make your RealAge 5.7 years older	Makes your RealAge 3.8 years older	4.7 years older

Why Are There Some Discrepancies between the Two Tests?

There are three reasons the two methods are not in perfect agreement:

- The writing and goals of the author differ from the specifics of the menus and recipes in the book.
- We used different criteria and weightings for the two tests. In the first test we placed more weight on the accuracy of the science and the ease of understanding and following the diets.
- We gave more weight to some nutritional factors (saturated fat, selenium, legumes, and meat, for example) in the first test than in the second.

Abandon or Switch Diets?

Our nutritional analyses of the diets, presented in Charts 3.2 through 3.13, have an additional benefit: They show you how to make each diet healthier. You can use each diet to make your RealAge younger. I will tell you how to do so.

Many of the bestseller diet books fall into one of three categories: high-protein diet, high-carbohydrate diet, or specialty diet. A high-protein diet is high in protein and (usually) fat and low in carbohydrates. A high-carbohydrate diet is usually low in fat and protein. A specialty diet is one that either restricts certain food groups or adheres to the author's own particular philosophy about food and diet.

High-Protein Diets

Since high-protein diets restrict carbohydrates, they rely largely on protein and fat to provide calories and nutrients. They are high-fat, low-carbohydrate food combinations. The philosophy behind high-protein diets is simple: Decrease your intake of carbohydrates, and you decrease your blood sugar levels, a condition that causes the pancreas to produce less insulin. With less insulin, your body cannot process and convert fat from food or convert the protein to sugar (as it would with normal carbohydrate intake) and thus is forced to burn fat reserves. This assumption—that lower insulin levels mean that your body will use its fat for energy—is *not* established scientifically. Nonetheless, this type of diet does promote weight loss. The appeal of these diets is that they tell you not to worry about fat grams at all. What relief for people who have been diligently counting fat grams and feel deprived.

The best known of the protein-rich, fat-laden diets are the Atkins diet, the Protein Power diet, the Carbohydrate Addict's diet, and the Sugar Busters diet. We will discuss how each falls short of the RealAge optimum, and how it can be modified to be healthier. But first a look at the effects of high-protein diets in general.

Why Do You Lose Weight?

In many cases, high-protein diets work simply by restricting calories. Look at the nutritional analyses of these diets in Charts 3.2 through 3.5. There are only about 2,000 calories per day in each of these diets! This is well below the 2,700 to 2,800 calories per day in the average American diet. Yet these diets say they *don't* restrict calories—and they allow you to eat calorie-laden foods.

How do you lose weight? When you eat fat, you feel fuller faster (that's why it's great to eat a little healthy fat before a meal), leading to less eating and restriction of calories.

Calorie restriction may not be the only reason your weight starts to drop. High-protein foods cause you to urinate frequently and lose a lot of water. In fact, usually about 70 percent of your weight loss during the first week of a high-protein diet is probably due to water loss.

Why High-Protein Diets Make Your RealAge Older

They Promote Ketoacidosis

Many high-protein diets encourage weight loss through a process that produces ketoacidosis (acidic blood). Although this process does cause weight loss, it can be extremely bad for your body. Ketoacidosis is a condition in which the blood is acidic because of the presence of high levels of ketones (toxic chemical compounds) that are produced when fat cells begin to break down. When you eat a diet low in carbohydrates, the body runs out of carbohydrates and looks for another source of fuel. Its major backup sources are protein (destroying such proteins as muscle to produce sugar) and fat. This process causes ketones to accumulate in the blood, which makes the blood acidic. Since it's important for the acid level of the blood to stay within a certain range for health, the body tries to get rid of the excess ketones by excreting them in the urine, and with them goes a lot of water. This is one reason why you may become dehydrated on a high-protein diet. Your body is producing a lot of urine. Other effects include shortness of breath, especially with some physical activity, and lack of stamina. You also begin to dislike the foods, since ketoacids disturb your sense of taste. In the next phase of the diet, you reduce calorie intake, further contributing to ketoacidosis. Once your body reaches the ketoacidosis state, your body's biochemical equilibrium is disturbed radically and you're putting yourself in jeopardy. When ketoacidosis gets to a certain point, it's a medical emergency, with a risk of abnormal heart rhythms and potential of loss of cardiac function.

They Lack Variety

Another big problem with high-protein diets is they limit the variety of foods you can eat and instead focus on meat, which is full of artery-aging saturated fats. Eating a diet that is full of variety is basic for health. In addition, because few people can stay away from almost all carbohydrates forever, you are at a higher risk of yo-yo dieting. Yo-yo dieting not only is discouraging and frustrating but also aging. In fact, these diets seem to inspire a false sense of security. "I can lose the weight any time I want on the Atkins diet. I tried it for two weeks two years ago and lost eleven pounds," Tom D. told me. He then gained 60 pounds in the following two years. He continued, "So why diet till I have to? I haven't had a heart attack yet, so I don't have to diet yet, do I?" Of course, he came to see me because of impotence and lack of energy, both caused by his artery-aging eating. This false sense of security from two weeks of success ("At that rate I can lose forty pounds in two months") was perpetuating aging behaviors while simultaneously causing the deterioration of his health. In addition to a lack of variety, the risk of yo-yo dieting, and loss of water in your urine, you can become dehydrated. As a result of dehydration and lack of fiber, high-protein diets often cause constipation and may increase the risk of colon cancer.

Dr. Atkins' New Diet Revolution, *by Robert Atkins, M.D.*

This is the diet my friend, Dr. Marks, called the "bacon diet": It seems to allow you to eat bacon all day long and still lose weight. Which he did. He stayed on the diet until he tired of it, and until he started to have a sour odor, despite the use of after-shave lotion. (The sour odor is a sign of ketoacidosis.)

What's the Theory?

The goal of the Atkins diet is to lose weight on a protein-rich, low-carbohydrate regimen that doesn't restrict calories. Dr. Atkins claims you'll lose weight even if you're eating the same quantity of calories that made you gain weight. What makes this possible? He provides numerous anecdotes (informal observations) about many people who have lost weight through the biological process of ketoacidosis, which follows from eating a high-protein diet.

Why Is It a Bestseller?

You can see why this is a popular book. Eat as much bacon, cream, and butter as you want, and still lose weight! Dr. Atkins asserts that if people replaced their cereal, banana, and skim milk with a ham and cheese omelet every day for thirty weeks, they would lose 51 more pounds of fat than if they stayed with cereal. It's a tempting diet, especially if nothing else has worked for you. Sales of the book and our own informal surveys indicate that this diet does cause weight loss, at least in the short term.

Will It Make You Younger or Older?

Of ninety people who had been on the Atkins diet and visited us over the years (mostly men chose this diet in our sample), eighty-one reported they had lost more than 10 pounds in their first two weeks on the diet. So, at first, there *is* weight loss. (The long-term effect of the diet in these ninety people will be discussed later.) Initially, you lose weight, because the lack of carbohydrates in your diet forces your body to use the glycogen stores in your muscles (glycogen is a carbohydrate your body uses to store energy). Since these stores also contain water, your muscles lose water and glycogen fast. A heavily muscled person will lose 7 pounds or more in the first three or four days. A less muscled person will lose 3 to 5 pounds.

Although Dr. Atkins claims you can eat the same number of calories as before and still lose weight, it's simply not true. One of the main causes of weight loss in this diet is simple calorie restriction. Even though you don't have to curb your calories, whenever you cut a major food group from your diet, you're bound to also cut calories. Finally, you eventually get bored with so much bacon, so you eat less food and consume fewer calories.

Dr. Atkins neglects to discuss the potentially harmful side effects of his diet. For example, ketoacidosis can cause weakness, dehydration, and even sudden death from disturbances in heart rhythm. It frequently results in a lack of stamina. He also overlooks the long-term effects of consuming a lot of saturated fat. Saturated fat can wreak havoc on your arteries: It increases your blood pressure and ages your arteries and immune system. Dr. Atkins claims his diet actually does not increase bad cholesterol levels or decrease healthy cholesterol levels, but those unhealthy consequences occur if you do not stay strictly on the diet and do not lose weight. For most patients, this much saturated fat increases your risk of arterial aging and its consequences—heart attacks, strokes, memory loss, impotence, and many other ill effects. But there are benefits.

There is no question that the Atkins diet works in the short term, but do the results last? Does this diet help change your eating habits so you keep the weight off? Our surveys indicate that most people do not stay on the diet. They end up yo-yo dieting.

What happens to your body if you have a carbohydrate binge while you're on the diet, or if you start eating carbohydrates again after being on the diet for a long time? Unfortunately, no scientific studies have been done on these situations. We do know that rapid weight fluctuations adversely affect your heart and cause your RealAge to become much older (see Chart 9.3).

The diet also makes your RealAge older because the recipes lack soluble fiber, monounsaturated and polyunsaturated fats, and sufficient nutrients. In fact, in a 1999 version of the Atkins diet, you're asked to take sixty-one pills a day! Taking sixty-one pills a day, at the right times, seems almost a full-time job and wasn't done by *any* of our ninety Atkins dieters, so we gave the diet a low rating for ease of use.

The Atkins diet also ages you because the recipes lack a lot of nutrients—appropriate amounts of fruit, lycopene, fish, legumes, water, calcium, folate, and nuts—and variety in the diet. It's also high in salt. All in all, this diet makes your RealAge 3.8 to 5.7 years older.

Would a RealAge benefit from weight loss offset the aging effect of this diet? Perhaps. If you have the effects of being overweight—high blood pressure, low back pain, high levels of bad cholesterol, etc.—and you're able to stay on the diet long enough to reduce your weight, lower your blood pressure, and alleviate back and joint pain so you can become more physically active, you could probably get younger with Dr. Atkins's prescription. But you may want to modify the Atkins diet to make yourself younger.

How to Make the Atkins Diet Healthier

Here's how you can modify the Atkins diet so it makes your RealAge younger:

- Eat fish, soy protein, nuts, olives, and other monounsaturated and poly-unsaturated fats as your proteins and fat.
- Avoid saturated and trans fats—avoid all four-legged fats—and substitute nuts, fish, and olive oil for beef jerky, meat, cream, and butter.
- Add four low-carbohydrate fruits (see Chart 4.3) to your daily diet as your carbohydrates.
- Use supplements to ensure you're getting all the fiber, minerals, and vit-amins you need.

Is it worth going on the Atkins diet to get a temporary weight loss? Maybe. But remember, the long- and short-term effects of going on an unmodified Atkins diet could make your RealAge more than 5 years older. Also remember

---

REALAGE CAFÉ TIP 3.1
Yo-Yo Dieting: The Facts

Yo-yo dieting, also called weight cycling, occurs when you lose and regain weight repeatedly. Typically, you jump into a fad diet all at once, feel food-deprived a couple of weeks or months into it, and then return to bad eating habits. Yo-yo dieting not only is frustrating, but is possibly more harmful than maintaining a steady weight, even if that weight is not ideal. This is true whether you lose 5 or 15 pounds and then regain it, or you lose more than 50 pounds.

That doesn't mean you shouldn't try to lose some weight if you need to. There is a difference between being overweight (weight up to 30 percent more than normal) and being obese (more than 30 percent over your normal weight). Being overweight, especially to the point of obesity, is extremely hard on your health and could lead to high blood pressure, cardiovascular disease, diabetes, and even cancer. Losing as little as an inch from your waist can give you big health benefits. Keeping your weight and body mass index at a desirable level can make your RealAge as much as 6 years younger.

Although many studies have suggested that repeated weight loss and gain may be linked to a shortened life span, the results are not yet conclusive. We do know that yo-yo dieting can be hard on your self-esteem, and this could lead to even more weight gain. If you tend to yo-yo diet, the problem may be the diet itself. For example, if your diet eliminates or severely restricts whole food groups, it's likely you won't be on that diet forever. Likewise, if you crash diet—skipping meals or not eating at all for long periods of time—this is not a lifestyle that you can or should maintain.

CHART 3.2

The Atkins Diet: Nutritional Contents of Ten Days of Recipes Randomly Selected from the Book

Age-Reducing Factor	What We Found in the Recipes:	RealAge Optimum
Calories per day (on average)	2,070	
Protein (g/day)	127	
Carbohydrates (g/day)	48	
Fat (g/day)	146.5	
% of calories that are fat	63.7	About 25%
% of fat that is saturated	43	Less than 33%
Saturated fat (g/day)	62.6	Less than 20*
% of fat that is monounsaturated	35.8	More than 40%
Cholesterol (mg/day)	1,087	Less than 150
Fiber (g/day)	10	25 or more
Sodium (mg/day)	2,570	2,400 or less
Potassium (mg/day)	2,653	3,000 or more
Iron (mg/day)	15.2	12–20
Calcium (mg/day)	599	1,200 or more
Folate (mcg/day)	360	700 or more
Vitamin E (IU/day)	12.5	400 or more
Vitamin C (mg/day)	56	1,200 or more
Fish (oz/week)	5.6	13 or more
Nuts (oz/week)	2.5	5 or more
Lycopene (servings/day)	1.4	1.5 or more
Flavonoids (mg/day)	4.1	30 or more

Note: Atkins, R. C. *Dr. Atkins' New Diet Revolution.* New York: Avon Books, 1997, and Atkins, R. C. *Dr. Atkins' Age-Defying Diet Revolution.* New York: St. Martin's Press, 2000. Robert Atkins, M.D., states that he is a cardiologist and internist. We could not determine if he was board certified in either of these American Board of Medical Specialty Societies. This chart does not include nutrients from the sixty-one supplement pills per day Atkins recommends.

*The RealAge optimum is less than 20 g per day of saturated and trans fat. This column lists only saturated fat, since few diets and menus use partially hydrogenated vegetable oils, or processed foods with partially hydrogenated vegetable oils.

that yo-yo dieting is aging. What happened to the ninety people who initially lost more than 10 pounds on the diet? Six lost 25 pounds or more and kept it off on a *modified* Atkins diet. Five are back to about their original weight. Most important, seventy-nine couldn't stay on the diet and now weigh an average of 11 pounds more than their original weight.

Protein Power, *by Michael Eades, M.D., and Mary Dan Eades, M.D.*

Another diet that limits carbohydrates and focuses on protein is the Protein Power diet, which is similar to the Atkins diet but offers more options. It makes your RealAge either slightly older or slightly younger.

What's the Theory?

The Protein Power diet, like the Atkins diet, claims to lower insulin levels. This is a benefit, the Eadeses say, because slightly lowering the level of insulin in the usual overweight person brings the insulin level into a normal range and helps the person lose weight. Not only that, but on this diet, if you're hungry, you're supposed to eat more protein. And, yet, no matter what your caloric intake is, you'll still lose weight.

Why Is It a Bestseller?

This diet is better than many of the other protein diets, because it doesn't require you to abstain completely from any major food group. Moreover, it encourages you to exercise, eat healthy monounsaturated fats, take a multivitamin, and drink water (almost all diets do that). All of these are attributes of eating the RealAge way.

Will It Make You Younger or Older?

The Protein Power diet lacks scientific evidence. The two anecdotal cases provided by the Eadeses are not definitive proof, because they were extreme cases of survival. I simply don't feel comfortable using such limited evidence when it comes to my health. Also, while reading the book, I found many medical discrepancies, and that makes me wonder about the accuracy of the rest of the book. For example, on page 12, the Eadeses write, "Reams of scientific studies, with more added to the stack daily, implicate excess insulin as a *primary* cause of a significant risk factor for high blood pressure, heart disease, obesity, elevated cholesterol and other blood fats, and diabetes."

Neither I nor the RealAge scientific team know of even *one* study that implicates excess insulin (in the ranges found in all but rare cases like the disease syndrome X) as a cause of high blood pressure.

On page 25, the Eadeses write, "Based on this reasoning and very little hard evidence, since no long term hypertensive control studies had ever been done, the push was to get Americans with high blood pressure diagnosed and medicated."

This statement is not only wrong but also dangerous. Physicians didn't start to treat hypertension aggressively until there were several solid studies (there are now more than nine) showing that treatment of even moderate hypertension prevented heart disease, stroke, kidney failure, and impotence. Nine randomized, controlled-intervention studies (the highest quality of studies) show that treatment of even mild hypertension slows arterial aging.

On page 151, the Eadeses write, "On our program the reduction in carbohydrate intake begins immediately to allow most ulcers and gastritis to heal."

Again, I know of no data that support this important claim; if there are such cases greater than the placebo effect, they would be important and worthy of scientific publication.

Despite such medical misstatements that make one worry about the scientific backbone of the book, we analyzed the book's nutritional advice and menus.

Although the Protein Power diet may make your RealAge significantly younger than the Atkins diet, it's a difficult diet to follow. Its recipes are high in salt and saturated fats (about twice as much as optimal) and low in nutrients; fiber; fruit; legumes; vitamins C, D, E, and folate; flavonoids; and nuts. They also lack variety.

What happens to your body in the long term? There are no good studies published showing sustained weight loss with this diet. My guess is that you might lose weight because the diet will make you restrict calories, but you'll probably regain it, because the diet is too complicated and strict to follow for a lifetime.

This diet could make your RealAge 0.9 to 3.8 years older. However, if you have low back pain, high blood pressure, and/or high levels of lousy cholesterol, triglycerides, and blood sugar all due to obesity, and you can stay on the diet long enough to lose weight and lower your blood pressure, blood sugar, triglycerides, and lousy cholesterol levels, you will be able to make your RealAge substantially younger.

How to Make the Protein Power Diet Healthier

You can make the Protein Power diet less aging by following the same recommendations we made for making the Atkins diet: Substitute fish for meat, nuts

CHART 3.3

The Protein Power Diet: Nutritional Contents of Ten Days of Recipes Randomly Selected from the Book

Age-Reducing Factor	What We Found in the Recipes:	RealAge Optimum
Calories per day (on average)	1,874	
Protein (g/day)	133	
Carbohydrates (g/day)	85	
Fat (g/day)	112	
% of calories that are fat	53.8	About 25%
% of fat that is saturated	33.8	Less than 33%
Saturated fat (g/day)	37.8	Less than 20
% of fat that is monounsaturated	45.2	More than 40%
Cholesterol (mg/day)	686	Less than 150
Fiber (g/day)	20	25 or more
Sodium (mg/day)	3,285	2,400 or less
Potassium (mg/day)	3,830	3,000 or more
Iron (mg/day)	15.4	12–20
Calcium (mg/day)	891	1,200 or more
Folate (mcg/day)	497	700 or more
Vitamin E (IU/day)	15	400 or more
Vitamin C (mg/day)	255	1,200 or more
Fish (oz/week)	12	13 or more
Nuts (oz/week)	1.4	5 or more
Lycopene (servings/day)	3	1.5 or more
Flavonoids (mg/day)	17.7	30 or more

Note: Eades, M. R., and Eades, M. D. *Protein Power: The High-Protein/Low Carbohydrate Way to Lose Weight, Feel Fit, and Boost Your Health—In Just Weeks!* New York: Bantam Books, 1996. Both Michael R. Eades, M.D., and Mary Dan Eades, M.D., practice bariatric (weight loss) medicine in Boulder, Colorado. The ten days of the Protein Power diet we analyzed included snacks, recommended desserts (one in ten days), and beverages (including seven cups of tea in the ten days, and wine). The Eadeses recommend supplementing with a multivitamin that contains twenty-two substances but considerably less than the RealAge optimum of calcium, magnesium, vitamin E, and vitamin D. We did not include the supplement in the nutritional analysis.

and low-carbohydrate fruits and vegetables for snacks, and olive oil for cream and butter. To make your RealAge even substantially younger on the Protein Power diet, you'd have to make these modifications and gradually lose weight until you reach the weight you were at age eighteen (women) or twenty-one (men).

The Carbohydrate Addict's Diet, *by Rachael Heller, Ph.D., and Richard Heller, Ph.D.*

What's the Theory?

This diet is very similar to the Protein Power diet in that its goal is to break your addiction to carbohydrates and decrease your insulin levels slightly so that you lose weight. This theory is not supported by any scientific evidence we know of. The hypothesis, as advanced by Atkins, the Eadeses, the Hellers, Barry Sears, and other authors, is that taking in fewer carbohydrates slightly lowers the insulin level in your blood. That part is established. The next part is what's in doubt: that having a slightly lower insulin level will decrease your appetite, make your body use its fat reservoirs, and lower the risk of heart disease. These assumptions have not been proven. The Carbohydrate Addict's diet requires you to avoid foods that increase your desire for carbohydrates, eat foods that decrease your addiction (especially at breakfast and lunch), and develop a positive attitude about controlling your addiction.

Why Is It a Bestseller?

The concept of breaking an addiction, growing thin, and improving your self-image is alluring, especially when food rewards are involved. An improved self-image is probably many people's main motivation for going on a diet. With the previous diets I've discussed, restricting a major food group will lead to consumption of fewer calories and, eventually, weight loss. I enjoyed the inspirational parts of the book but was dismayed to find only anecdotal reports and little supporting scientific evidence, even though the Hellers seem to be substantial scientists.

Will It Make You Younger or Older?

The Carbohydrate Addict's diet will make your RealAge about 3.3 years younger, if you follow it; however, this diet is harder than the Atkins diet to implement. Using the Hellers' criteria for carbohydrate addiction, most people will test positive. One of our researchers gave the test to fifty people, and *all* of them tested at least moderately positive as carbohydrate "addicts." Perhaps this

CHART 3.4

The Carbohydrate Addict's Diet: Nutritional Contents of Ten Days of Recipes Randomly Selected from the Book

Age-Reducing Factor	What We Found in the Recipes:	RealAge Optimum
Calories per day (on average)	2,244	
Protein (g/day)	123	
Carbohydrates (g/day)	149	
Fat (g/day)	134	
% of calories that are fat	53.7	About 25%
% of fat that is saturated	33.6	Less than 33%
Saturated fat (g/day)	45	Less than 20
% of fat that is monounsaturated	45.5	More than 40%
Cholesterol (mg/day)	735	Less than 150
Fiber (g/day)	19.7	25 or more
Sodium (mg/day)	2,414	2,400 or less
Potassium (mg/day)	2,974	3,000 or more
Iron (mg/day)	19.6	12–20
Calcium (mg/day)	1,017	1,200 or more
Folate (mcg/day)	576	700 or more
Vitamin E (IU/day)	16.5	400 or more
Vitamin C (mg/day)	216	1,200 or more
Fish (oz/week)	5.6	13 or more
Nuts (oz/week)	1.4	5 or more
Lycopene (servings/day)	3.5	1.5 or more
Flavonoids (mg/day)	24.5	30 or more

Note: Heller, R. F., and Heller, R. F. *The Carbohydrate Addict's Lifespan Program: A Personalized Plan for Becoming Slim, Fit, and Healthy in Your 40s, 50s, 60s, and Beyond.* New York: Penguin Books, 1998. Both Rachael F. Heller, Ph.D., and Richard F. Heller, Ph.D., are retired research scientists at Mount Sinai Hospital School of Medicine and the Department of Biomedical Sciences at City University of New York. One is a health psychologist, and the other is a research pathologist. The ten days of the Carbohydrate Addict's Lifespan Program we analyzed included tea (sixteen cups in ten days) and desserts. There was no mention of supplements.

is the point. Everyone needs some amount of carbohydrates to live. Does that mean that everyone needs to go on this particular type of diet? I'm not sure.

How to Make the Carbohydrate Addict's Diet Healthier

As I've mentioned, throughout *The Carbohydrate Addict's Diet* we found substantial medical misstatements that disturb us. For example, the information on hormones, nutrients, and drugs is either misleading or flat-out wrong in important places. Even worse, the sample meals don't follow their own diet plan. They're long on salt and saturated fat; short on fruit and variety; and a little short on potassium, fiber, legumes, nuts, fish, and vitamins (if you do not use supplements). You can make this diet healthier by adding the missing elements. If you read the book to gain inspiration, wonderful. If you're looking to change your eating habits for life, this diet could make your RealAge as much as 3.4 years younger.

Sugar Busters!, *by H. Leighton Steward and Others*

What's the Theory?

Steward and his co-authors claim you will get slimmer and healthier by avoiding foods that quickly break down into simple sugars (high-glycemic foods). This claim is supported by science. However, the Sugar Busters diet also aims to limit the production of insulin, claiming that this will cause weight loss. No science currently proves this. Although this diet isn't a true high-protein diet, it does encourage consumption of foods that are high in protein and saturated fat. Even though the diet probably won't work based on its scientific claims, you may lose weight because of restricted intake of carbohydrates and therefore calories; the menus provide only 1,375 calories a day, as Chart 3.5 shows.

Why Is It a Bestseller?

This is a very appealing diet. People rave about this diet and want to go on it, because it lets you eat butter, eggs, bacon, sausage. The only villain is simple sugar? The diet has a great name! With menus of less than 1,400 calories a day, you will lose weight. And it was developed in one of the taste capitals of the world, New Orleans. If you could eat great in New Orleans style for only 1,400 calories a day, the diet would be great.

Will It Make You Younger or Older?

The Sugar Busters diet will probably make your RealAge older. For starters, no attention is paid to the health effects of eating the amount of foods high in

CHART 3.5

The Sugar Busters Diet: Nutritional Contents of Ten Days of Recipes Randomly Selected from the Book

Age-Reducing Factor	What We Found in the Recipes:	RealAge Optimum
Calories per day (on average)	1,375	
Protein (g/day)	88	
Carbohydrates (g/day)	128	
Fat (g/day)	60.2	
% of calories that are fat	39.4	About 25%
% of fat that is saturated	33.7	Less than 33%
Saturated fat (g/day)	20.3	Less than 20
% of fat that is monounsaturated	42.7	More than 40%
Cholesterol (mg/day)	282	Less than 150
Fiber (g/day)	20.2	25 or more
Sodium (mg/day)	1,654	2,400 or less
Potassium (mg/day)	2,981	3,000 or more
Iron (mg/day)	13.3	12–20
Calcium (mg/day)	718	1,200 or more
Folate (mcg/day)	326	700 or more
Vitamin E (IU/day)	10.7	400 or more
Vitamin C (mg/day)	163	1,200 or more
Fish (oz/week)	8	13 or more
Nuts (oz/week)	3	5 or more
Lycopene (servings/day)	4.5	1.5 or more
Flavonoids (mg/day)	7.5	30 or more

Note: Steward, H. L., Bethea, M. C., Andrews, S. S., Brennan, R. O., and Balart, L. A. *Sugar Busters! Cut Sugar to Trim Fat.* New York: Ballantine Books, 1998. Leighton Steward has a master's of science degree in geology from Southern Methodist University in Dallas, Texas, and was the CEO of a Fortune 500 energy company. As an environmental activist, he has written a booklet about the destruction of the lower Mississippi River wetland system. Morrison C. Bethea is a board-certified cardiovascular surgeon practicing in New Orleans. Samuel S. Andrews and Luis A. Balart are physicians practicing at Louisiana State University. The ten days of the Sugar Busters diet we analyzed included snacks, desserts, and tea (about three cups in ten days). There was no mention of supplements.

saturated fats (eggs, sausage, bacon, and butter) that this diet advocates. In the long run, the positive or negative effects on your health, and on your rate of aging, of a diet that is 40 percent fat are simply not known. But getting 13 or 14 percent of your overall calories from saturated fat will cause aging.

I like some of the recipes and love New Orleans, but the recipes are a little short on fiber, fruit, flavonoids, legumes, calcium, and nuts. Again, it's a gamble. Will the benefits of weight loss make up for the direct aging effects of the food? Based on the information they give us, the Sugar Busters diet will, without modification, make your RealAge 0.9 years younger to 0.8 years older.

How to Make the Sugar Busters Diet Healthier

You can make it healthier by substituting fish for meat and adding four additional pieces of fruit, an ounce of nuts, and some bright-colored vegetables like broccoli and spinach to the menu every day. You'll still be under 2,000 calories a day, and still losing weight, but the effects of the diet will be age reducing.

High-Carbohydrate Diets

The second group of books we analyzed takes an opposing stance to the high-protein diets. These include *Total Health Makeover, Everyday Cooking with Dr. Dean Ornish,* and *The Pritikin Principle.* All of these books recommend that you eat low-fat, high-carbohydrate foods and avoid meats.

Some of these books are written for those who want to reverse arterial aging. The Ornish and Pritikin diets definitely succeed in doing that if you can stay on them. When I tried to eat the Pritikin recipes for two weeks—I did that with each of the diets—I found I couldn't force myself to like the food. And my palate was already used to a diet low in saturated fat. But I didn't give the Pritikin diet eight weeks. These diets may help you lose weight in the short term, but you are likely to feel deprived of the foods you like and want. You might end up eating more, and gaining weight, to make up for the lack of enjoyable taste (for me) in some of these Pritikin recipes.

Also, by eliminating a major food group—most fat—you're putting yourself at risk of nutrient deficiencies (*Total Health Makeover* doesn't have this problem), since your body may not absorb fat-soluble vitamins well. Yes, multivitamins or supplements can help balance out your diet (if taken with some fat), but most nutritionists believe the best nutrients come from food, and a bit of fat is needed to absorb optimally the vitamins from food (or pills).

Can this lack of dietary fat lead to neurological or psychiatric disorders, as some large-scale studies report? The data are not yet clear.

Let's look at each high-carbohydrate bestseller diet individually.

Total Health Makeover, *by Marilu Henner*

What's the Theory?

Henner claims that the body is always seeking balance between three food categories: animal foods, plant foods, and plant derivatives. She says you should avoid animal foods (milk and milk products, cheese, eggs, fish, chicken, and meat) and avoid such plant derivatives as drugs, alcohol, and sugar. What does that leave? Plants. Yes, this is basically a vegetarian-focused diet.

Why Is It a Bestseller?

I'm not sure. The author bases the diet on her own experience, which is a personal approach that many people find inspiring. She is very attractive, appears fit, and was a star on the TV show *Taxi*. The stories about her life and the men she dated are interesting and fun. The main reason for weight loss in this diet is the elimination of a major food group: You are likely to limit calorie intake and lose weight if you eliminate or severely limit all animal and plant-derived products. The menus as written, on average, provide only 904 calories a day, so plenty of calorie room remains to add nutrients to make the diet healthier. Many of the recipes I tested tasted great.

Will It Make You Younger or Older?

Some facets of the Total Health Makeover diet, such as its emphasis on the monounsaturated and polyunsaturated fats, vegetables, water, and fish, make your RealAge younger. This diet is likely to be short-lived, however, and may make your RealAge older because of the effects of yo-yo dieting.

For starters, the directions are complicated. I believe it's difficult to make this diet a lifestyle change. For example, Henner suggests that you not eat proteins and starches together; that you not mix fruit with proteins, starches, or vegetables; that you eat fruit only with other fruit; that you always eat melons alone; and that you not mix acid or subacid fruits with sweet fruits at the same meal (she tells you which fruit belongs in each group). The list of strict instructions would require considerable concentration and discipline to follow. If you don't make the regimen a lifestyle change, you are bound to gain the weight back as soon as you return to old eating habits. Only a dedicated

CHART 3.6
The Total Health Makeover Diet: Nutritional Contents of Ten Days of Recipes Randomly Selected from the Book

Age-Reducing Factor	What We Found in the Recipes:	RealAge Optimum
Protein (g/day)	74.7	
Carbohydrates (g/day)	99	
Fat (g/day)	25.8	
% of calories that are fat	25.7	About 25%
% of fat that is saturated	18.6	Less than 33%
Saturated fat (g/day)	4.8	Less than 20
% of fat that is monounsaturated	48	More than 40%
Cholesterol (mg/day)	131	Less than 150
Fiber (g/day)	15.5	25 or more
Sodium (mg/day)	921	2,400 or less
Potassium (mg/day)	2,732	3,000 or more
Iron (mg/day)	9.4	12–20
Calcium (mg/day)	310	1,200 or more
Folate (mcg/day)	274	700 or more
Vitamin E (IU/day)	16.5	400 or more
Vitamin C (mg/day)	216	1,200 or more
Fish (oz/week)	60	13 or more
Nuts (oz/week)	0	5 or more
Lycopene (servings/day)	2	1.5 or more
Flavonoids (mg/day)	15	30 or more

Note: Henner, M. *Total Health Makeover.* New York: Reganbooks, 1998. Besides being the author of several books, Marilu Henner is a popular actress best known for her roles in the television sitcoms *Taxi* and *Evening Shade* and the Broadway musical *Chicago.* The ten days of the Total Health Makeover diet we analyzed included snacks and juice and tea (about sixteen cups in ten days). Also, Ms. Henner says that you can take a supplement, but she doesn't say how much or which one.

lifestyle change is going to help you lose weight and maintain a low weight for life, helping you to make your RealAge younger.

The other thing that concerns me is that the diet is short on fruit, folate, flavonoids, legumes, calcium, and other minerals. It also lacks variety. Without considering the benefits of losing weight and lowering blood pressure, etc., this diet could make your RealAge 1.0 to 3.5 years older.

How to Make the Total Health Makeover Diet Healthier

This diet is easy to make healthier: Add four fruits a day, an ounce of nuts a day, five bright-colored vegetables a day, and a multivitamin with calcium just after the nuts.

Everyday Cooking with Dr. Dean Ornish, by Dean Ornish, M.D.

What's the Theory?

This plant-based diet takes you one step further than the Total Health Makeover diet, because it restricts all fat. The Ornish diet is designed specifically for people with severe cardiovascular disease, people who are rehabilitating from a heart attack, and people who have had severe angina (chest pain) due to heart disease. For these people the diet is great: It reverses arterial disease with good to excellent taste, if you've trained your palate to like very low fat foods. Do not judge the food the first week you try it—you'll need to train your palate to enjoy food with less fat. However, if your health is average to good and you've not yet had *overt* arterial aging (a heart attack, stroke, or heart disease), restricting all fats may not make your RealAge younger.

Why Is It a Bestseller?

Not many Americans are willing to become vegetarians for life, so why is this book a bestseller? Because the diet doesn't count calories. Instead, it restricts fat and allows you to eat as many complex carbohydrates as you want, supplemented with moderate amounts of nonfat dairy products and egg whites. Dr. Ornish claims that your appetite will be satisfied before you eat too many calories, and thus you'll lose weight (the average day has 1,360 calories as the menu is written). He also asserts that the diet reduces the incidence of osteoporosis, Type II (adult-onset) diabetes, hypertension, obesity, and other illnesses. Who doesn't want to lower the risk of these conditions?

What does science say about the Ornish diet? This diet was examined in three published medical studies, more scientific attention than any other diet I know of has received. The statistics show that intensive lifestyle changes—getting no more than 10 percent of your calories from fat, eating whole foods, eating a vegetarian diet, exercising, reducing stress, and stopping smoking—

lead to a decrease in the size of coronary artery plaques. After five years, a further decrease in coronary atherosclerosis can occur. Fantastic! These changes will help your heart.

The Ornish diet is based in science and is intended for people who have had *overt* arterial aging events and are very motivated. Except for the severity of fat and food restrictions, this program is similar to the RealAge program. My estimate is that following the Ornish regimen would prevent at least 70 percent of arterial aging and its consequences.

But It May Make Your RealAge Older

Although many of Dr. Ornish's assertions are a big part of eating healthfully, some are open to question for people who do not have overt coronary heart disease. For example, he states that the more olive oil you eat, the worse your cholesterol levels and the greater your weight gain will be. However, there are strong indications that moderate amounts of olive oil actually help raise your blood levels of healthy (HDL) cholesterol. Furthermore, healthy fats help your body absorb important nutrients such as antioxidants that protect you from cancer and effectively reduce your risk of cardiovascular disease. Finally, eating a tiny bit of this good kind of fat at the beginning of your meal will help you feel full, so that you don't consume as many calories during your meal.

Also, as you may guess, it's a difficult diet to stick to for the long term. In fact, one study notes that despite the motivation of life-threatening heart disease, only a little more than half of patients who needed either the diet or a major operation were able to continue the diet. Nevertheless, that's about 45 percent more than any other diet.

The diet is light on healthy fats, fish, nuts, and variety, but it hits almost all the other RealAge goals for nutrients. Again, if you tend to go on and off strict diet plans, this diet is probably not for you; you could make your RealAge older. If you can stick with it, the Ornish diet may make your RealAge as much as 0.7 to 5.8 years younger by itself. Then add the additional benefits of lower blood pressure and more activity.

How to Make the Everyday Cooking Diet Healthier

The Everyday Cooking diet is a great diet for those for whom it was designed: people with overt coronary artery disease. If you did not have overt artery aging, this diet could make you younger if you added fish, nuts, onions, apples, tea, wine, avocados, and olive oil. Personally, I found that these simple changes made the diet much tastier.

CHART 3.7A
The Ornish Everyday Cooking Diet: Nutritional Contents of Ten Days of Recipes Randomly Selected from the Book

Age-Reducing Factor	What We Found in the Recipes:	RealAge Optimum
Calories per day (on average)	1,360	
Protein (g/day)	61	
Carbohydrates (g/day)	239	
Fat (g/day)	25	
% of calories that are fat	16.4	About 25%
% of fat that is saturated	32.8	Less than 33%
Saturated fat (g/day)	8.2	Less than 20
% of fat that is monounsaturated	28.2	More than 40%
Cholesterol (mg/day)	63	Less than 150
Fiber (g/day)	34.5	25 or more
Sodium (mg/day)	946	2,400 or less
Potassium (mg/day)	3,985	3,000 or more
Iron (mg/day)	17	12–20
Calcium (mg/day)	895	1,200 or more
Folate (mcg/day)	453	700 or more
Vitamin E (IU/day)	17.6	400 or more
Vitamin C (mg/day)	287	1,200 or more
Fish (oz/week)	0	13 or more
Nuts (oz/week)	0	5 or more
Lycopene (servings/day)	7	1.5 or more
Flavonoids (mg/day)	13.3	30 or more

Note: Ornish, D. Everyday Cooking with Dr. Dean Ornish: 150 Easy, Low-Fat, High-Flavor Recipes. New York: HarperPerennial, 1997. Dean Ornish, M.D., is an internist and cardiac researcher who is president and director of the Preventive Medicine Research Institute in Sausalito, California. He is a board-certified internist on the faculty at the University of California at San Francisco. The ten days of the Everyday Cooking diet we analyzed included fruit for dessert. There was no mention of supplements.

CHART 3.7B

The Ornish Eat More, Weigh Less Diet: Nutritional Contents of Five Days of Recipes Randomly Selected from the Book

Age-Reducing Factor	What We Found in the Recipes:	RealAge Optimum
Calories per day (on average)	1,758	
Protein (g/day)	67	
Carbohydrates (g/day)	358	
Fat (g/day)	14	
% of calories that are fat	7.2	About 25%
% of fat that is saturated	29.6	Less than 33%
Saturated fat (g/day)	4.2	Less than 20
% of fat that is monounsaturated	22.8	More than 40%
Cholesterol (mg/day)	22	Less than 150
Fiber (g/day)	50	25 or more
Sodium (mg/day)	1,842	2,400 or less
Potassium (mg/day)	6,615	3,000 or more
Iron (mg/day)	21	12–20
Calcium (mg/day)	1,235	1,200 or more
Folate (mcg/day)	703	700 or more
Vitamin E (IU/day)	9	400 or more
Vitamin C (mg/day)	441	1,200 or more
Fish (oz/week)	0	13 or more
Nuts (oz/week)	0	5 or more
Lycopene (servings/day)	3.8	1.5 or more
Flavonoids (mg/day)	23	30 or more

Note: Ornish, D. *Eat More, Weigh Less : Dr. Dean Ornish's Life Choice Program for Losing Weight Safely While Eating Abundantly.* New York: HarperPerennial, 1993. Dean Ornish, M.D., is an internist and cardiac researcher who is president and director of the Preventive Medicine Research Institute in Sausalito, California. He is a board-certified internist on the faculty at the University of California at San Francisco. There are seven days of recipes in his meal plan; we used five for these analyses. The days of the Eat More, Weigh Less diet we analyzed included fruit for dessert. There was no mention of supplements.

What about Dr. Ornish's Other Books?

A few of my scientific reviewers worried that *Everyday Cooking with Dean Ornish* had a diet different from the diet in his earlier books. Dr. Ornish has authored a number of other bestsellers, the most popular being his 1993 *Eat More, Weigh Less*. To ensure we were not biased in our analyses, we analyzed the recipes of five days of menus in that earlier book. The Eat More, Weigh Less diet has more calories, less fat, and more flavonoids than the Everyday Cooking diet and will make your RealAge even younger—5.1 years. Adding the same changes we recommend for the Everyday Cooking diet will make the Eat More, Weigh Less diet even healthier. We show the similarities and differences in the two Ornish diets in Charts 3.7A and 3.7B.

The Pritikin Principle, *by Robert Pritikin*

What's the Theory?

The Pritikin diet is yet another low-fat, high-carbohydrate eating plan. The aim is to shed fat, lower your cholesterol, and stay fit. All are excellent goals.

Why Is It a Bestseller?

The Pritikin Principle is probably a bestseller because it claims to prevent or treat many serious health conditions. It also lets you snack between meals.

Will It Make You Younger or Older?

This diet may make your RealAge older. The foods that are recommended are great suggestions. For the most part, the off-limits list includes anything with fat in it. In reality, many of the off-limit foods won't do a great deal of harm to your RealAge if you eat them in moderation. Also, the Pritikin diet, like the Ornish diet, is supported by much scientific evidence.

What's the problem? Unfortunately, there is little hard evidence that this diet sustains long-term weight loss or health. Pritikin doesn't include any evidence of long- or short-term adherence for patients who do not have heart-threatening arterial aging. Although my palate is pretty well trained to prefer low-fat food, I found it tough to stay on the diet for even two weeks. Even if someone cooks the food for you and gives it to you free, it's hard to stay on this diet. Even if you did, the recipes are a little short on fiber, fruit, lycopene, flavonoids, legumes, nuts, and healthy fats that help you absorb fat-soluble age-reducing nutrients. However, if everything the book says is true and you

CHART 3.8

The Pritikin Diet: Nutritional Contents of Ten Days of Recipes Randomly Selected from the Book

Age-Reducing Factor	What We Found in the Recipes:	RealAge Optimum
Calories per day (on average)	1,224	
Protein (g/day)	65	
Carbohydrates (g/day)	188	
Fat (g/day)	23	
% of calories that are fat	16.7	About 25%
% of fat that is saturated	27.7	Less than 33%
Saturated fat (g/day)	6.4	Less than 20
% of fat that is monounsaturated	29.4	More than 40%
Cholesterol (mg/day)	97	Less than 150
Fiber (g/day)	24	25 or more
Sodium (mg/day)	984	2,400 or less
Potassium (mg/day)	3,933	3,000 or more
Iron (mg/day)	12.8	12–20
Calcium (mg/day)	740	1,200 or more
Folate (mcg/day)	387	700 or more
Vitamin E (IU/day)	60	400 or more
Vitamin C (mg/day)	257	1,200 or more
Fish (oz/week)	10	13 or more
Nuts (oz/week)	0	5 or more
Lycopene (servings/day)	3.8	1.5 or more
Flavonoids (mg/day)	6.2	30 or more

Note: Pritikin, R. *The New Pritikin Program: The Easy and Delicious Way to Shed Fat, Lower Your Cholesterol, and Stay Fit.* New York: Pocket Books, 1991. Robert Pritikin is director of the Pritikin Longevity Center and the son of its founder, Nathan Pritikin. The ten days of the Pritikin diet we analyzed included snacks, nonfat milk, and three cups of tea for the ten days. Pritikin states that no supplement is needed because the right amounts of vitamins C, E, and B (including folate) and selenium are already included.

are able to stick to the diet, you could make your RealAge 2.3 to 3.4 years younger by the direct effect of the diet.

How to Make the Pritikin Diet Healthier

As with the Total Health Makeover diet, there is plenty of calorie room in the Pritikin diet to make it healthier. I needed more olive oil, avocados, and nut oils to make it palatable to eat. Then adding more garlic, onions, tea, wine, fruit, fish, and brightly colored vegetables plus some nuts to start most meals would add to its ability to make the RealAges of those without arterial aging younger.

Specialty Diets

The diet books in the third group tend to have one thing in common: For the most part, they eliminate certain groups of foods. The problem? There is no scientific evidence that this is a good thing to do. Only when you eat a highly varied diet will you be getting all the nutrients that your body needs to stay healthy and strong.

Eat Right for Your Type, *by Peter D'Adamo, N.D.*

What's the Theory?

I know you've heard of this one. It's usually called the "blood type diet." It claims that proper dietary selections, *based on your blood type,* may help assist in the avoidance of illness. Your blood type, D'Adamo theorizes, indicates your anthropologic background: hunter, cultivator, nomad, or enigma.

Why Is It a Bestseller?

It's a fascinating gimmick! And it's written in an entertaining style. The history of the different foundations of our ancestors is compelling. The only plausible explanation for any success this diet might produce is that the restriction of foods (and therefore calories) is a mechanism for weight loss. The four diets average about 1,785 calories a day, 800 to 1,000 less than Americans usually eat. So you'll lose 1.5 to 2 pounds a week by following this diet.

Will It Make You Younger or Older?

The lack of virtually any supporting scientific evidence is readily apparent. Each blood type plan is a diet that restricts certain types of foods and calories. The long and confusing lists of Dos and Don'ts that are specific to each blood

CHART 3.9A

The Eat Right for Your Type Diet, Blood Type A: Nutritional Contents of Ten Days of Recipes Randomly Selected from the Book

Age-Reducing Factor	What We Found in the Recipes:	RealAge Optimum
Calories per day (on average)	1,767	
Protein (g/day)	83.8	
Carbohydrates (g/day)	250.8	
Fat (g/day)	56.8	
% of calories that are fat	28.9	About 25%
% of fat that is saturated	22.4	Less than 33%
Saturated fat (g/day)	12.7	Less than 20
% of fat that is monounsaturated	46.3	More than 40%
Cholesterol (mg/day)	125	Less than 150
Fiber (g/day)	27.8	25 or more
Sodium (mg/day)	1,984	2,400 or less
Potassium (mg/day)	4,168	3,000 or more
Iron (mg/day)	23.5	12–20
Calcium (mg/day)	1,109	1,200 or more
Folate (mcg/day)	554	700 or more
Vitamin E (IU/day)	12.5	400 or more
Vitamin C (mg/day)	276	1,200 or more
Fish (oz/week)	17	13 or more
Nuts (oz/week)	2.1	5 or more
Lycopene (servings/day)	0	1.5 or more
Flavonoids (mg/day)	33	30 or more

Note: D'Adamo, P. J. *Eat Right for Your Type: The Individualized Diet Solution to Staying Healthy, Living Longer, & Achieving Your Ideal Weight.* New York: G.P. Putnam's Sons, 1996. Peter J. D'Adamo is a naturopathic physician, researcher, and lecturer. Since only three days of menus were included, we used each day three times (and chose the tenth randomly) to calculate our ten-day nutritional analysis of the diet. The days of the Eat Right for Your Type diet for blood type A that we analyzed included two to four cups of tea a day, other beverages, desserts, and snacks. D'Adamo mentions that if you suffer from anemia, you may want a small supplement of folic acid. He also states that this diet may need to be supplemented with vitamin C (500–1,000 mg), vitamin E (400 IU), and calcium (300–600 mg).

CHART 3.9B

The Eat Right for Your Type Diet, Blood Type B: Nutritional Contents of Ten Days of Recipes Randomly Selected from the Book

Age-Reducing Factor	What We Found in the Recipes:	RealAge Optimum
Calories per day (on average)	1,917	
Protein (g/day)	81.2	
Carbohydrates (g/day)	251.8	
Fat (g/day)	70.0	
% of calories that are fat	32.9	About 25%
% of fat that is saturated	29.6	Less than 33%
Saturated fat (g/day)	20.7	Less than 20
% of fat that is monounsaturated	39.4	More than 40%
Cholesterol (mg/day)	286	Less than 150
Fiber (g/day)	20.2	25 or more
Sodium (mg/day)	1,760	2,400 or less
Potassium (mg/day)	3,678	3,000 or more
Iron (mg/day)	13.1	12–20
Calcium (mg/day)	1,202	1,200 or more
Folate (mcg/day)	356	700 or more
Vitamin E (IU/day)	11.7	400 or more
Vitamin C (mg/day)	196	1,200 or more
Fish (oz/week)	17	13 or more
Nuts (oz/week)	3	5 or more
Lycopene (servings/day)	0	1.5 or more
Flavonoids (mg/day)	28.9	30 or more

Note: Since only three days of menus were included, we used each day three times (and chose the tenth randomly) to calculate our ten-day nutritional analysis of the diet. The days of the Eat Right for Your Type diet for blood type B that we analyzed included snacks, desserts, and beverages including two to four cups of tea a day. D'Adamo also states that in some instances 300–600 mg of magnesium may be needed.

CHART 3.9AB

The Eat Right for Your Type Diet, Blood Type AB:
Nutritional Contents of Ten Days of Recipes Randomly Selected from the Book

Age-Reducing Factor	What We Found in the Recipes:	RealAge Optimum
Calories per day (on average)	1,714	
Protein (g/day)	82.3	
Carbohydrates (g/day)	199.6	
Fat (g/day)	71.5	
% of calories that are fat	37.5	About 25%
% of fat that is saturated	17.7	Less than 33%
Saturated fat (g/day)	12.6	Less than 20
% of fat that is monounsaturated	48.8	More than 40%
Cholesterol (mg/day)	237	Less than 150
Fiber (g/day)	20.9	25 or more
Sodium (mg/day)	972	2,400 or less
Potassium (mg/day)	3,678	3,000 or more
Iron (mg/day)	18.8	12–20
Calcium (mg/day)	1,113	1,200 or more
Folate (mcg/day)	509	700 or more
Vitamin E (IU/day)	14	400 or more
Vitamin C (mg/day)	204	1,200 or more
Fish (oz/week)	16	13 or more
Nuts (oz/week)	2.2	5 or more
Lycopene (servings/day)	0.9	1.5 or more
Flavonoids (mg/day)	12.6	30 or more

Note: Since only three days of menus were included, we used each day three times (and chose the tenth randomly) to calculate our ten-day nutritional analysis of the diet. The days of the Eat Right for Your Type diet for blood type AB that we analyzed included the nutrients in recommended snacks, desserts, and beverages, including one to two cups of tea a day. D'Adamo mentions that this diet may need to be supplemented with 500–1,000 mg of vitamin C.

CHART 3.90

The Eat Right for Your Type Diet, Blood Type O: Nutritional Contents of Ten Days of Recipes Randomly Selected from the Book

Age-Reducing Factor	What We Found in the Recipes:	RealAge Optimum
Calories per day (on average)	1,742	
Protein (g/day)	98.5	
Carbohydrates (g/day)	164	
Fat (g/day)	82.6	
% of calories that are fat	42.7	About 25%
% of fat that is saturated	27.6	Less than 33%
Saturated fat (g/day)	17.4	Less than 20
% of fat that is monounsaturated	42.9	More than 40%
Cholesterol (mg/day)	419	Less than 150
Fiber (g/day)	26.1	25 or more
Sodium (mg/day)	894	2,400 or less
Potassium (mg/day)	3,804	3,000 or more
Iron (mg/day)	18.6	12–20
Calcium (mg/day)	474	1,200 or more
Folate (mcg/day)	465	700 or more
Vitamin E (IU/day)	6.2	400 or more
Vitamin C (mg/day)	215	1,200 or more
Fish (oz/week)	13	13 or more
Nuts (oz/week)	5	5 or more
Lycopene (servings/day)	0.9	1.5 or more
Flavonoids (mg/day)	26.9	30 or more

Note: Since only three days of menus were included, we used each day three times (and chose the tenth randomly) to calculate our ten-day nutritional analysis of the diet. The days of the Eat Right for Your Type diet for blood type O that we analyzed included nutrients from snacks, dessert, and beverages, including two to four cups of tea a day. D'Adamo also mentions that this diet may need to be supplemented with calcium (600–1,100 mg) and vitamin C (500 mg).

type make the diets difficult to follow. And what do you do if you, your husband, and one of your children have different blood types, say, A, B, and AB? Not only that, but D'Adamo claims that within each blood type, people of different ethnic backgrounds vary still further in their nutritional needs. You are left with a confusing kaleidoscope of dietary recommendations.

I'm afraid that these diets and the confusing directions will lead their followers to unbalanced eating habits. To stay healthy, lose weight, and maintain a good weight for a long time, you must eat a variety of nutritious foods that you enjoy every day; you must also exercise regularly. Diet AB, the diet for blood type AB, contains fruit, flavonoids, nuts, and lycopene and doesn't avoid simple sugars. Diet A is short on lycopene and nuts and doesn't avoid simple sugars. Diet B misses fruit, lycopene, legumes, and flavonoids and is higher in simple sugars and salt. For the average person, attempting the blood type diet could make your RealAge as much as 4.2 years older or 5 years younger, with an average of about 0.8 years older.

How to Make the Eat Right for Your Type Diet Healthier

These diets are peculiar, but not bad. I suggest finding your blood type in the table and then adding foods with the nutrients that are missing. For example, for blood type A, I'd add nuts and tomatoes and eliminate foods with simple sugars.

Suzanne Somers' Get Skinny on Fabulous Food, by Suzanne Somers

What's the Theory?

This book has a terrific mission: To reprogram your metabolism to burn fat, providing you with a constant source of energy and therefore a positive and healthy family atmosphere. As an inspirational book, it works, but as a diet that's going to make you healthier, I have my doubts.

Why Is It a Bestseller?

Suzanne Somers is a famous TV star who overcame an addiction. She is still highly visible, seems to be a nice person, and her attractiveness and popularity over the years are bound to make her a role model for many of us. Her stories about family and friends make her book much more enjoyable to read than the usual nutritional information that most diet books provide.

Will It Make You Younger or Older?

The Get Skinny diet may make your RealAge older. It begins by eliminating a small list of foods, including sugar, white flour, alcohol, caffeine, and potatoes—she calls them "funky foods." She mentions that these foods are bad for your system but doesn't explain why. She also specifies everyday food combinations that must be followed and might be difficult to adhere to. For example, the diet demands eating fruit alone or on an empty stomach. Protein and fat, Somers says, should be eaten with vegetables. She also says that they should not be eaten within several hours of eating carbohydrates, a confusing contradiction, given that most vegetables are largely carbohydrates.

The evidence offered as proof that this eating regimen works consists of anecdotes, testimonials, and endorsements from numerous people who have tried her diet and lost weight. The overall health of such individuals is not mentioned in a long-term context. Even Somers admits that when she goes off the diet, even a little, she gains weight and feels lousy. There are no long-term studies showing that her diet actually reduces weight, maintains weight loss, or even promotes health.

Somers doesn't claim she has any scientific data to support her diet. In fact, some of her statements indicate a very basic misunderstanding of metabolic processes. For example, she says that when proteins and carbohydrates are eaten together, their enzymes "cancel each other out," halting the digestive process and causing weight gain. This idea is not supported by any scientific data. The body contains many enzymes that have highly specific functions, and they do not cancel each other out.

Furthermore, even if you overlook the lack of scientific evidence and analyze the recipes, the diet plan is short on suggesting eating fat first, fiber, fruit, fish, flavonoids, and folate and lacks sufficient quantities of legumes, nuts, and healthy fats for optimal health. It also has too much saturated fat for the RealAge optimum. If you do manage to stick to this diet, your RealAge could become 0.6 to 2.9 years older.

How to Make the Get Skinny Diet Healthier

This diet can be made healthier if you substitute fish, olive oil, nut oils, and more fruits, vegetables, and food with flavonoids, such as onions, apples, strawberries, cranberries, grapes, broccoli, tomatoes, and garlic, for meat, butter, and cream. Of course, eating folate-rich cereal and adding fruit to it may change the nature of the diet, but it will make your RealAge younger. Though the science may not be valid, the menus look health promising (see Chart 3.10). The "science" in the

CHART 3.10
The Suzanne Somers Get Skinny Diet: Nutritional Contents of Ten Days of Recipes Randomly Selected from the Book

Age-Reducing Factor	What We Found in the Recipes:	RealAge Optimum
Calories per day (on average)	1,787	
Protein (g/day)	92	
Carbohydrates (g/day)	99	
Fat (g/day)	113	
% of calories that are fat	56.9	About 25%
% of fat that is saturated	33.6	Less than 33%
Saturated fat (g/day)	38	Less than 20
% of fat that is monounsaturated	47.7	More than 40%
Cholesterol (mg/day)	520	Less than 150
Fiber (g/day)	16.3	25 or more
Sodium (mg/day)	2,024	2,400 or less
Potassium (mg/day)	3,033	3,000 or more
Iron (mg/day)	12.5	12–20
Calcium (mg/day)	696	1,200 or more
Folate (mcg/day)	271	700 or more
Vitamin E (IU/day)	11.1	400 or more
Vitamin C (mg/day)	172	1,200 or more
Fish (oz/week)	4.3	13 or more
Nuts (oz/week)	0.4	5 or more
Lycopene (servings/day)	6.8	1.5 or more
Flavonoids (mg/day)	13	30 or more

Note: Somers, S. *Suzanne Somers' Get Skinny on Fabulous Food.* New York: Crown, 1999. Besides publishing several books and successfully promoting fitness products, Suzanne Somers is a popular actress best known for her appearances on QVC and HSN and her roles in the TV shows *Three's Company* and *Candid Camera.* The days of the Get Skinny diet that we analyzed included desserts (three days of ten) and beverages. No mention of supplements was made.

book made two of the reviewers on the RealAge team very annoyed. If you look past the "science" in the book, the diet and plans can be made quite good, and some of the recipes we tasted were delicious.

The Anti-Aging Zone, *by Barry Sears, Ph.D.*

What's the Theory?

The Zone diet is based on keeping certain hormonal systems within a proper range—"the Zone." This diet is not about losing weight, but rather views food as a drug that influences insulin secretion.

Why Is It a Bestseller?

What's really happening with this diet is that you are controlling the percentages of fat, protein, and carbohydrates in your diet to 30, 30, and 40 percent, respectively, and you are restricting calories. The menus miss these 30/30/40 percentages by a little. The diet recommends excellent food choices and encourages exercise, so you should lose weight safely on this diet.

Will It Make You Younger or Older?

We are concerned that the book asserts a number of claims without any scientific evidence to substantiate them. This diet may lead to healthier eating habits, but the other anti-aging promises are unsubstantiated. In the end, the Zone diet would make your RealAge at least 1.8 and maybe 6.7 years younger.

How to Make the Anti-Aging Zone Diet Healthier

Analyses of the Zone menus indicate that this diet is long on fat and salt and short on nuts, fish, and flavonoids (see Chart 3.11). Adding two more fish dishes a week, especially if cooked with roasted onions and pecans, for example, can make the Zone even healthier. Eliminating salt with greater use of herbs and garlic and replacing some fat with other choices can make this essentially a RealAge diet.

CHART 3.11

The Anti-Aging Zone Diet: Nutritional Contents of Ten Days of Recipes Randomly Selected from the Book

Age-Reducing Factor	What We Found in the Recipes:	RealAge Optimum
Calories per day (on average)	1,655	
Protein (g/day)	129	
Carbohydrates (g/day)	158	
Fat (g/day)	65.2	
% of calories that are fat	35.5	About 25%
% of fat that is saturated	28.2	Less than 33%
Saturated fat (g/day)	18.4	Less than 20
% of fat that is monounsaturated	46.6	More than 40%
Cholesterol (mg/day)	228	Less than 150
Fiber (g/day)	35.6	25 or more
Sodium (mg/day)	3,374	2,400 or less
Potassium (mg/day)	6,170	3,000 or more
Iron (mg/day)	25.5	12–20
Calcium (mg/day)	935	1,200 or more
Folate (mcg/day)	779	700 or more
Vitamin E (IU/day)	15.5	400 or more
Vitamin C (mg/day)	475	1,200 or more
Fish (oz/week)	3.5	13 or more
Nuts (oz/week)	2.1	5 or more
Lycopene (servings/day)	11	1.5 or more
Flavonoids (mg/day)	25	30 or more

Note: Sears, B. *The Anti-Aging Zone.* New York: HarperCollins, 1998. Barry Sears, Ph.D. (microbiology), is a widely published scientist and researcher who serves as president of Eicotech Corporation, a biotechnology company. His Ph.D. is in microbiology. The ten days of the Anti-Aging Zone diet that we analyzed included five desserts. He also says that you may need to supplement the diet with vitamin E (100–400 IU), vitamin C (500–1,000 mg), magnesium (250 mg), vitamin B_3 (20 mg/day), vitamin B_6 (5–10 mg/day), folic acid (500–1,000 mcg/day), zinc (15 mcg/day), selenium (200 mcg/day), chromium (200 mg/day), lycopene and lutein (3–5 mg), CoQ10 (5–10 mg/day), antioxidants such as oligoproanthocyanidins or polyphenolics (5–10 mg/day), and fish oils (200–400 mg/day).

The Omega Diet, *by Artemis Simopolos, M.D., and Jo Robinson*

What's the Theory?

The goal is to inform the reader about the influence of healthy fats as a dietary tool to improve health. Dr. Simopolos and Jo Robinson discuss seven rules that foster good health. The first rule is to enrich your diet with omega-3 fatty acids, as opposed to the omega-6 family of fatty acids. The book advises the reader to use mostly monounsaturated oils (olive oil and canola oil); to eat seven or more servings of fruits and vegetables every day; to consume more vegetable proteins, including peas, beans, and nuts; and to avoid saturated fat by choosing lean meat and low-fat over full-fat milk products. The authors emphasize the ratio of omega-6 to omega-3 fatty acids and tell us which fats have the best ratios. The data supporting the benefits of striving for the best omega-3 to omega-6 ratio is all inferential, however. The benefits of the ratio, in my analyses, are not supported as well as is the assertion that mono- and polyunsaturated fats are healthier than saturated fats. Dr. Simopolos does present the data that saturated fat consumption leads to ill health. This part of the science is solid. Though omega-3s may be the secret to health, this has not been scientifically established yet.

Why Is It a Bestseller?

We know that the Mediterranean area had the least disease and disability of anywhere in the world in the 1950s. This book approximates the diet of that area at that time. The lure of discovering what a diet "tested" over decades actually includes has made this a bestseller. It is chock-full of great charts and excellent data on fats.

Will It Make You Younger or Older?

The Omega diet has the lure of omega fats, a substantial body of food information, and the Mediterranean diet. It aims for you to have 35 percent of your calories from fat. The book has a series of good recipes and substitutions. In analyzing the recipes, we found a shortage of fruits, lycopene, and even nuts in the diet, and there is no elimination of simple sugars. Almost 40 percent of your calories will come from fat, most of it healthy fat. Is that much fat, even healthy fat, advisable or health promoting? We just do not know. From what we do know, the diet, by itself, will make your RealAge 6.7 years younger to 2.6 years older. The recipes we randomly selected do not seem to closely match the general description of the diet. This inconsistency was observed

CHART 3.12

The Omega Diet: Nutritional Contents of Ten Days of Recipes Randomly Selected from the Book

Age-Reducing Factor	What We Found in the Recipes:	RealAge Optimum
Calories per day (on average)	1,363	
Protein (g/day)	84	
Carbohydrates (g/day)	131	
Fat (g/day)	58.5	
% of calories that are fat	38.6	About 25%
% of fat that is saturated	26.3	Less than 33%
Saturated fat (g/day)	15.5	Less than 20
% of fat that is monounsaturated	45.5	More than 40%
Cholesterol (mg/day)	270	Less than 150
Fiber (g/day)	18	25 or more
Sodium (mg/day)	1,576	2,400 or less
Potassium (mg/day)	2,671	3,000 or more
Iron (mg/day)	11.7	12–20
Calcium (mg/day)	488	1,200 or more
Folate (mcg/day)	223	700 or more
Vitamin E (IU/day)	7.9	400 or more
Vitamin C (mg/day)	126	1,200 or more
Fish (oz/week)	12	13 or more
Nuts (oz/week)	1.5	5 or more
Lycopene (servings/day)	3.4	1.5 or more
Flavonoids (mg/day)	5.6	30 or more

Note: Simopolos, A. P., and Robinson, J. *The Omega Diet: The Lifesaving Nutritional Program Based on the Diet of the Island of Crete.* New York: HarperCollins, 1998. Artemis P. Simopolos, M.D., is a world authority on essential fatty acids and was nutritional adviser to the Office of Consumer Affairs at the White House. Jo Robinson is author of *The Healing Diet* and the editor-in-chief of *World Review of Nutrition and Dietetics.* We chose five days from their 1,500-calorie-a-day diet and five from their 1,200-calorie-a-day diet. Our nutritional analyses included the recommended snacks. Simopolos and Robinson suggest the diet be supplemented with calcium if you don't get enough milk products. They also say you should take antioxidant and vitamin supplements if you are not eating seven or more servings of fruits and vegetables a day. In addition, they recommend supplementing the diet with fish oil or flaxseed oil and taking at least 100 IU of vitamin E every day.

even in a second random selection of menus. If you succeed in staying on the diet, you can add the other benefits of weight loss and lower blood pressure.

How to Make the Omega Diet Healthier

You need more fiber, fruit, flavonoids, folate, and nuts. Adding a whole grain pasta dish laden with onions, tomatoes, a few nuts, and vegetables, plus some extra fruit two or three times a week, would increase potassium intake to make the menus RealAge healthier.

Eating Well for Optimum Health, *by Andrew Weil, M.D.*

What's the Theory?

This book aims to provide the basics of human nutrition so you can make informed decisions about weight reduction and diet aids. Great! That's also what the RealAge Diet is about. Dr. Weil teaches you to read labels and presents menu plans, recipes, and guidance in eating. He says that there is no one right way to eat (bravo, for someone who tells it like it is!) and that your nutritional needs may change over time. Many of the food choices he advocates are similar to ours. The book is laced with references from the peer-reviewed literature, and although Dr. Weil does not use the great amount of evidence-effect data that we use to determine RealAge effects, he comes to very similar conclusions.

Our only objection is that he goes beyond what the study data allows. For example, he has a specific prejudice for fish that are rich in omega-3 fatty acids, as opposed to fish in general. No one really knows if it's the omega-3s that make fish better: It may be the protein or some other specific component of fish, and not the omega-3s. Dr. Weil also doesn't take into account ways you can make eating healthier and more fun, for example, eating a little healthy fat before you eat a high-glycemic food, to turn it into a low-glycemic food.

In a set of tables, Dr. Weil lists dietary changes that are good for certain diseases. Though some of these (for example, the recommendations for allergies) seem logical, some of them (for example, the recommendations for arthritis, bronchitis, inflammation, and thyroid conditions) seem not to rely closely on the scientific basis that runs throughout the rest of the book.

Following this diet will make your RealAge between 3.3 and 9 years younger.

How to Make the Eating Well Diet Healthier

Although the menus indicate that 534 of your average 1,565 calories a day will come from fat, mostly monounsaturated, the menus are high in fat and deficient in nuts, folate, and flavonoids. They do have plenty of fiber, fish, and fruit.

CHART 3.13

The Eating Well for Optimum Health Diet: Nutritional Contents of Ten Days of Recipes Randomly Selected from the Book

Age-Reducing Factor	What We Found in the Recipes:	RealAge Optimum
Calories per day (on average)	1,565	
Protein (g/day)	68.6	
Carbohydrates (g/day)	206	
Fat (g/day)	59.3	
% of calories that are fat	34.1	About 25%
% of fat that is saturated	17.9	Less than 33%
Saturated fat (g/day)	10.7	Less than 20
% of fat that is monounsaturated	50.2	More than 40%
Cholesterol (mg/day)	138	Less than 150
Fiber (g/day)	33.8	25 or more
Sodium (mg/day)	1,128	2,400 or less
Potassium (mg/day)	3,931	3,000 or more
Iron (mg/day)	18.7	12–20
Calcium (mg/day)	544	1,200 or more
Folate (mcg/day)	390	700 or more
Vitamin E (IU/day)	10.7	400 or more
Vitamin C (mg/day)	202	1,200 or more
Fish (oz/week)	34	13 or more
Nuts (oz/week)	0.8	5 or more
Lycopene (servings/day)	9	1.5 or more
Flavonoids (mg/day)	15	30 or more

Note: Weil, A. *Eating Well for Optimum Health: The Essential Guide to Food, Diet, and Nutrition.* New York: Alfred Knopf, 2000. Andrew Weil, M.D., is a clinical assistant professor of medicine and the director of the Program in Integrative Medicine at the University of Arizona. The ten days of the Eating Well diet that we analyzed included recommended snacks and desserts. The nutritional data did not include milk. Weil also suggests the diet be supplemented with a B-complex supplement (400 mcg of folic acid), vitamin C (200 mg/day), a capsule of mixed carotenoids, vitamin E (400–800 IU), vitamin D (400 IU) for those at risk for osteoporosis, calcium for those who take in less than 1,200–1,500 mg of calcium daily, and selenium (200 mcg) with vitamin E.

Adding a few more vegetables rich in calcium, like broccoli, parsley, turnips, and kale, plus almonds and a low-fat dairy substitute supplemented with calcium, would make the diet still healthier. Also a whole grain cereal or pasta that is loaded with folate would make your RealAge even younger. Even so, this is a great book and presents wonderfully tasty recipes that will make your RealAge younger.

What's the Bottom Line on the Popular Diets?

In most of the bestseller diets we tested, health is promoted by weight loss. Major health benefits can accrue by steadily approaching the weight you want to achieve. This loss is created by whatever means of calorie restriction is advocated, with little regard for the long-term health effects of that restriction or the foods you end up eating because of the restriction. Exceptions are the Weil, Simopolos, Ornish, Pritikin, and Sears diets. As a result of omitting certain foods, and sometimes entire food groups, many of these bestseller diets are deficient in such major nutrients as fiber, carbohydrates, or protein, as well as in vitamins and minerals. The Anti-Aging Zone diet does not completely eliminate any one food group and is unique in that respect.

As a result, the following diets could make your RealAge older: Eat Right for Your Type, Total Health Makeover, Dr. Atkins' New Diet Revolution, Protein Power, and Suzanne Somers' Get Skinny.

The Everyday Cooking with Dr. Dean Ornish, the Anti-Aging Zone, the Eating Well for Optimum Health, and, surprisingly, the Carbohydrate Addict's diets make your RealAge the youngest.

Although all diets claim different mechanisms for weight loss and maintenance, in essence they all use the same fundamental principle: calorie restriction. As shown in Charts 3.2 through 3.13, which present the nutrition in the menus and recipes from each diet, these four diets average 1,600 calories a day. The average American now consumes 1,000 to 1,200 calories a day more than that, so the average American would lose about 2 pounds per week on these diets (you lose a pound if you take in 3,500 fewer calories in food than you use). Each diet is calorie restricted. The authors may deny this, but many of these diets create calorie restriction through an illusion of science. In reality, they either eliminate a major food group altogether or eliminate a different group at each eating period. Some bestseller diets are better than others. For example, the books by Weil, Sears, Ornish, and the Hellers contain diets that, with small changes, can be made very similar to a RealAge optimum. Why agonize over a

CHART 3.14

The RealAge Diet Plan: Nutritional Contents of Ten Days of Recipes from Plan 2 in This Book

Age-Reducing Factor	What We Found in the Recipes:	RealAge Optimum
Calories per day (on average)	1,640	
Protein (g/day)	70	
Carbohydrates (g/day)	270	
Fat (g/day)	46	
% of calories that are fat	24	About 25%
% of fat that is saturated	31	Less than 33%
Saturated fat (g/day)	14.5	Less than 20
% of fat that is monounsaturated	42	More than 40%
Cholesterol (mg/day)	89	Less than 150
Fiber (g/day)	30.2	25 or more
Sodium (mg/day)	2,201	2,400 or less
Potassium (mg/day)	3,530	3,000 or more
Iron (mg/day)	14.9	12–20
Calcium (mg/day)	710	1,200 or more
Folate (mcg/day)	527	700 or more
Vitamin E (IU/day)	11.1	400 or more
Vitamin C (mg/day)	202	1,200 or more
Fish (oz/week)	14.5	13 or more
Nuts (oz/week)	12	5 or more
Lycopene (servings/day)	4	1.5 or more
Flavonoids (mg/day)	31	30 or more

Note: Since only five days of recipes are provided, we used each recipe twice. The ten days of the RealAge Plan we analyzed recommended snacks, tea, and two days with desserts. Supplements are not included (recommendations regarding supplements are given in Chapter 5).

temporary, short-term diet when you can change your eating habits for life, and enjoy your food each step of the way?

When you're evaluating a diet, or your own food choices, just remember the fundamental RealAge principles and ask yourself, "Is it a nutrient-rich, calorie-poor diet? Do the recipes taste world-class great? Does it advocate healthy fats, fruits, vegetables, lycopene, legumes, fiber, fish, flavonoids, and the right vitamins and minerals in the right amounts? If not, what can I change about the diet to make it so?"

Many of us could benefit by shedding a few pounds, but it is not easy to lose weight and keep it off. Although your weight is important in determining your rate of aging, it is not as important as avoiding medical conditions that can age you even more. You can easily learn to substitute and choose foods that keep your RealAge young and you healthy and energetic.

What's the bottom line? None of these bestseller diets provides any evidence of successful long-term weight loss. Nor do we. Those data do not exist. If you want to choose foods that retard aging and lose weight slowly, find out which diet, when modified as we suggest in this chapter, provides food choices you can enjoy for the rest of your life. It's your health. It's your call.

4

The Magic of the RealAge Diet

It's as Simple as an Hourglass

Eating well means feeling great, and that's what staying young is all about. It's about having the energy to live an active life and to do the things you want to do. Healthy eating can increase your endurance and help you stay fit. Whether you're a weekend warrior or a mom on the go, or you just want to boost your general level of energy, eating the right kinds of food recharges your batteries and revitalizes your daily life.

How I Know This Diet Works

How do I know the RealAge Diet works? I live it. Years ago, I was the typical, busy professional who did not like to cook. I often ate standing up, and I was not above munching from vending machines. I was either on the go, eating fast food, or dining with co-workers several times a week in restaurants.

Though I have always been an active person—I even play competitive squash—my weight tended to go up and down, depending on whether it was squash season or not. In squash, quickness counts, and I'm quicker when I'm lighter. The extra weight was slowing me down.

Not only did my weight fluctuate, but so did my energy level. Typically, at the start of the squash season, I had to battle an extra 20 pounds to get back into competitive shape. Back then, I had no idea that this yearly cycling was accelerating my rate of aging.

In 1993, I started learning about factors that affect RealAge, one being year-round physical conditioning, which could keep my arteries young and my energy level up. Slowly, I started to keep up my level of physical activity throughout the year, instead of being somewhat sedentary during the off-season. I stayed in better overall shape. Still, my weight fluctuated and, as the years went on, it got harder to get down to my ideal playing weight when squash season started.

As I continued to learn more about what could make my RealAge younger, I realized that a good diet—one rich in nutrients but poor in calories—could slow my rate of aging, and I began to change the foods I ate. As my palate changed, I was surprised to find myself genuinely enjoying the whole grains, fruits, and fish on my new diet. I learned that healthy food could taste world-class great. I even started to cook. Every year it got easier to maintain my optimal weight. Most important, I feel great. I have more energy than I've had in years—enough to socialize, play sports, and spend time with my family, even with a demanding schedule.

Imagine what *you* could do with extra energy. Picture yourself playing the sports you used to love. Or imagine spending more quality time with your children, because you have extra energy, even after a long day at the office. These are the payoffs for eating the RealAge way. All it takes are a few simple, delicious changes in the way you eat.

In a nutshell, there are five keys to keeping your weight down and your RealAge younger:

- Think nutrient rich, calorie poor, and delicious.
- Eat healthy fat and fiber first.
- Be the CEO any time you eat out, and any time you pay for food.
- Make eating and every place you eat a special pleasure, and a special place.
- Remember the principles embodied by the RealAge hourglass.

The Hourglass

The hourglass (Figure 4.1) is my symbol for the RealAge Diet. It's a visual reminder that you'll slow the sands of time if you follow the principles embodied by the RealAge hourglass. For example, you'll slow your rate of aging if you eat only small amounts of the foods in the middle of the hourglass.

FIGURE 4.1   A DAY'S WORTH OF REALAGE-SMART EATING.
USE THE HOURGLASS TO REMEMBER THE REALAGE
DIET AND MAKE AGING STAND STILL.

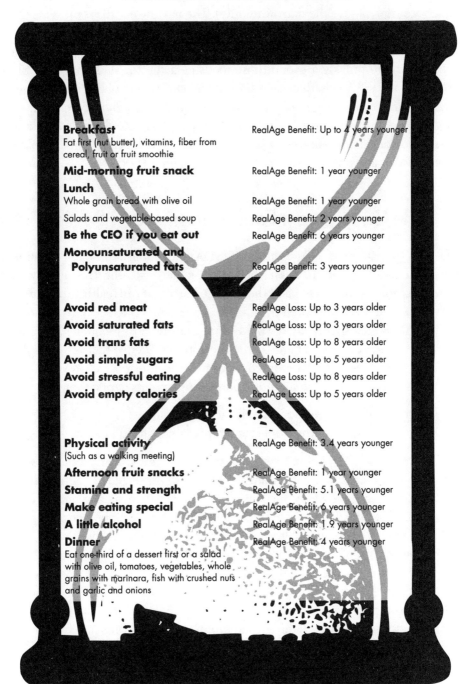

Breakfast   RealAge Benefit: Up to 4 years younger
Fat first (nut butter), vitamins, fiber from
cereal, fruit or fruit smoothie

Mid-morning fruit snack   RealAge Benefit: 1 year younger

Lunch
Whole grain bread with olive oil   RealAge Benefit: 1 year younger

Salads and vegetable-based soup   RealAge Benefit: 2 years younger

Be the CEO if you eat out   RealAge Benefit: 6 years younger

**Monounsaturated and
  Polyunsaturated fats**   RealAge Benefit: 3 years younger

Avoid red meat   RealAge Loss: Up to 3 years older

Avoid saturated fats   RealAge Loss: Up to 3 years older

Avoid trans fats   RealAge Loss: Up to 8 years older

Avoid simple sugars   RealAge Loss: Up to 5 years older

Avoid stressful eating   RealAge Loss: Up to 8 years older

Avoid empty calories   RealAge Loss: Up to 5 years older

Physical activity   RealAge Benefit: 3.4 years younger
(Such as a walking meeting)

Afternoon fruit snacks   RealAge Benefit: 1 year younger

Stamina and strength   RealAge Benefit: 5.1 years younger

Make eating special   RealAge Benefit: 6 years younger

A little alcohol   RealAge Benefit: 1.9 years younger

Dinner   RealAge Benefit: 4 years younger
Eat one-third of a dessert first or a salad
with olive oil, tomatoes, vegetables, whole
grains with marinara, fish with crushed nuts
and garlic and onions

Imagine in the midportions of the upper and lower bulbs of the hourglass are the foods and nutrients that you can eat in moderation with little effect on aging: complex carbohydrates, insoluble fiber, diet sodas, coffee, and dark chocolate (right above the narrow middle). The narrow middle represents the foods you want very little of: red meat, trans fat, saturated fat, and simple sugars. If you eat too many of these foods, the middle widens, making the sands of time pass more quickly. Beyond those foods near the top and bottom of the hourglass are the foods that have flavonoids and carotenoids—fruits, vegetables, tomato sauce, legumes, and nuts, followed by fish and cereal. These foods retard or even reverse aging. In the base of the hourglass is something we should consider a real treat: physical activity, be it for strength, flexibility, or stamina, or any physical activity at all (see Chapter 9).

The Government Food Pyramid, and Politics

The U.S. Department of Agriculture (USDA) has published a food pyramid for about twenty years. In 2000, the USDA joined with the U.S. Food and Drug Administration (FDA) and the U.S. Department of Health and Human Services to publish an updated pyramid.

You'd think that the pyramid would represent the most recent and reliable information on nutrition. There is much scientific evidence that supports the pyramid. All of the USDA reports on diet rely on an extensive review of the scientific literature, and the literature consistently points to one thing:

A nutrient-rich, calorie-poor diet is the best regimen for overall health and longevity. The goal is to eat healthfully for a lifetime.

The trouble is, the pyramid gets polluted by politics. Sugar producers and soft drink manufacturers don't want soft drinks to be excluded; cattle ranchers, hog farmers, and dairy farmers don't want red meat and milk to be excluded. So lobbying can apparently change this blue ribbon panel's pronouncements to the point of altering good science, it seems. Nevertheless, the nutritional groups of the pyramid are a useful place to learn about foods.

At the bottom of the pyramid are **bread, cereal, rice, and pasta.** Grain products, especially whole grains, are excellent sources of nutrients, vitamins, minerals, complex carbohydrates, and fiber.

Fruits and vegetables are the second group. Although fruits and vegetables vary in the amount of vitamins, minerals, and other nutrients they contain, as a general rule, they are good sources of vitamin C and fiber. Some contain significant amounts of folic acid, potassium, vitamin B$_6$, calcium, magnesium, and selenium. Moreover, most contain loads of the age-reducing antioxidant flavonoids and carotenoids.

The third group consists of **dairy, meat, and eggs,** and I consider it the protein group: Milk, yogurt, cheese, meat, poultry, fish, dry beans, eggs, and nuts all belong to this group. Meats, nuts, legumes, and dairy products can be great sources of protein if you choose low-fat, nonfat, or, even better, healthy fat varieties.

At the top of the pyramid are **fats, oils, and sweets.** These are not classified as a food group, because the USDA says you should eat these foods only in very small amounts, mostly to add taste and flavor to meals. However, we now know that healthy fat makes you younger. So I haven't found the pyramid as helpful as the RealAge hourglass in reminding me what to eat.

A Serving Size—How Much Is That?

It will take you a couple of weeks to learn the serving sizes for your favorite foods, shown in Chart 4.1. When I first started eating the RealAge way, I copied the chart, carried it around, and referred to it when I was in doubt. I soon knew the serving sizes for most foods and didn't need it anymore.

CHART 4.1
What Is a Serving Size?

Food	Serving Size	Calories
DAIRY:		
Low-fat (1%) milk	1 cup	119
Fat-free (skim) milk	1 cup	99
Low-fat cottage cheese	1 cup	163
Fat-free cottage cheese	1 cup	123
Low-fat cheeses	2 oz (two standard packaged slices)	160
Natural cheese	1 1/2 oz (1" cube)	160
Processed cheese	2 oz (two standard packaged slices)	140
Low-fat yogurt	1 cup	150
Nonfat yogurt	1 cup	120

(continued)

Food	Serving Size	Calories
GRAINS:		
Bread	One slice	80
Pita bread	One 4"	165
Bagel	Half a small (about 3") bagel	98
English muffin	Half a small (about 3") muffin	75
Yeast breads (wheat, rye)	One slice	80
Corn tortillas	One 7"	54
Low-fat flour tortillas	One 7"	150
Plain cereal, dry	1 oz (1 cup)	100–200
Plain cereal, cooked	1/2 cup	150
Saltines, soda crackers, low sodium, unsalted	Five to six small	65
Graham crackers	Three to four large	105
Animal crackers	Nine	90
Popcorn	2 cups (air popped)	65
Rice (brown, white)	1/2 cup (cooked)	100
Pasta (noodles, spaghetti)	1/2 cup (cooked)	100
MEAT AND EGGS:		
White meat chicken/ turkey, skinless	2–3 oz (deck of cards)	140
Fish, not battered	2–3 oz (deck of cards)	130
Lobster or shrimp	1/4 cup (deck of cards)	39
Beef, round or sirloin	2–3 oz (deck of cards)	150
Extra lean ground beef	2–3 oz (deck of cards)	230
Pork tenderloin	2–3 oz (deck of cards)	230
Lunch/deli meats, 95% fat free	2–3 oz (deck of cards)	78
Eggs	One	75
FRUITS:		
Apples	One medium (tennis ball)	81
Bananas	One medium	120

Food	Serving Size	Calories
Oranges	One medium (tennis ball)	65
Pears	One small	51
Peaches	One medium (tennis ball)	37
Grapefruit	Half	37
Apricot	One large (tennis ball)	74
Dried fruits	1/4 cup	60
Cherries	1/2 cup (eleven cherries)	61
Strawberries	1/2 cup (five large or seven medium)	23
Blueberries	1/2 cup (fifty large blueberries)	41
Raspberries	1/2 cup (thirty large raspberries)	31
Raisins	1/2 cup	219
Plums	1 1/2 medium (small fist)	51
Grapes	1/2 cup (twelve grapes)	30
Cantaloupe	One-fourth medium	50
Honeydew melon	One-eighth medium	30
Mango	1/2 cup (one-half medium)	68
Papaya	1/2 cup (one-fourth medium)	30
Kiwi	One large	55
Olives	Five medium	45
Figs	1/2 cup	75
Pomegranates	1/2 cup	52
Guava	1/2 cup	42
Pineapple, fresh or canned	1/2 cup	75
Frozen blueberries	1/2 cup	41
Frozen raspberries	1/2 cup	31

VEGETABLES:

Food	Serving Size	Calories
Broccoli	1 cup (three raw florets or two cooked spears)	44
Peas	1/2 cup	34
Cauliflower	1/2 cup	14
Red/green pepper	1/2 cup (eight rings)	13
Squash (summer)	1/2 cup (one-third of the squash)	18

(continued)

Food	Serving Size	Calories
Green beans	1/2 cup	17
Spinach	1 cup	42
Romaine lettuce	1 cup (four leaves)	8
Cabbage	1 cup	32
Artichokes	1/2 cup (one artichoke heart)	60
Cucumber	1/2 cup (one-third medium cucumber)	13
Asparagus	1/2 cup	22
Mushrooms	1/2 cup	21
Carrots	1/2 cup (seven to eight sticks)	40
Celery	1/2 cup (two stalks)	20
Onions	1/2 cup	46
Potato	One medium baked (the size of a computer mouse)	124
Sweet potato	3/4 cup	117
Corn	1/2 cup (one medium ear)	88
Tomatoes	1/2 cup	10
Tomato/spaghetti sauce	1/2 cup	40
Bok choy	1/2 cup	10
Seaweed	1/2 cup	16
Bean sprouts	1/2 cup	8

VEGETABLE PROTEIN:

Food	Serving Size	Calories
Lentils	1/2 cup (cooked)	40
Black beans	1/2 cup (cooked)	90
Red beans (kidney beans)	1/2 cup (cooked)	112
Navy beans	1/2 cup (cooked)	129
Pinto beans	1/2 cup (cooked)	117
Black-eyed peas	1/2 cup (cooked)	90
Tofu (bean curd)	1/2 cup (deck of cards)	94
Beans	1–1 1/2 cups	339
Nuts and seeds	1/3 cup	300
Peanut butter	2 tablespoons	188
Fava beans	1/2 cup (cooked)	93

Food	Serving Size	Calories
Italian white beans	1/2 cup (cooked)	125
Chickpeas (garbanzo beans)	1/2 cup	110
Canned bean soup	1 cup	95

Now let's turn to each food group. Chart 4.2 shows how important it is to your RealAge to include all the major food groups in your diet. What makes each choice an important part of your diet? How can you eat from each food group to improve your health, reach your ideal weight, and reduce needless aging?

CHART 4.2
The RealAge Effect of Diversity in Your Diet

	1–2 food groups eaten from each day	3–4 food groups eaten from each day	5 food groups eaten from each day
Calendar Age		RealAge	
MEN			
35	38.3	34.8	34.7
55	59.4	54.8	54.5
70	75.3	69.8	69.3
WOMEN			
35	38.3	34.8	34.7
55	59.4	54.8	54.5
70	75.3	69.8	69.3

Note: The five food groups are milk and milk substitutes, grains, protein (meat, eggs, nuts, beans, etc.), fruits, and vegetables.

Carbohydrates

Most complex carbohydrates are found in whole grain breads, cereals, rice, and pasta, so this food group can be an important part of your diet, no matter what your nutrition goals—losing weight, reducing your bad cholesterol, increasing your healthy cholesterol, controlling high blood pressure or blood sugar levels, or just plain making yourself younger.

REALAGE CAFÉ TIP 4.1
What's the Scoop on Energy, Diet, and Cereal Bars?

You have to read the label to tell. Most bars have 150 to 250 calories and are relatively nutrient poor for that amount of calories. Granola bars, cereal bars, and even diet bars tend to have more simple sugar than age-reducing whole grains, fruits, nuts, raisins, and flavonoids in them. That makes them calorie dense and nutrient poor, the exact opposite of the RealAge ideal!

The goal of these bars is to fill you up with only a few calories. A 200-calorie bar is supposed to provide all the nutrition and satisfaction of an entire meal. The bars aim to be convenient to use, nutritious, and so satisfying you won't want to eat for another four hours. Although we couldn't find any bars that were as good as a meal, some are relatively healthy.

The 1- to 1.5-ounce versions of Health Valley Fruit Bars, Barbara's Nature's Choice Bars, and Jenny Craig Oatmeal Raisin Bars all have fewer than 150 calories, almost no saturated or trans fat, a little healthy (monounsaturated) fat, and some whole grains. However, all of these bars have too much sugar. Sugar in small quantities is not necessarily bad, but the sugar is out of proportion to the nutrients.

And those are some of the best bars. The SlimFast Apple Cobbler Meal-on-the-Go Bar has 220 calories and 4 grams (g) (one-fifth your daily total) of artery-aging, saturated fat. The Atkins Diet Advantage Bar has 230 calories and 7 g of artery-aging fat. On the other hand, the 2.1-ounce Atkins Almond Brownie Diet Advantage Bar has 230 calories but only 3 g of saturated fat and no sugar. This Atkins bar may be one of the better bars.

The Zone Perfect Almond Crunch and the Zone Chocolate Almond Bar are each 1.5 ounces with about 190 calories, 2 g of saturated fat, and a lot of simple sugar. So are most of the cereal bars. Power Bars have more calories than these and more fiber and less protein than many other bars.

If you find you can have a bar on the go and not eat for four hours, these bars are relatively healthy snacks, but not, of course, compared with fruit. From a RealAge standpoint, the bars are much better than Pop Tarts, Cinnabons, or Krispy Kreme doughnuts, if those are *your* alternatives. On the other hand, bars are generally nutrient-poor substitutes for fruit or a meal.

The answer to the sugar question is to read the label and then find out if you want that particular bar. I think a few nuts and a piece of fruit are a much better alternative.

The best grains are whole grains. They have not been stripped of their outer layers, the source of many key nutrients, and they have not been refined and so retain most of their vitamins and minerals. Whole grains are significant sources of B vitamins, iron, zinc, calcium, selenium, and magnesium. Whole grains are also an enjoyable source of chromium, a mineral that is reported in some studies to be important in balancing blood sugar levels. Grain products, in particular whole grains, contain high amounts of fiber, important for preventing arterial aging and reducing the risk of cancer. Common whole grains are wheat, rice, corn, oats, rye, and barley.

If you are concerned about lowering your cholesterol, focus on the grains that have primarily soluble fiber—for example, oats—since it helps your cholesterol profile more than insoluble fiber. Most of the grains consumed in the United States are refined and have been stripped of many important nutrients and much of their fiber. Products made with highly refined grains, such as white bread, white flour, most white pastas, and white rice, although not *bad* for you, have little nutritive value or fiber.

Breads

Although whole wheat bread and other whole grain breads contain more nutrients and fiber than white bread, don't assume that simply because the package says "wheat bread" that it's rich in whole grains. Many so-called wheat breads contain mostly enriched white flour with a little wheat flour thrown in, and many contain needless sugar. To be sure, read the ingredients label. Unless the label says specifically that the bread is 100 percent whole wheat, the bread may contain flour that has been highly refined, with caramel coloring added to give it that dark, "good-for-you" look. Whole wheat flour should be the first flour in the list of ingredients (I like Natural Oven breads).

Consider choosing dark breads, such as rye and pumpernickel. These often contain lots of fiber. Multigrain breads contain oats, oat bran, barley, sunflower seeds, and nuts, which are all good RealAge choices.

 REALAGE CAFÉ TIP 4.2
Where's the Whole Grain?

Ever wonder how much whole grain is actually in the "whole grain" products you buy? Since August 1999, figuring out which foods on the grocery shelf provide the health benefits of whole grains has been as simple as reading the label. Since then, foods that are at least 51 percent whole grains have been permitted to carry the following claim: "Diets rich in whole grain foods and other plant foods and low in total fat, saturated fat, and cholesterol may reduce the risk of heart disease and cancer."

Wheat and wheat products do have a high glycemic index. If you are concerned about blood sugar levels, eat whole wheat breads (oat bran, pita, whole rye, and mixed-grain breads) with food that enters your bloodstream more slowly, such as peanut butter, almond butter, or a slice of roasted turkey.

Chart 4.3 shows the glycemic indices for a variety of foods.

CHART 4.3
Glycemic Indices of Various Foods

The higher its glycemic index (GI), the more quickly a food is absorbed by the body, if the food is eaten alone. To slow the emptying of your stomach so the food is not absorbed quickly and your blood sugar level doesn't soar, try to eat a little healthy fat before consuming any food that has a GI of 75 or higher. Here are the glycemic indices for various foods:

BAKERY PRODUCTS:	GI:
Cake	
angel food	95
banana, made with sugar	79
banana, made without sugar	67
flan	93
pound	77
sponge	66
Croissant	96
Crumpet	98
Doughnut	108
Muffins	88
Pastry	84
Pizza, cheese	86
Waffles	109

BEVERAGES:	GI:
Soy milk	43
Orange cordial	94

	GI:
Lucozade glucose energy drink	136
Fanta soft drink	97

BREADS:	GI:
Bagel, white	103
Barley-flour bread	95
Barley-kernel bread	55
Bread stuffing	106
Linseed rye bread	78
Fruit loaf	67
Hamburger bun	87
Kaiser rolls	104
French baguette	136
Melba toast	100
Mixed-grain bread	69
Oat kernel bread	93
Oat-bran bread	68
Pita bread, white	82
Pumpernickel	71
Rye-kernel bread	66

Rye-flour bread	92	Rice Chex		127
Semolina bread	92	Rice Krispies		117
Wheat bread		Shredded Wheat		99
white	101	Special K		77
high fiber	97	Team		117
WonderWhite	112	Total		109
gluten-free	129	Wheat Biscuit		100
wholemeal flour	99	Kelloggs'		
Whole wheat snack bread	105	All Bran Fruit 'n Oats		57
		Guardian		52
		Honey Smacks		99
BREAKFAST CEREALS:	**GI:**	Just Right		84
All-Bran	60	Mini-Wheats		101
Bran Buds	75			
Bran Chex	83			
Breakfast bar (many varieties—see RealAge Cafe Tip 4.1)	109	**CEREAL GRAINS:**		**GI:**
		Barley, cracked		72
Cheerios	106	Barley, pearled		36
Cocoa Pops	110	Barley, rolled		94
Corn Bran	107	Buckwheat		78
Corn Chex	118	Bulgur		68
Corn Flakes	119	Couscous		93
Cream of Wheat	100	Cornmeal		98
Crispix	124	Corn, sweet		78
Golden Grahams	102	Corn taco shells		97
Grapenuts	96	Millet		101
Grapenuts Flakes, Post	114	Rice		
Life	94	white		83
Muesli	80	brown		79
Nutri-Grain	94	Sunbrown Quick		114
Oat Bran	78	Calrose		124
Porridge (oatmeal)	87	instant, boiled 6 min		128
Puffed Wheat	105	instant, boiled 1 min		65
Rice Bran	27	parboiled		68

(continued)

Rye	48	Milk + 30 g bran	38
Tapioca, boiled with milk	115	Milk + custard + sugar	61
Wheat kernels	59	Yogurt	
Wheat, quick cooking	77	low fat, sweetened with fruit sugar	47
		low fat, artificially sweetened	20
COOKIES:	GI:	unspecified	51
Arrowroot	95		
Graham Wafers	106	LEGUMES:	GI:
Oatmeal cookies	79	Baked beans, canned	69
Rich tea cookies	79	Beans, dried, not specified	40
Shredded Wheatmeal	89	Black-eyed peas	59
Shortbread	91	Broad beans (fava beans)	113
Vanilla Wafers	110	Butter beans	44
		+ 5 g sucrose	53
		+ 10 g sucrose	64
CRACKERS:	GI:	+ 15 g sucrose	77
Breton Wheat Crackers	96	Chickpeas (garbanzo beans)	47
Jatz	79	Haricot/navy beans	54
Puffed Crispbread	116	Kidney beans	42
Rice cakes	110	Lentils	
Rye crispbread, high-fiber	93	green	42
Stoned Wheat Thins	96	red	36
Water crackers	102	Lima beans, baby, frozen	46
		Pinto beans	55
		Romano beans	65
DAIRY FOODS:	GI:	Soybeans	25
Ice cream	87	Split peas, yellow, boiled	45
Ice cream, low fat	71		
Milk		PASTA:	GI:
full fat	39	Capellini	64
skim	46	Fettuccine	46
chocolate, sweetened with sugar	49	Gnocchi	95
		Instant noodles	67
chocolate, artificially sweetened	34	Linguine	65

Macaroni	64	SNACK FOODS AND SWEETS:	GI:
Macaroni and cheese	92	Jelly beans	114
Ravioli, durum, meat-filled	56	Life Savers	100
Spaghetti		Chocolate	70
protein-enriched	38	Mars Bar	97
white	59	Muesli Bars	87
boiled 5 min	52	Popcorn	79
durum	78	Corn chips	105
wholemeal	53	Potato chips	77
Spirali, durum	61	Peanuts	21
Star pastina	54	Pretzels	116
Tortellini, cheese	71	Mars Chocolate (Dove)	63
Vermicelli	50	Mars M&Ms (peanut)	46
Rice pasta, brown	131	Mars Skittles	98
		Mars Snickers Bar	57
ROOT VEGETABLES:	GI:	Mars Twix Cookie Bars (caramel)	62
Beets	91		
Carrots	101	SOUPS:	GI:
Parsnips	139	Black bean	92
Potatoes, instant	118	Green pea, canned	94
Potato		Lentil, canned	63
baked	121	Split pea	86
new	81	Tomato	54
boiled, mashed	104		
canned	87	SUGARS:	GI:
white, not specified, boiled	80–90	Honey	104
		Fructose	32
mashed	100	Glucose	137
steamed	93	Glucose tablets	146
microwaved	117	Maltose	150
French fries	107	Sucrose	92
Sweet potato	77	Lactose	65
Swede (rutabaga)	103	Maltodextrin	137
Yam	73	High-fructose corn syrup	89

(continued)

VEGETABLES:	GI:		
Peas, green	68	Paw Paw	83
Pumpkin	107	Peach	
Sweet corn	78	fresh	60
		canned	67
		Pear	
		fresh	53
FRUITS AND FRUIT PRODUCTS:	GI:	canned	67
Apple	54	Pineapple	94
Apple juice	58	Pineapple juice	66
		Plum	55
Apricots	44	Raisins	91
Banana	77	Watermelon	103
Cantaloupe	93		
Cherries	32	MEXICAN:	GI:
Fruit cocktail	79	Black beans	43
		Brown beans	54
Grapefruit	36		
Grapefruit juice	69	MISCELLANEOUS:	GI:
Grapes	66	Fish fingers	54
Kiwi fruit	75	Sausages	40
Mango	80	Nutella (Ferrero)	46
		Power Bar (Powerfoods)	82
Orange	63	VO2 Max Energy Bar	
Orange juice	74	(chocolate; Mars)	69

Note: This table was compiled by the RealAge team from many sources.

Cereals

A bowl of cereal in the morning is the easiest way to add fiber to your diet. Certain cereals contain almost half the recommended daily amount of fiber. Add strawberries or another high-fiber fruit, and your first meal will provide most of the fiber you need for the day.

Cereals are also a great source of vitamins. Approximately 90 percent of the cereals today have been fortified with vitamins and minerals (fortified indicates that extra nutrients have been added to the natural food). Some cereals are even made with soy protein and whole grains. Try Kashi cereals for extra soy and extra vitamins.

Be aware that many of the cereals sold in the United States today are made of highly refined flour, and many also contain a ton of sugar. Read the nutritional labels, and look for cereals in which a whole grain or part of the grain (for example, bran) is the first item in the ingredient list (enriched means that nutrients have been added back after the natural food has had some or all nutrients removed by refining).

Pastas

Fresh whole grain pastas can be good sources of immune-building antioxidant vitamins and minerals. Choose whole wheat, spinach, and high-protein varieties over white pasta. Whole wheat pasta is made from whole wheat flour and is a great source of fiber. It also contains folate, vitamin B_6, magnesium, phosphorus, potassium, zinc, copper, and manganese. Vegetable-based pastas— spinach and tomato pastas, for example—usually have more dietary fiber than plain pasta does.

Try to limit or stay away from pastas filled with cheese (tortellini or ravioli). Instead, add a variety of vegetables, some olive oil, and some fresh garlic to your pasta for extra cancer-fighting nutrition. A little tomato sauce will also give you a dose of lycopene, an antioxidant that is present in tomato products and has been shown in many studies to be associated with a decreased rate of cancer.

Oats and Oatmeal

Oats have one of the highest fiber contents of all the grains. Studies have shown that just 2 ounces of oats a day may help lower cholesterol. Several

---

REALAGE CAFÉ TIP 4.3
Superhealthy Soba

Most noodles that fill your plate do little to fill your nutritional needs. Unless those noodles are soba. Soba is made from a blend of wheat and buckwheat flours and has more nutrients than the typical white-flour noodles. In fact, several studies indicate that buckwheat boasts two cancer-fighting antioxidants, quercetin and rutin. Soba is also a powerhouse of virtually fat-free protein.

Soba has been a Japanese staple for centuries. In Japan, the thin noodles are eaten winter and summer, served either hot in broth or cold in dipping sauce. The noodles come in several varieties, including green cha soba (chasoba), which is made with green tea; nama soba; and hashiwari soba, which is particularly rich in buckwheat flour. You can now find soba in many supermarkets, as well as in Asian food stores.

cereals feature oats, the most popular being oat bran, granola, and rolled oats. Although oat bran contains the most fiber, all are good sources of fiber. Chart 4.4 shows how important fiber is to your RealAge.

The easiest way to incorporate oats into your diet is with a morning bowl of oatmeal. Oatmeal with fruit, oatmeal pancakes, homemade granola (baked oats and other grains with raisins and nuts) with yogurt, and breakfast fruit shakes are all excellent choices. Oats can also be used in stuffing, in baked goods such as muffins and breads, or as a breading for poultry or fish.

Rice

Rice is a common side dish. Unfortunately, refined white rice is what's typically served. When choosing rice, opt for brown. Brown rice is unrefined and therefore retains most of its fiber, vitamins, and minerals. Wehani, Black Japonica, and wild rice are good enough to eat all by themselves.

CHART 4.4

The RealAge Effect of the Amount of Fiber You Eat Each Day

Calendar Age	RealAge				
	MEN				
	Less than 5.2 g	5.2– 11.1 g	11.2– 17.1 g	17.2– 24.9 g	More than 24.9 g
35	35.7	35.3	35	34.5	34.1
55	55.9	55.4	55	54.1	53.5
70	71.0	70.5	70	68.9	68.1
	WOMEN				
	Less than 3.2 g	3.2– 9.1 g	9.2– 15.1 g	15.2– 24.9 g	More than 24.9 g
35	36.7	35.7	35	34.1	33.5
55	57.3	56.0	55	53.6	52.8
70	72.7	71.1	70	68.1	67.2

Note: Soluble fiber is preferable.

Fruit

Fruits—sweet-tasting, brightly colored—provide fiber and a harvest of age-reducing antioxidant vitamins, carotenoids, flavonoids (see Charts 4.5 and 4.6), and other plant chemicals that help prevent needless aging. As a rule, the more brightly colored your choices, the more nutritious. So, pick a spectrum of colors—deep purples, bright reds, brilliant oranges, and sunshiney yellows—to get the full antioxidant spectrum. Citrus fruits, berries, and melons provide a significant boost in the antioxidant vitamin C. Red and yellow fruits, including apricots, peaches, and mangoes, contain beta-carotene. Pink and red fruits are generally rich in lycopene, a substance that has been linked to reduced aging of the immune system and perhaps arteries. You should eat at least two servings of fruit a day, but eating four or five servings (and a citrus fruit) a day is even better and will make your RealAge as much as 4 years younger.

Eat fresh, well-washed fruits that are unpeeled when possible (if peeled, you'll lose much of the fiber). Although fruit juices count as a serving of fruit, most lack the fiber found in whole fruits, so don't make juice your main source of fruit.

Don't worry about the sugar in fruits. Even though fruits contain a great deal of sugar, it's in a form called fructose, or "fruit sugar," which is converted to glucose—the kind of sugar that your body burns at a slow rate. Thus, most fruits have relatively low glycemic indices (see Chart 4.3). Fruits that have high glycemic indices include fresh apricots, bananas, cantaloupe, kiwi, mango, watermelon, pineapple, and raisins. If you are worried about your blood sugar levels but want to eat these fruits, mix them with other foods that have a lower glycemic index and thus slow the emptying of the stomach. Try a banana with some peanut butter, or eat raisins as part of a trail mix with low-fat granola and nuts. Or, just eat a few nuts before you eat a fruit to slow the emptying of the stomach.

Apples

Long criticized as nutritional weaklings, apples are making a justified comeback. High in fiber and containing a respectable amount of vitamin C, apples, it's now thought, may also reduce the risk of cancer. A recent study in the journal *Nature* indicates that the combination of plant chemicals (phytochemicals) found in the skin and flesh of fresh apples may act as a powerful antioxidant to help make your immune system younger. Apples contain both flavonoids and polyphenols. The phytochemicals in fresh apples inhibited the

CHART 4.5
What's Your Flavonoid Intake?

To get a rough estimate of your daily flavonoid intake, write down the number of servings of each food you eat per day, multiply by the flavonoid content per serving, write the resulting number in the Total column, and add all of the totals.

Food	Serving Size	Servings per Day	Flavonoid Content per Serving	Total
Cranberries	1 cup		13.0 mg	
Cranberry juice	8 oz		13.0 mg	
Tea (not herbal)	8 oz		7.2 mg	
Tomato juice	8 oz		7.2 mg	
Apples	One medium		4.2 mg	
Applesauce	1 cup		4.2 mg	
Strawberries or grapes	1 cup		4.2 mg	
Broccoli	1 cup		4.2 mg	
Onions	1 cup or one small		3.0 mg	
Red wine or grape juice	One 5-oz glass		3.0 mg	
Tomato	One medium		2.6 mg	
Orange juice and mixtures (e.g., pineapple-orange)	8 oz		2.4 mg	
Oranges and tangerines	One medium		2.4 mg	
Tomato sauce	1 cup		1.8 mg	
Peaches	One medium		1.4 mg	
Vegetable soups (e.g., minestrone, tomato)	1 cup		1.3 mg	
Coleslaw/cabbage	1 cup		0.9 mg	
Green peppers	1 cup		0.9 mg	
Green leafy vegetables	1 cup		0.9 mg	
Peas	1 cup		0.9 mg	
Ketchup or salsa	1 tblsp		0.45 mg	

TOTAL: _____

CHART 4.6

The RealAge Effect of the Amount of Flavonoids You Eat Every Day

Calendar Age	0–19 mg	19.1–29.9 mg	30 mg or More
		RealAge	
MEN			
35	36.0	34.2	33.9
55	56.4	53.9	53.2
70	71.6	68.3	67.7
WOMEN			
35	35.9	34.3	34.1
55	56.1	53.9	53.5
70	71.4	68.9	68.0

growth of colon cancer cell cultures grown in a laboratory and, in other experiments, acted as antioxidants to neutralize free radicals.

Choose from a broad array of apples—Granny Smiths, MacIntoshes, Golden Delicious, Fujis, and more. Drink fresh cider to get a great-tasting antioxidant punch.

Apricots, Peaches, and Nectarines

These fruits of summer are rich in vitamin C, vitamin A, and beta-carotene. All that deep yellow flesh means they are brimming with nutrients. Mix them with your breakfast yogurt, granola, or cereal or, for a delicious dessert, bake them and top them with almond liqueur and cinnamon.

Avocados

Avocados are called the "vegetable fruit" because of their unusual taste. They're just about the only fruits that are high in fat; even so, they're good for you. Avocados are rich in monounsaturated fats, which raise healthy (HDL) cholesterol levels. This spreadable fruit is also a great source of folate and potassium. To top it off, new research indicates that the avocado contains an antioxidant,

REALAGE CAFÉ TIP 4.4

Fruit Smoothies

Want a quick, easy, and healthy addition to breakfast? Make a fruit smoothie. Add ice, orange juice, a banana, and any other fruit you want—strawberries, mangoes, peaches, kiwis—to the blender and mix. You get a low-calorie, nutrient-packed drink rich in vitamin C, potassium, and carotenoids to start the day off right. You also get at least two servings of fruit in one glass. And, unlike most juices, which have the fiber strained out, a smoothie gives you all the benefits of eating a full piece of fruit. Or try the Triple Berry Blender Blaster (see Chapter 11) for breakfast.

RealAge Benefit: Eating breakfast can make your RealAge as much as 1.1 years younger.

glutathione, believed to help fight heart disease and cancer. Avocados also contain significant amounts of magnesium and vitamin C. Plus, they taste great!

Since they're fattening, eat avocados in moderation, but do eat them. "Florida" avocados taste less creamy and have half the fat and two-thirds the calories of "California" avocados, but the "California" variety contains more antioxidant vitamins and minerals. Try adding a couple slices of avocado instead of mayo to a veggie or turkey sandwich or put them in a salad. Or use avocado in a guacamole appetizer to be served with low-fat, baked tortilla chips, soft corn tortillas, or vegetables for dipping.

Eating avocado at the beginning of a meal is a great way to get a world-class taste of healthy fat and reduce your overall caloric consumption.

Bananas

Bananas, the most popular fresh fruit in America, are a potassium powerhouse, and potassium makes your RealAge younger (see Chapter 5). A favorite among athletes, bananas have a low water content and a high carbohydrate content. This makes them a quick source of energy and a good way to refuel the body's potassium loss after exercise. Bananas provide almost 600 milligrams (mg) of potassium, along with good doses of magnesium and vitamin C. They are a good source of folate, and, even better, their folate is easily used by the body. Bananas make a great breakfast-on-the-go. Add them to hot or cold cereal, to low-fat yogurt or cottage cheese, or to waffles or pancakes as a topping. They're also great in fruit smoothies. For an age-reducing banana split, slice a banana, add low-fat or no-fat chocolate frozen yogurt, and top it with fresh sliced strawberries and toasted walnuts. Or just put a sliced banana

REALAGE CAFÉ TIP 4.5

Beyond Bananas

Ask anyone for a good source of potassium, and you'll probably be told, "bananas." Potassium is key to proper nerve and muscle function and helps your cells maintain correct fluid levels.

Although bananas are a potassium treasure trove, containing about 600 milligrams (mg) each, plenty of other foods provide potassium, too. Each of the following foods contains more than 350 mg of potassium per serving:

1 cup of cantaloupe or honeydew melon	2 tablespoons of tomato paste
Half a medium baked potato	1/2 cup of cooked spinach
1 glass of orange juice	1/2 cup of skim milk

---

in the freezer for thirty minutes to an hour and serve as dessert. It tastes amazingly creamy. Try it!

Berries

Berries are virtual antioxidant pills, containing more antioxidants per ounce than almost any other fruit. Anthocyanins—the same nutrients that give blueberries their deep blue color—repair free-radical damage in your body. Just a half cup of blueberries gives you as much antioxidant power as five servings of almost any other fruit or vegetable.

All berries—strawberries, blueberries, and raspberries—contain a compound called ellagic acid. Preliminary research suggests that this substance may help prevent certain types of cancers. Plus, berries are loaded with vitamin C and fiber. Strawberries are runaway vitamin C winners. Mix them with your yogurt or cereal in the morning, or have them as an after-dinner dessert. Take a few handfuls to work for a delicious mid-afternoon snack.

Citrus Fruits

C is for citrus—and vitamin C. As you may already know, all citrus fruits are a great source of vitamin C and fiber. Most citrus fruits also contain moderate amounts of potassium, magnesium, calcium, thiamin, niacin, and folate, not to mention a ton of colorful carotenoids. Although oranges are the most popular citrus fruit, tangerines, clementines, tangelos, lemons, limes, and grapefruit are also delicious. Blood oranges, which make their appearance in late winter, are a delicious source of lycopene, the carotenoid that gives them their deep red color.

REALAGE CAFÉ TIP 4.6

Just Juicy

Eating whole fruit is generally better for you than drinking juice. Fiber is lost during the juicing process, and, ounce for ounce, juices pack more calories than whole fruit does. A small orange has about 60 calories, while a glass of orange juice has about 110. Nonetheless, drinking juice can be a quick way to get one of your daily servings of fruit. Each 6-ounce glass of pure juice counts as a full serving of fruit.

And ounce for ounce, orange juice has the most vitamins, minerals, and fiber of all the juices, followed by grapefruit, prune, and pineapple juices. When buying juice, look at the label to make sure it's 100 percent juice. Many products may look juicy, but really contain lots of sugar and little juice.

Try using citrus fruits in a variety of ways. Orange or tangerine slices make great additions to salads. Or, add a little lemon and lime. Grapefruit offers an excellent supply of cholesterol-lowering fiber and blood pressure–lowering potassium. Half a grapefruit provides 40 mg of vitamin C. The red varieties of grapefruit are loaded with immune-boosting vitamin C and beta-carotene. They also are an important source of lycopene.

An important note for lovers of grapefruit juice: Grapefruit and grapefruit juice interact with many medications, even herbal ones, so if you want to add grapefruit or grapefruit juice to your food choices, check with your physician first. Grapefruit can also decrease the effectiveness of calcium channel blockers, medications used to control high blood pressure. However, don't assume you have to forego grapefruit—it's a wonderful, nutrient-rich food. Consult your physician to see if the dosage of your medicine can be adjusted so that the effects of grapefruit are taken into consideration and the medicine remains its most effective.

Dried Fruits

Want a snack on the go? Try dried fruit. Loaded with nutrients, dried fruits are an ideal snack food. Apricots, dates, pears, and more are good-for-you alternatives to candy, chips, or cookies. Remember, however, that just because the water's gone, the calories aren't. A piece of dried fruit contains about the same calories as a fresh piece of the same fruit. To fight the temptation to eat a whole bag, think about how many pieces of the fruit you would eat if it were fresh. If you would normally eat two fresh apricots at a sitting, you probably shouldn't eat ten dried ones. Dried fruits are good just to carry around for quick snacks, but they can also be great desserts, salad toppings, and additions to cooked meats and fishes.

Dates supply significant amounts of potassium, about 60 percent more than bananas, but are slightly higher in fat. Approximately twelve dates, or 3.5 ounces, provide 650 mg of potassium, as well as magnesium and many other vital nutrients.

Figs, like dates, are known for their sweet taste, potassium, and magnesium content. They provide even more calcium than skim milk but, unfortunately, are higher in calories.

Prunes (dried plums) are a concentrated source of fiber and contain vitamin A, beta-carotene, vitamin E, copper, potassium, magnesium, manganese, and many other minerals.

Raisins have about the same nutrients as prunes. Mix raisins with granola and nuts to make a high-energy trail mix, or use them to sweeten low-fat yogurt or cottage cheese, hot cereal, muffins, and cookies.

Grapes

Grapes are a great snacking fruit, too. You can easily take them in your car or add them to salads. Or, have them waiting in a bowl for your mid-morning or mid-afternoon snack. Full of fiber, grapes are a super alternative to chips. Or, as explained in Chapter 1, you can freeze them and add them to drinks to cool the temperature, add beauty, and boost nutrients. Grapes, purple grape juice, and red wine provide a considerable dose of flavonoids, at least 4 mg per cup. One of these flavonoids is quercetin. However, the substance in grapes believed to be the most beneficial is resveratrol, a flavonoid found in all grape skins. A number of studies have found that resveratrol reduces aging of the immune system and arteries in animals and thus reduces cancer, stroke, memory loss, and heart disease. At least five groups of researchers are now studying resveratrol in humans.

If resveratrol is found to provide that wonderful extra benefit, grapes, purple grape juice, and red wine will prove even more youth-promoting than we now think. However, the alcohol in red wine confers an extra anti-aging benefit not provided by grapes and purple grape juice.

Melons

Melons, especially cantaloupes, are another great source of antioxidants. The orange color of cantaloupe comes from beta-carotene. Melons also contain significant amounts of vitamin C. Treat yourself to a melon salad mixed with mangoes, grapes, and berries for a real age-reducing treat. Because of its potassium, melon is another good fruit choice for people with high blood pressure. Watermelon is a good source of lycopene, the antioxidant linked to a reduction in cancer rates. Slices of cantaloupe, watermelon, or honeydew are great additions to morning meals, as afternoon snacks, or as after-dinner desserts. At restaurants, ask for a fresh fruit plate with melon.

Two of the biggest surprises I've had in doing RealAge research are the discoveries of the benefits of two compounds I didn't even know about in 1995: lycopene and resveratrol. Now I enjoy grapes, watermelon, and tomatoes even more, knowing they are making me younger.

Tomatoes

Grow younger with tomatoes, a cancer-fighting food that we should eat all year round. Studies have found that people who eat just one serving of tomatoes a week have a 40 percent reduction in esophageal cancer. Also, a high tomato intake reduces the risk of eleven cancers by as much as 50 percent.

The reason appears to be the antioxidant power of tomatoes. An antioxidant found in tomatoes—lycopene—retards or reverses the aging of the cells in the prostate that can promote cancer growth. The prostate is especially vulnerable to damage from environmental factors and damage by free radicals. Lycopene is one of several kinds of carotenoids known for their antioxidant properties. Cooking the tomato makes it easier for the body to absorb the lycopene, so cooked tomato sauce and cooked salsa are even better for you than whole fresh tomatoes. You need a little fat to absorb the lycopene, so have some olive oil with your tomato.

Use Chart 4.7 to determine how much lycopene you're getting and then Chart 4.8 to figure out the effect it's having on your RealAge.

Tropical Fruits

Although many of us don't often think of eating them, tropical fruits are among the most age-reducing fruits. Pineapples, mangoes, guavas, kiwifruits, and other tropical fruits are packed with vitamins and antioxidants. The only tropical fruit you want to stay clear of is coconut, since it is chock-full of artery-aging saturated fats.

Guava contains nearly 50 percent more cancer-fighting lycopene than the tomato. This tropical fruit, which can be found at many grocery stores and

CHART 4.7

How Many Servings of Lycopene Do You Eat in a Week?

Copy this chart and add up your tomato servings. Estimate how many servings of each food you ate last week or eat during a typical week.

Food	Serving Size	Servings per Week
Salsa, tomato sauce, tomato paste	1 tblsp when eaten with fat *or* 4 tblsp when eaten without fat	
Pizza	One slice	
Guava	One medium	
Tomato	Two large, when eaten with some fat; one-half cooked when eaten with with some fat	
Watermelon	One-fourth medium-sized watermelon	
Red pepper	2 cups	
Red grapefruit	2 cups	
Tomato soup	1 cup	

TOTAL: _____

 REALAGE CAFÉ TIP 4.7

Tomato Temptations

The humble tomato is a rich source of lycopene, an antioxidant that appears to reduce the risk of cancer. However, on their own, tomatoes are not enough. Our bodies cannot absorb lycopene except in the presence of fat. So, drinking tomato juice on its own or eating slices of raw tomato without salad dressing won't do the trick.

Here are some things you can do to be sure you get all the protective benefits of lycopene without adding too much saturated fat to your diet:

- Add salsa to meats or salad.
- Have roasted tomatoes with a little olive oil.
- When eating pasta, choose a tomato-based sauce rather than a cream-based sauce.
- Nibble on a few nuts when drinking tomato juice.
- Have pizza with a flavorful low-fat cheese or even without cheese. There's enough fat in the crust to ensure absorption of the lycopene.

CHART 4.8

The RealAge Effect of the Number of Servings of Lycopene-Rich Tomato Sauce You Eat Each Week

Calendar Age	Less than 1 serving	1–3 servings	4–7 servings	8–10 servings	More than 10 servings
			RealAge		
			MEN		
35	35.4	35.1	35	34.8	34.7
55	55.8	55.3	55	54.6	54.0
70	71.1	70.5	70	69.4	68.8
			WOMEN		
35	35.4	35.1	35	35.0	34.9
55	55.7	55.2	55	54.9	54.6
70	70.8	70.3	70	69.8	69.5

Note: A serving is a tablespoon of tomato sauce or the amount of tomato paste on one slice of pizza.

most specialty produce stores, is also a great source of fiber, containing more than 9 grams of fiber per cup.

Another tropical splendor is the brilliant green kiwifruit. It contains twice as much vitamin E as an avocado, nearly twice as much vitamin C as an orange (per ounce), and a number of carotenoids, making it an excellent choice to keep your immune system young. Two kiwifruits contain about one-and-a-half times as much potassium as a medium-sized banana.

Mangoes are another super source of cancer-preventive antioxidants. Mangoes contain substantial levels of beta-carotene, vitamin C, and vitamin E. Best of all, they're delicious. Add them to smoothies and fruit salads. It's no wonder Hawaiians live three years longer than the average American.

Vegetables

Vegetables are another age-reducing part of the RealAge hourglass. They are the best first steps in the fight against aging, containing more than one hundred

REALAGE CAFÉ TIP 4.8
Eat Your Greens. And Yellows. And Reds.

Eating a diet rich in vegetables has been shown to reduce the risk of a number of cancers, including breast, prostate, and bladder cancers—and now ovarian cancer. A recent study found that a diet rich in leafy green vegetables might help reduce the risk of ovarian cancer, a disease that has a high mortality rate. Women who included vegetables such as spinach, kale, broccoli, and mustard greens in their diets at least six times a week had about half the risk of ovarian cancer as women who ate these vegetables twice a week or less.

Both women and men can benefit from eating lots of vegetables. Although starchy vegetables (such as potatoes) have not been shown to have an anticancer effect, dark green vegetables and colorful vegetables (such as carrots and tomatoes) have been linked to a reduction in a variety of cancers. These vegetables are rich in carotenoids, flavonoids, and other antioxidants that are believed to protect the body from cancer cells.

RealAge Benefit: Eating a diverse diet that includes five servings of vegetables a day can make your RealAge as much as 6 years younger.

---

vitamins and minerals that can protect the body. You can eat the USDA minimum of three servings of vegetables a day, but you'll make your RealAge younger with five. Five servings a day can make your RealAge as much as 6 years younger. Even if you don't have an elevated risk for arterial aging, eating certain vegetables can decrease your risk of hypertension and cardiovascular disease.

Try to eat some kind of dark green leafy vegetable and one serving of a cruciferous vegetable (for example, broccoli, cauliflower, watercress, or cabbage) every day. Although it's important to eat plenty of vegetables every day, remember that some contain a small amount of carbohydrate. Starchy carbohydrates such as potatoes, carrots, beets, parsnips, sweet potatoes, corn, and yams can raise your blood sugar if you eat them first in the meal (they have high glycemic indices), but you can make them RealAge healthy by eating them after having a little monounsaturated fat first. Almost all other vegetables have very low to moderate glycemic indexes and a high fiber content (see Chart 4.3).

Some vegetables are best eaten raw, but many vegetables taste good cooked or can only be eaten cooked. Steaming lightly and roasting at high temperature are two great ways to cook vegetables, sealing in all the nutrients and bringing out loads of flavor. Be careful about adding creamy sauces, since they can be poison to your arteries if they contain a lot of bad fats. Also, many restaurants use sauces that are high in sodium, like soy sauce, so when you are eating out, be the CEO (see Chapter 7) and ask that your vegetables be prepared in a little olive oil and salt-free spices. If you don't like steamed or roasted vegetables, you can grill, boil, sauté, or microwave them.

Increasing Your Vegetable Consumption

To help bring your RealAge to its youngest, you should eat five or six servings of vegetables a day. This may seem like a lot, but it's not. One serving is a fifth of an onion, a tablespoon of tomato sauce or tomato paste, half a red pepper, or three stalks of celery. If you make vegetables your new snack food, you'll reach your goal very easily. Bags of precut baby carrots, broccoli, and other vegetables are good to have on hand because they're ready to eat. Cucumbers, celery, peppers, radishes, and even mushrooms all make great snacks, too. Eaten raw, and with a few nuts, they are handy and delicious. Vegetable drinks and veggie burgers are also good sources for vegetables.

There are many great-tasting vegetables that fit the nutrient-rich, calorie-poor RealAge Diet goal—in fact, almost all vegetables do. Although we do not have enough space to celebrate all of them here, they occupy an important place in the RealAge hourglass.

ReALAGE CAFÉ TIP 4.9
Easy Vegetables

Do you find it hard to get five servings of vegetables every day? This weekend, make it easy on yourself. If you have a barbecue, throw veggies on the grill. Brush them lightly with olive oil and place them right on the grill. Or, you can toss them with garlic, pepper, and a drizzle of olive oil and wrap them in aluminum foil. If you don't want the added fat, use balsamic, red wine, or rice wine vinegar after grilling.

Artichokes

Many people shun the artichoke, because you have to use your hands and it takes a little effort to eat it. However, the wonderful taste and texture of artichokes, plus their high vitamin C, copper, manganese, and fiber content, certainly make them worth the effort.

Artichokes also enhance the flavor of other foods eaten with them. Because they contain cynarin, a substance that stimulates the sweetness receptors in the taste buds, when you eat an artichoke, all the other foods taste a little sweeter. If you want to dip the artichoke leaves in a sauce, try an olive oil vinaigrette or a low-fat dip of roasted garlic cloves, olive oil, and lemon juice. You can't go wrong with this powerful age-reducing combination.

Asparagus

Asparagus is full of the antioxidant vitamins C and E, as well as copper and manganese. Toss chopped asparagus into a salad or pasta dish, or lightly sprinkle cooked asparagus with olive oil and a little Parmesan cheese. Use leftover asparagus to make a low-fat cream-of-asparagus soup or, my favorite, a low-fat guacamole.

 REALAGE CAFÉ TIP 4.10
The Joy of Soy

If you're battling to lower your lousy (LDL) cholesterol levels, you probably know that eating less saturated fat is a key factor in reducing your risk of cardiovascular disease. What you may not know is that consuming soy protein rather than animal protein significantly decreases blood levels of total cholesterol and LDL cholesterol.

Furthermore, as little as 25 grams of soy protein a day has been found to be effective in those people who are at the highest risk. In other words, the higher your starting levels of total cholesterol and LDL cholesterol, the greater the reduction from soy protein.

If soy foods such as tofu and soy milk are scary territory for you, consider taking a good-quality soy supplement, or try edamame (pronounced eh-DAH-mah-may). You don't have to be a sushi fan to enjoy this staple of Japanese cuisine. For the uninitiated, edamame are fresh soybeans, and they're loaded with heart-healthy plant protein but are low in fat and calories.

Edamame have become so popular that they're available now in many larger grocery stores, as well as specialty food stores. For the most savory tasting soybeans, lightly steam or boil edamame in their pods and serve while still warm.

Beans

Beans are of two types: vegetable and legume. The vegetable beans are the beans in the shell, for example, green beans and wax beans.

All three varieties of shell beans contain significant amounts of fiber, along with iron, potassium, and folate. Folate (also called folic acid) helps reduce homocysteine levels in the blood, a key cause of arterial aging. Soybeans can be eaten as an appetizer (soybeans are popular in Japanese restaurants, where they are called edamame), served as a side dish, roasted as nuts, or added to soups and salads.

Foods such as lentils, kidney beans, and black-eyed peas are considered legumes and are discussed later in this chapter.

Beets

Beets, known for their sweetness, are brimming with a compound called beta-cyanin. This substance gives beets not only their deep crimson color but also a potent cancer-fighting power. Researchers who tested beet juice and other vegetable and fruit juices against some common cancer-causing chemicals found that beet juice ranked close to the top in preventing cell mutations that are commonly linked to cancer.

Carrots

We all know how good carrots are for the eyes—no, it's not a myth!—but they have other benefits as well. One is that they can help lower the amount of lousy cholesterol in the blood. Carrots contain calcium pectate, a type of soluble fiber that has been shown in many studies to reduce levels of lousy cholesterol.

Corn

Although not as RealAge beneficial as some other vegetables, corn contains soluble fiber. Corn is also an excellent source of lutein, an antioxidant that may reduce your risk of colon cancer and age-related vision problems. Also, like beans, corn contains an abundance of the B vitamin folate, which helps prevent birth defects and aging of the arteries. A single ear of sweet corn contains only 80 calories. Consuming the right amount of folate every day (700 micrograms) makes your RealAge 1.4 years younger. Eating corn with butter and salt offsets the RealAge benefits of corn, so instead season it with lemon juice, pepper, Tabasco, herbs, or a little olive oil and vinegar. Popcorn is also a favorite, and Simon, the first-ever RealAge patient, taught me how to make it RealAge healthy and give it world-class taste (see RealAge Café Tip 4.12).

REALAGE CAFÉ TIP 4.11
Can You Say Cruciferous?

Add bladder cancer to the list of diseases that may be prevented by a vegetable-rich diet. A recent study revealed that men who ate seven or more servings a week of cruciferous vegetables, including broccoli, cabbage, cauliflower, and Brussels sprouts, cut their risk of bladder cancer in half compared with men who ate one serving or less per week. These vegetables have also been found to help reduce the risk of other gastrointestinal cancers. Try adding cruciferous vegetables to pasta sauces, pizzas, salads, omelets, and stir-fries. Cabbage has also been found to contain a number of chemicals that have anti-cancer effects in test tube experiments and animals. Two compounds in particular—indole-3-carbinol and sulforaphane—make cabbage an especially potent cancer fighter in animals.

Cucumbers

Another great salad addition is the cucumber. Cucumbers are a refreshing, low-calorie addition to salads and sandwiches. They are even great eaten alone or with other raw vegetables. A medium-sized cucumber has approximately 12 percent of the minimum daily recommended amount of fiber.

Garlic and Onions

In ancient times, people thought garlic gave them strength and courage. In modern times, our beliefs aren't quite as bold. Although the exact benefits of garlic are debated, most experts believe it has substantial health benefits. It can help lower blood pressure and prevent the formation of blood clots. It also contains an agent that has important anti-cancer effects in animals and may have a similar effect in humans. Furthermore, garlic contains calcium, potassium, and vitamin C, so adding a little fresh garlic flavor to your food may add youthful years to your life.

Garlic does cause nausea and bloating in about one in seven people; if you are one of them, try onions. Onions are thought to have many of the same capabilities as garlic, since they also contain a substance that interferes with the formation of blood clots. They are also a great source of flavonoids, the antioxidant that helps prevent aging of the arteries and immune system. Onions and garlic not only make food taste great but also make you younger.

REALAGE CAFÉ TIP 4.12

Simon's RealAge Popcorn

Simon, the first RealAge patient (see *RealAge: Are You as Young as You Can Be?*), taught me how to have great-tasting popcorn—even with a butter flavor—with virtually none of the calories and aging effects of butter. He taught me something new about popping popcorn: You can do it without oil and without an air popper. Take a microwavable glass container of ample size, put in a cup of popcorn kernels, and put the top on it. Find out how long popcorn takes to pop in your microwave by using various times. Believe it or not, nonmicrowavable popcorn (regular popcorn kernels) will pop without oil in a glass container in a microwave. It takes about 5 minutes in our microwave. A microwave that has a turning platform lets all of the popcorn kernels get equal heat. After it's popped, put the popcorn on a cookie sheet and spray it lightly with PAM—you can use the olive oil PAM, or the butter-flavored PAM, or whatever your favorite flavor is. Do this very quickly and then spray on your favorite salt accompaniment. I use garlic salt or any other salt flavor I feel like having. One of my friends uses a cinnamon flavor. Then toss the popcorn into a paper bag with the flavoring, close the bag, and shake it. Place the popcorn into a container for eating, and you've made Simon's RealAge popcorn—nutrient rich, calorie poor, and world-class delicious.

Greens and Leafy Vegetables

Dark green leafy vegetables contain a host of cancer-fighting nutrients. Arugula, beet greens, broccoli, chard, collard greens, kale, mustard greens, romaine lettuce, spinach, turnip greens, and watercress contain significant amounts of the carotenes and vitamin C, as well as riboflavin, folate, iron, calcium, magnesium, and potassium. Spinach and kale, along with two less commonly consumed vegetables—fennel and okra—are loaded with calcium, magnesium, potassium, and vitamins. Grilling fennel and okra makes them sweeter. These vegetables make great side dishes to any meal, and spinach salads make good starters or lunches.

Mushrooms

Mushrooms add great taste and texture to many food dishes and are delicious even by themselves. They are loaded with potassium: 4 ounces of shiitake mushrooms provide more than 2,500 mg of potassium. The usual button mushrooms are also bountiful in potassium, with 1 cup providing 300 mg—nowhere near the shiitake, but still very RealAge healthy.

Potatoes

Potatoes are a popular side dish in many restaurants, and you usually have the choice of how you want them prepared. The best choice? From a cholesterol-lowering perspective, it's the baked potato, with its high-fiber skin. Ask for your condiments on the side and use them sparingly, unless they are salsa, ketchup, low-fat cottage cheese with chives, steamed broccoli, fresh herbs, nonfat or low-fat yogurt, or low-fat sour cream.

Water Chestnuts

Water chestnuts, that staple of Chinese food, are good low-calorie sources of dietary fiber. Water chestnuts complement any salad or stir-fry, adding great eye appeal and crunchiness.

Dairy Products and Eggs

Do you avoid fats by avoiding dairy? If so, you're missing a terrific source of protein, calcium, and other nutrients. One half cup of nonfat milk contains approximately 15 percent of the daily recommended amount of calcium for adults. All low-fat and nonfat dairy foods, with the exception of foods with added sugars, such as ice cream, are great choices for maintaining blood sugar levels.

The fat problem? No problem. Simply choose low-fat and nonfat versions of milk and yogurt, and low-fat cheese. They provide just as many nutrients, vitamins, and minerals as their whole-fat versions. Once you've retrained your palate, these products will taste great, too. If you don't like dairy or are lactose-intolerant, don't worry. You can get the nutrients elsewhere.

Cow's Milk (Skim, Please)

Milk is an old nutrition standby, offering nearly one-third of your daily calcium and one-fourth of your daily vitamin D in a single glass. Also, ounce for ounce, milk is an excellent source of protein. Choose 1 percent milk or nonfat milk for your cereal, for your coffee, and in your cooking.

Cheese

Despite its high calcium content, cheese is not a diet winner. High in calories, sodium, and saturated fats, cheese should be eaten sparingly. I like *tiny* amounts of full-fat cheese. If you want more than a pinch of cheese, and the greatest benefit from calcium-rich cheese, go for the low-fat, low-sodium varieties. Don't make cheese a major part of any meal. Some types of cheeses, such as ricotta, naturally have less sodium than others.

When you do eat cheese, get the most nutrients possible by choosing natural, unprocessed cheese. Processed cheeses, such as American cheese, are higher in sodium and lower in vitamin A, calcium, iron, and protein than natural cheeses.

Good cheese choices include low-fat versions of mozzarella, ricotta, string cheese, cheddar, Monterey jack, and Swiss. Cottage cheese—nonfat or low fat, of course—is an excellent choice. With only 0.5 grams (g) of fat and an amazing 19.5 g of protein per half cup, it's by far the healthiest cheese *and* dairy product. You can spice up your pasta and vegetables dishes with a little bit of authentic, high-quality Parmesan and Romano cheeses but, again, do so sparingly.

Many pizza restaurants now offer pizza with low-fat cheese. Try a vegetable pizza with low-fat mozzarella. You'll love it and probably will learn to love the taste of the lower-fat cheese.

REALAGE CAFÉ TIP 4.13
Cheese Head

The more cheese you eat, the higher your tyramine intake. If you notice that your migraines hit after eating cheese, tyramine may be the cause. Consider reducing your aged cheese intake. People sensitive to tyramine, a natural chemical found in many types of aged cheese, may experience dilated blood vessels and increased blood pressure in the brain, conditions that can lead to migraines. In general, the longer a cheese has aged, the greater its tyramine content. Cheeses high in tyramine include blue, cheddar, feta, Gorgonzola, mozzarella, Muenster, Swiss, Parmesan, and Brie. Soft cheeses, such as cottage, farmer's, ricotta, and cream cheese, contain the lowest levels of tyramine.

Yogurt

The best source of calcium? Low-fat or nonfat yogurt offers more calcium per serving than any other dairy food. Look for a low sodium content, too—less than 100 mg per serving (1 cup). Yogurt is great in the morning mixed with fruit and granola, as a salad dressing, as a topping on a baked potato, or as a dessert.

Frozen yogurt can be a healthy treat if you choose the low-fat or nonfat versions. Keep the toppings healthy, too. One healthful after-dinner dessert is nonfat chocolate frozen yogurt topped with walnuts. It still contains significant amounts of sugar but has approximately half the calories of ice cream. And it tastes great!

REALAGE CAFÉ TIP 4.14
More Good News about Dairy Products

Most people know that calcium helps prevent bone loss and osteoporosis, but new studies show that calcium—or some *other* nutrient in low-fat dairy foods—might help prevent aging of the arteries and immune system. A study recently published in the *Journal of the American Medical Association* shows that people who consume an abundance of low-fat dairy products have a lower incidence of the precancerous cells that can lead to colon cancer. Older data shows that a high intake of low-fat dairy products might help reduce high blood pressure.

Eggs

So, what's the scoop on eggs? For extra protein and vitamin E, include eggs, or especially egg whites, in your diet. Eggs also provide vitamin B_{12} and iron. It's true that one medium-sized egg has about 213 mg of cholesterol. However, most people who have high levels of cholesterol in their blood have had a lot of *saturated fat* in their diet; they may not necessarily have had a lot of *cholesterol* in their diet. That's because most of the cholesterol in our body does not come from the cholesterol we eat. Instead, our bodies use saturated fat to manufacture most of the cholesterol in our bodies.

Eggs are high in cholesterol, but they are low in calories, not too high in fat (about 5 g), and fairly high in protein. An egg has 6 g of protein, just as much as 1 ounce of low-fat cheese. So, one egg every Saturday morning is probably not going to put your cholesterol levels through the roof. However, remember that the yolks are high in cholesterol and fat, so don't overdo it. A great way to cut down on the cholesterol and fat but still get much of the protein and nutritional benefits of the egg is to mix a couple egg whites with one full egg. An omelet made of two egg whites, one egg, broccoli, spinach, or asparagus, and low-fat cheese, along with some fruit, is an excellent way of keeping your immune system younger (about 170 calories without the cheese, 215 with a small amount of cheese).

If your doctor has put you on a low-fat, low-cholesterol diet, you might skip on egg yolks altogether and try a liquid egg alternative, which is mostly egg whites. This product has the same amount of protein as regular eggs but less than half the fat and no cholesterol. When you're eating an omelet made from this product, you might not even notice the difference. An omelet of egg whites, tomato, onion, peppers, and a touch of ground pepper makes a terrific breakfast (and with two egg whites alone is less than 90 calories).

 REALAGE CAFÉ TIP 4.15
Eggs-ceptionally Good

Not only are eggs a lot better for you than they were once thought to be, but a special group of them may be exceptionally good for you.

In addition to a variety of healthful nutrients, some eggs now contain omega-3 fatty acids. The hens that lay these enriched eggs are fed a diet that includes fish oil, fishmeal, or flax, all sources of omega-3s. Few of us get enough of these good-for-you fats, which have been shown to lower cholesterol levels and blood pressure. These eggs have no more calories or fat than standard eggs.

Many supermarkets and grocery stores now carry a brand of these extra-ordinary eggs; the egg carton indicates "omega-3 enriched eggs." If your local grocery store doesn't, consider asking your grocer to order these. You can expect to pay more for such enriched eggs, but a little more for health may be worth it for you.

Meats, Poultry, and Fish

The biggest problem with eating meat is that most Americans eat too much and, as a result, consume far more saturated fat than they should. When it comes to cutting down on meat, there's no one right strategy. Some people eliminate meat from their diets entirely. Others eat the right kinds of meats and in appropriate quantities. You have to make the choice that's right for *you*. As long as you make plant foods the centerpiece of your diet, you can eat meat on rare occasions and still be quite healthy. However, try not to eat red meat (including pork) more than once a week, relying, instead, on such sources of protein as fish, poultry, nuts, and legumes.

Protein usually supplies somewhere between 10 and 60 percent of your total daily calories. We don't yet know what the least-aging percentage is, but most nutrition experts aim for 15 percent. However, there's no data to support that choice.

Protein-rich foods contain important and essential protein building blocks, or amino acids, minerals, and other nutrients. Although meat and poultry can be valuable sources of protein, don't forget that they are the primary sources of saturated fats in our diets. Meat-heavy diets make your arteries and immune system older.

In 1996, a study published in the *Journal of the American Medical Association* indicated a possible link between eating red meat and some forms of cancer. The study of thirty-five thousand older women showed that those who ate a lot of meat and animal fat, especially hamburgers, had twice the risk of certain kinds of cancer. Colon cancer, the third greatest cancer killer in the United States, has also been strongly linked with a diet that's high in animal fat and low in fruits, vegetables, and whole grain products.

The way you prepare meat affects how much fat—and aging—you're adding to your diet. Avoid fried meats and, when roasting, make sure the fat drips away from the meat. Use marinades and sauces that are low in sodium, for example, olive oil and wine, and lots of herbs and salt-free spices. Try to steer clear of prepared bottled sauces, or use small amounts. Stir-frying meats and adding meats to kebabs with a touch of olive oil and spices are great ways to flavor beef without getting the unwanted sodium that comes in bottled sauce. Many other types of processed meats, including deli meats, contain large amounts of sodium and should be avoided. A serving of brisket, corned beef, salami, bologna, bacon, or ham can contain more than your entire day's allotment of sodium. Instead opt for low-sodium roasted turkey (turkey prepared fresh at the deli counter that has no added sodium and no added seasoning solution listed on the label) or fresh tuna.

Beef

Although red meat is high in protein, making it your main source of protein can make your RealAge years older. Red meat is in the narrow middle of the RealAge hourglass (Figure 4.2). Think of it this way: Because red meat has loads of saturated fat, eating it is like widening the neck of the hourglass, causing the sands of time to run faster. Even when you cut off the fatty white edges, you're still getting a large dose of saturated fat.

When you do eat meat, limit your portion to 3 ounces—about the size of a pack of playing cards. Make meat a side dish or a condiment for the meal. The rest of your plate should be filled with as many colorful vegetables and whole grains as possible.

FIGURE 4.2 THE KEY OF THE NECK.

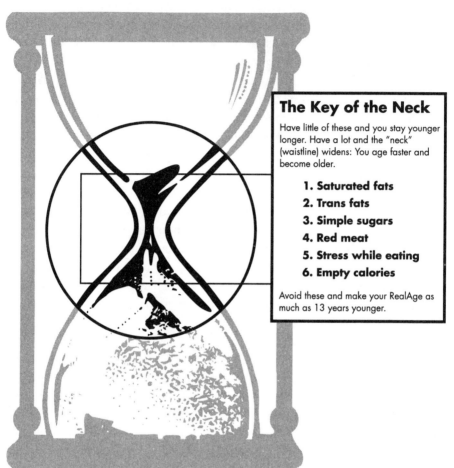

The Key of the Neck

Have little of these and you stay younger longer. Have a lot and the "neck" (waistline) widens: You age faster and become older.

1. **Saturated fats**
2. **Trans fats**
3. **Simple sugars**
4. **Red meat**
5. **Stress while eating**
6. **Empty calories**

Avoid these and make your RealAge as much as 13 years younger.

Which meat is the absolute worst for your heart and arteries? It's the big nationwide favorite: hamburger. Even lean ground beef has more total and saturated fat than all the other cuts of beef, and that's before it's grilled in trans fat. The white spots in raw hamburger are fat that's been ground into the beef. You can't cut it off and you can't cook it out. If you try, the burger will be dry.

Even beef that's 7 percent fat has 7 g of fat (reduced from 16.7 g) per 100 grams of hamburger, or a little more in a quarter pounder. The average reduced-fat burger has 7 g of fat, or one-third of your total daily desirable amount of saturated fat. Although you get a good dose of protein with a hamburger, it's not really worth it. A 3-ounce patty of the usual burger contains about 16 g of saturated fat. That's minus the bun, sauces, and whatever fat the

CHART 4.9
The RealAge Effect of the Percentage of Your Total Calories You Consume as Saturated Fat

Calendar Age	Less than 10%	10–14%	15–20%	More than 20%
		RealAge		
		MEN		
35	34.7	35	35.6	36.9
55	54.6	55	55.8	57.5
70	69.5	70	71	73.1
		WOMEN		
35	34.7	35	35.6	36.9
55	54.6	55	55.8	57.5
70	69.6	70	70.9	73.2

hamburger was fried in. Chart 4.9 shows how the consumption of saturated fat affects your RealAge, fast-forwarding your arteries to old.

Flank steak, also called London broil, is a much better bet than hamburger. Round steak has three of the leanest cuts available—eye of the round, top round, and round tip. Short loin also has lean cuts—top loin and tenderloin. Other lean choices are sirloin steaks.

Following the RealAge Diet Plan doesn't mean depriving yourself of the things you love. In the long run, deprivation can cause effects that make your RealAge older. So, if you love red meat, by all means serve yourself a side dish of it on occasion. Just remember, meat should be a side dish!

Pork and Lamb

Lamb and pork, though good sources of protein and other nutrients, are not, as the advertisement claims, "the other white meat" in terms of health. Lamb and pork tend to be high in saturated fat and cholesterol. If they are your favorites, save them for very special occasions. And choose the leanest cuts. Loin cuts of pork are the leanest and are comparable to beef in overall fat content. Spareribs are very fatty and should be eaten infrequently. If you buy ham, choose lean or extra lean varieties. When you buy lamb, remember that the foreshank is the leanest part.

Chicken

For protein, chicken is generally a better choice than red meats, because it is usually leaner. Choose the leanest parts (for example, the breast) and remove the skin. Beef and chicken have the same quality protein and the same amount of vitamins and minerals, except that beef contains slightly more iron and zinc. White breast meat contains moderate levels of magnesium and many other nutrients.

> If you're thinking fast-food fried chicken, you'd be better off with a steak dinner. Fried chicken—or any chicken with the skin left on, or fried, for that matter—contains a great deal of fat. If you include the skin in your meal, 50 percent of your calories will come from fat, and you'll be eating three times more fat than if you didn't eat the skin.

Whether you skin your poultry before or after cooking is up to you. I tell my patients that if they must eat fried chicken, they should take the skin off after frying. Grilling, broiling, or roasting skinless chicken can make the meat very dry.

Is one type of chicken better than another from a RealAge perspective? No. Most fresh chicken at your grocery store is the same. There is a difference between white meat and dark meat, however. White meat has less fat than dark meat, so it's a better RealAge choice. Although some people believe that free-range chickens—chickens that have not been raised in cages—are better for your health than commercially raised chickens, no evidence supports this theory. Intuitively, however, we assume that buying chickens that haven't been fed growth-promoting hormones or antibiotics is probably a more sensible thing to do than buying chickens that have been given those substances. Look for USDA-certified organic chicken that hasn't been basted (injected with butter, fat, broth, stock, or water) or given antibiotics or added hormones.

Turkey

Turkey is the healthiest and leanest of all the meats and poultry and contains significant amounts of magnesium, a boon if you are trying to keep your bones and arteries young. Most prepared turkeys, especially processed, prepackaged deli turkey, are high in sodium. Read the labels to find low-sodium versions. Roast a fresh turkey, instead of ham or brisket, for holidays or parties. You can look for USDA-certified organic turkey, just like you can for other poultry. Replace your beef burgers with low-fat turkey burgers or vegetable burgers.

Duck and Game

If turkey is the leanest of poultry, duck is one of the fattiest. If you're trying to watch the saturated fats, avoid duck. Game, however, is significantly lower in fat and cholesterol than other meats, and quail, venison, and buffalo are some of the leanest meats of all.

REALAGE CAFÉ TIP 4.16

Is a Vegetarian Diet OK?

Are there any risks from a vegetarian or virtually vegetarian diet? Not if you're careful to get important vitamins, amino acids, and minerals from other sources. If you include a variety of whole grains (such as barley and rye) and soy (or fish and low-fat dairy products) in your diet, you are largely covered. In addition, meat does contain significant amounts of iron, zinc, vitamin B_6, and vitamin B_{12}, so if you don't eat meat, it's important to find other sources of these vitamins and minerals, such as a supplement.

Salmon, soy burgers, low-fat dairy products, and lima and kidney beans are good sources of protein. Those foods, plus fortified breakfast cereals, spinach, and raisins, can be nutrient-rich additions to your diet, especially if you don't eat meat. Zinc can be found in nonmeat sources such as wheat germ, wheat bran, crab, tofu, sunflower seeds, almonds, and canned tuna. Vitamin B_6, though mostly found in foods of animal origin, can also be found in whole grains, nuts, and legumes. Peanut butter, green beans, bananas, artichokes, whole wheat spaghetti, and sunflower seeds are also good sources of vitamin B_6. You can get vitamin B_{12} from salmon, shrimp, nonfat yogurt, and eggs (mainly the yolks, unfortunately). Make sure to get a variety of protein-rich foods, since any nonmeat source of protein tends to have a smaller range of essential nutrients and amino acids than meat.

If you are a complete vegetarian and eat no animal products whatsoever, consider talking to a registered dietitian to ensure you are getting the full spectrum of nutrients.

Fish

Fish has all the protein of beef and less than half the fat. That alone is reason enough to eat fish. In addition, the fat in fish may even be good for you. Most of the fish we eat contains omega-3 fatty acids, a type of fat that increases healthy cholesterol and decreases bad cholesterol in the blood; it may also reduce triglyceride levels. Lowering triglycerides appears to lower blood pressure and decrease the risk of atherosclerosis, the hardening and aging of the arteries.

No one knows precisely how omega-3s work. Many experts believe they help prevent fatty buildup along the arterial walls. Another theory is that they help stabilize the heartbeat, reducing the irregular heart rhythms that are associated with heart attacks and sudden death. Omega-3s also appear to make platelets less sticky, which decreases the risk of clotting.

In addition, preliminary research from the University of California, Los Angeles, suggests that omega-3 fatty acids may help maintain healthy breast tissue and reduce your risk of breast cancer. Fish oils may also be potent in reducing the incidence of colon cancer. In one study, participants who supplemented their diet with fish oils produced less of a carcinogen associated with colon cancer than did a group that was not supplementing their diet with fish oil.

Omega-3 fatty acids may even help with anti-inflammatory conditions of the immune system. In studies of patients with rheumatoid arthritis, consumption of fish oils appeared to decrease joint stiffness and swelling. In a study of patients with Crohn's disease, an inflammatory bowel disease, participants who took the equivalent of 3 g of fish oils a day stayed symptom free.

> The fish that are highest in omega-3 fatty acids are primarily cold water fish, including salmon, trout, tuna (fresh and canned), Atlantic mackerel, sardines, Pacific herring, and most shellfish. We really do not know if it's the omega-3s or something else in fish that is age reducing. The data indicate that any fish, not just the fatty fish, make your RealAge younger. Since fish are rich in different proteins compared to other sources of protein, perhaps it's that ratio of proteins, and not the omega-3s, that is beneficial. Whatever the reason, eating 13 ounces of fish a week makes your RealAge 1.6 to 3.4 years younger (see Chart 4.10).

It is fairly easy to incorporate fish in your daily diet. Lox (smoked salmon) and bagels is a popular breakfast combination. One of my favorite breakfasts when I eat out is an egg white omelet with a side of salmon. It makes me younger and tastes great. For lunch, you can't go wrong with canned tuna on multigrain bread. Just mix it with vinegar and a little olive oil, low-fat or nonfat mayonnaise, or mustard to cut down on your saturated fat intake. Remember, eating fish makes the sands of time slow down in the RealAge hourglass.

Shellfish are low in fat and also have cholesterol-lowering qualities.

CHART 4.10

The RealAge Effect of Your Weekly Intake of Fish

	Less than 1 oz	1–6.9 oz	7–13.0 oz	More than 13.0 oz
Calendar Age		RealAge		
		MEN		
35	36.2	35.1	34.9	34.3
55	56.6	55.1	54.8	53.9
70	71.9	70.2	69.8	68.5
		WOMEN		
35	36.0	35.1	34.9	34.4
55	56.3	55.1	54.9	54.0
70	71.6	70.2	69.4	68.7

It's commonly believed that shellfish are high in cholesterol, but in fact most shellfish have only 50 to 70 mg of cholesterol per 3.5 ounces. That's even lower than chicken or turkey. Shrimp is one exception. It has almost twice the amount of cholesterol as the same-size serving of lean beef.

However, you should be concerned more about the amount of saturated fat rather than cholesterol in your diet, since saturated fat has the greater impact on cholesterol levels in your blood.

 REALAGE CAFÉ TIP 4.17
No Fish Fry

Fish makes us younger, but many of the ways we cook it do not. How you cook fish is important if you want to avoid adding unnecessary years to your RealAge.

Avoid breaded fish or fish with other coatings, since they are generally loaded with fat. Instead, broil, bake, sauté, or grill your fish.

Avoid seasoning fish with butter or sauces that contain butter, cream, or margarine. Instead, for a Mediterranean flair, try poaching fish in white wine and capers or roasting a filet with tomatoes, onions, and peppers.

Other Protein Sources

Meats and fish are not your only sources of protein, and some other sources are even better at slowing your rate of aging. For example, legumes and nuts not only are rich sources of protein but also contain important nutrients and minerals that help regulate and lower blood pressure and cholesterol. Most of the common types of beans—black, pinto, kidney, red, soy, lima, and navy beans—contain differing levels of calcium, magnesium, and potassium. Eat a variety of different beans, all of which are packed with calcium and fiber.

Legumes (dried beans and peas) are great nonmeat sources of many cancer-fighting vitamins and minerals, including iron, zinc, and B vitamins. You can add black beans, kidney beans, pinto beans, red beans, navy beans, and lentils to almost any meal. Hummus (a dip made from chickpeas, olive oil, lemon, garlic, and sesame seeds), commonly served in Mediterranean restaurants, is a great source of immune-building legume nutrients.

In the morning, top your low-fat yogurt or cottage cheese with some heart-healthy walnuts; add some sunflower seeds to your salad; snack on a few pistachios and some fruit for an afternoon lift; or toss some toasted, sliced almonds into your brown rice or pasta.

Legumes

Dried beans, peas, and lentils—a class of vegetable called legumes—are good sources of protein, fiber (both soluble and insoluble), and many other nutrients, including complex carbohydrates, B vitamins, zinc, potassium, magnesium, calcium, and iron. Studies have shown that a diet high in legumes can lower cholesterol levels significantly.

Legumes can be added to salads, soups, casseroles, and sandwiches, or they can be eaten alone. Combining black beans and brown rice makes an easy cholesterol-lowering meal. I even add beans to all my stir-fry dishes for that extra boost of fiber.

In particular, lentils are loaded with folate. In fact, no other unfortified food contains more of this key B vitamin, which helps lower heart disease and the risk of cancer and certain birth defects. A cup of cooked lentils in a stew or soup gives you 90 percent of the daily folate that you need. And preparing lentils couldn't be easier, because you don't have to soak them overnight or boil them for hours, like you do for dried beans.

Legumes have an unusually low glycemic index (see Chart 4.3). In fact, they can also lower the glycemic indices of other foods, because they have a

REALAGE CAFÉ TIP 4.18

Can I Cook the Protein and Other Nutrients Away?

People often hear that cooking destroys nutrients in foods. This is a concern primarily with regard to the B vitamins and vitamin C, which are broken down by prolonged heating. And some nutrients—especially the water-soluble B vitamins and vitamin C—are transferred ("lost") into the water in which they are cooked. Most other nutrients are not affected adversely by cooking. In fact, cooking improves the digestibility of most proteins, because high heat "denatures" protein, that is, partially breaks down the structure of the protein before you eat it.

Fresh vegetables versus cooked? Sometimes, frozen or canned vegetables have higher nutrient content than fresh vegetables do, because today "fresh" no longer means "just picked." Produce bought in a supermarket is often picked weeks before the consumer gets it. Some vitamins decline. Mineral content and calorie content do not change. While boiling in water can remove some minerals, the amount is usually not nutritionally significant. If you are concerned about this, steaming is a good option.

---

high soluble-fiber content and an enzyme that impairs the digestion of starch. When black beans are eaten with rice, for example, the glycemic index of the rice, usually high, decreases significantly because of the beans. Similarly, adding kidney beans to a pasta dish lowers the glycemic effect of the meal. Add a little olive oil or a few nuts first, and your blood sugar level will barely budge.

Nuts and Seeds

Nuts are a very good source of protein and are rich in vitamin E, thiamin, niacin, riboflavin, magnesium, zinc, copper, and selenium. Some seeds, including sunflower, pumpkin, and sesame seeds, also contain potassium and phosphorus. Both nuts and seeds have a lot of fiber as well.

In addition, nuts contain specific proteins that are especially rich in arginine, an amino acid that may provide a heart-healthy benefit. Arginine is part of an enzyme that helps dilate the blood vessels, allowing blood to flow more freely. This means the heart doesn't have to work as hard to deliver blood (oxygen) and hence energy to your body. Peanuts (a legume), walnuts, almonds, and hazelnuts are good sources of arginine. Although you shouldn't go overboard eating nuts, since they're high in calories, eating an ounce of nuts or nut products five times a week can make your RealAge as much as 3.4 years younger.

Yes, nuts, like fish and legumes, make the sands of time slow down or even reverse upward in your RealAge hourglass.

 REALAGE CAFÉ TIP 4.19
Sunflower Power

Good news for all you sunflower-seed snackers: The crunchy little kernels contain loads of anti-aging nutrients. Studies show that sunflower seeds are a superior source of phenolic acid, an antioxidant that helps counteract cell-damaging free radicals in the body. In fact, preliminary research found that the seeds contain a whopping 1,000 milligrams of phenolic acid per serving.

Sunflower seeds also supply a high dose of artery-friendly monounsaturated and polyunsaturated fats. Moreover, the seeds contain vitamin E and the mineral selenium, which are thought to play a role in preventing heart disease and cancer.

Eating a few nuts at the start of a meal makes you feel fuller sooner, so you'll eat less. One study showed that eating nuts may help with weight loss. One group of participants ate a standard low-fat, weight-reducing diet in which 20 percent of their calories came from fat. A second group ate a diet higher in fat, and most of the fat came from tree nuts, peanuts, olives, and olive oil. At first, both groups lost the same amount of weight. After eighteen months, only 20 percent of the first group was still on the diet, whereas over 50 percent of the second group, the nut eaters, had stayed on their diet and had lost more weight.

Another plus for nuts is that they lower lousy (LDL) cholesterol levels and increase healthy (HDL) cholesterol levels. Studies have confirmed the benefit for your heart and arteries. For example, in the Iowa Women's Health Study, women who ate nuts two to four times a week had less than half the arterial aging of those who ate almost no nuts. Another group studied healthy men with normal cholesterol levels who obtained 20 percent of their calories from walnuts. Their bad cholesterol levels decreased by as much as 15 percent, and, even more important, their healthy cholesterol levels increased by as much as 10 percent.

Most health food markets have many varieties of unsalted nuts and unsalted peanut butter. Almonds, Brazil nuts, pecans, cashews, chestnuts, peanuts, macadamia nuts, pistachios, sunflower seeds, and walnuts are all great nuts to try. Chestnuts are the only nuts that have vitamin C. They also contain significant amounts of vitamin B$_6$, which is important for people who don't eat meat.

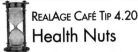

REALAGE CAFÉ TIP 4.20
Health Nuts

In 1993, a study reported in the *New England Journal of Medicine* showed that walnuts were beneficial in reducing blood cholesterol levels and protecting against heart disease. Perhaps it's because they are 70 percent poly-unsaturated fatty acids and 18 percent monounsaturated fatty acids, both of which are age reducing. Walnuts also contain other nutrients that may prove beneficial.

More recent studies have also shown the benefits of eating nuts. For example, researchers found that eating a few pecans may be as beneficial to your blood vessels as cooking with cholesterol-friendly olive oil. Pecans are high in fat, it's true, but almost 90 percent of the fat in pecans is healthy to your arteries. Pecans have a high concentration of a fatty acid that's found in olive oil and other monounsaturated fats. These monounsaturated fats can help lower bad cholesterol and preserve the healthy cholesterol that helps fight heart disease and all forms of aging of the arteries.

Tofu and Soy Products

Tofu, which is made from soy milk, is a great alternative to meat, because consuming soy protein rather than animal protein significantly decreases total cholesterol and bad (LDL) cholesterol levels. The higher your initial levels of total and LDL cholesterol, the more the consumption of soy protein will lower them.

For a fast and healthy Asian favorite, stir-fry your tofu with vegetables. Blend silken tofu for puddings, dips, and sauces. Baked, seasoned tofu is good for main dishes. Try soy ice cream for dessert, and soy burgers for lunch, or even a snack. And fresh soybeans, boiled and shelled, are a great snack.

Fats

Some fat is essential. The problem is not that we eat fat, but that we eat too much of it. It is equally essential to eat the right fats and to time our consumption of fats correctly. The importance of these habits is discussed in Chapter 1.

How Much Fat Should You Eat?

Your fat intake should be around 25 percent of your total calorie intake, with saturated fat comprising less than 10 percent. Focus on foods that are high in poly- and monounsaturated fats, such as salmon, tuna, olive oil, nuts, peanut butter, and avocados. Remember, fats have more than twice as many calories per gram as carbohydrates or proteins have, so eat them sparingly.

REALAGE CAFÉ TIP 4.21

High Blood Sugar and Fats

If you have high blood sugar, your choice of fats is even more important than usual. Higher amounts of monounsaturated fats—the fat found in olive and canola oils, nuts, and avocados—can help regulate insulin and help control the rise in triglyceride levels, a typical side effect of blood sugar problems and diabetes.

Oils

If you're like most people, you probably use oils fairly regularly in your food preparation. If so, you should know that different types of oils contain different types of fats and that some of these fats can be detrimental to your cholesterol levels, while others may be beneficial (see Charts 4.11 through 4.13).

Olive, canola, sunflower, and safflower oils contain significant amounts of unsaturated fats, along with small amounts of saturated fats. Unsaturated fats can lower your bad cholesterol and even increase your healthy cholesterol. So, choose your oils wisely. In restaurants, always request that the kitchen go light on the oil in cooking your foods, and ask what type of oil is used. Then ask for canola or olive oil.

In addition, certain oils have shown to be beneficial in lowering the risk of cancer. So, oils that contain a lot of unsaturated fat should replace butter and less healthy oils in your diet. The best oils are olive and canola. Remember, though, like all fats, even these "good" oils are high in calories, so consume them in moderation.

Our best advice is to cut as much saturated and trans fats from your diet as possible. Use liquid vegetable oils whenever a recipe calls for butter or margarine. Avoid stick margarine with hydrogenated oils and shortenings. If you decide to eat margarine, buy "tub" or liquid margarine. The first ingredient on

---

CHART 4.11

Which Fats Are Healthy, and Which Are Aging?

A large percentage of the fats in these oils (which are mixtures) fit in the following categories:

FATS THAT ARE HEALTHY

MONOUNSATURATED: USE IN MODERATION

Avocado oil

Canola oil, cold-pressed

Cod liver oil

Nut oils, most

Olive oil

Peanut oil

POLYUNSATURATED: PROBABLY HEALTHY

Corn oil

Cottonseed oil

Fish oils, most

Flaxseed oil

Grapeseed oil

Primrose oil

Safflower oil

Sesame oil

Soybean oil

Sunflower oil

Walnut oil

FATS THAT ARE AGING

SATURATED: STAY AWAY

Animal fats

Butter and milk fats

Coconut oil

Lard

Palm and palm kernel oils

TRANS: TERRIBLE

Hydrogenated oils

Margarines that are hard at room temperature

Partially hydrogenated vegetable and other oils, including partially hydrogenated canola or soybean oil, or vegetable shortening

The usual oil used for fast-food frying of fries, onions, chicken, etc.; also found in the glaze on doughnuts, in cookies and crackers meant to have a long shelf life, and in other packaged goods in grocery stores

---

CHART 4.12
The RealAge Effect of the Percentage of Your Total Calories You Get from Trans Fats

Calendar Age	Less than 1.5%	1.5–1.85%	1.86–2.2%	2.3–2.65%	More than 2.65%
			RealAge		
MEN					
35	33.6	34.2	34.7	35.1	36.2
55	52.4	53.4	54.4	55.6	56.7
70	67.1	67.9	69.1	70.7	72.0
WOMEN					
35	34.2	34.5	34.8	35.1	35.7
55	53.1	53.9	54.6	55.1	56.6
70	67.6	68.5	69.4	70.2	71.9

CHART 4.13
The RealAge Effect of the Percentage of Your Total Calories You Get from Polyunsaturated Fats

Calendar Age	Less than 3%	3.1–4%	4.1–4.8%	4.9–6.1%	More than 6.1%
			RealAge		
MEN					
35	36.0	35.5	35	34.9	34.8
55	56.4	55.7	55	54.9	54.6
70	71.6	70.8	70	69.8	69.5
WOMEN					
35	35.8	35.4	35	34.9	34.8
55	56.1	55.5	55	54.9	54.7
70	71.3	70.7	70	69.8	69.6

the product labels should be water and vegetable oil/vegetable oil blend (both are unsaturated fats). Or try one of the new margarines that contain plant extracts (for example, Benacol and Take Control), since they may actually lower your level of bad cholesterol.

> When it comes to oil, a little goes a long way. When cooking, spray the pan with an oil mister, as opposed to dumping in a couple of tablespoons. Or put some oil on a paper towel and smear it around the pan quickly. Instead of pouring salad dressing on your salad, dip the tines of your fork in the dressing before you scoop up a bite of lettuce. That way, you can get all of the flavor, with a lot fewer calories.

Other Food Concerns

Alcohol

Studies show that moderate amounts of alcohol may help reduce aging of your arteries. Even more recent studies show that those who are at the greatest risk of arterial aging, such as people with diabetes, benefit substantially from a moderate daily amount of alcohol intake. Moderation is the key for everyone, as large quantities of alcohol age your immune system. Drink only if you have no risk and no personal history or family history of alcohol or drug abuse.

Women can make their RealAge younger with one-half to one drink a day; men, with one or two drinks a day.

REALAGE CAFÉ TIP 4.22
The Best of the Reds? Pinot Noir!

You may already know that having a glass of red wine with dinner can help prevent heart disease. But did you ever wonder if all red wines protect the heart equally? Studies from the University of California at Davis and Cornell University suggest that resveratrol, an antioxidant found in all wine but particularly in red, is the reason red wine provides more protection from aging of the arteries than other alcoholic drinks. Resveratrol may even protect us from cancer.

Pinot noir is thought to contain twice as much resveratrol as cabernet franc, cabernet sauvignon, or merlot. Wines produced in humid climates, such as Napa, Sonoma, Burgundy, and Bordeaux, contain more resveratrol than wines produced in dry climates. But I like many red wines, and some is certainly better than none. The resveratrol is in the skin, so table grapes, whether green, blue-black, or red, also contain resveratrol.

Salt

The association between dietary sodium (salt) and high blood pressure has been debated but appears well documented. Salt (sodium chloride) is the main form of sodium found in food or added to food. There are other types of sodium, such as MSG (monosodium glutamate), onion salt, sea salt, garlic salt, and soy sauce. Although most of us experience a small but definite increase in blood pressure and arterial aging from too much salt, some people are "sodium-sensitive," and a diet high in sodium can contribute to making their RealAge much older.

The recommended daily allowance for sodium is no more than 2,400 mg a day.

 REALAGE CAFÉ TIP 4.23

The Potassium–Salt Balance

If your diet includes a lot of processed foods and few fresh foods, you may be at risk of a sodium–potassium imbalance. The average person consumes 2,000 to 3,000 milligrams of potassium a day. The upper end of that range is usually enough. In addition to being required for normal nerve and muscle function, potassium also regulates the amount of water that enters your cells, thereby enabling them to function normally. If your sodium intake is too high, however, you may need to increase the amount of potassium you consume. Why? Because potassium excretion is directly related to sodium excretion. The more excess sodium your body has to excrete, the more potassium you lose along with it.

To counteract this aging effect, limit your intake of processed foods to reasonable amounts. Better yet, make yourself younger by enjoying three potassium-rich foods a day: for example, orange juice, bananas, shiitake mushrooms, potatoes, and whole grain breads and cereals.

Sugar

Cutting back on your overall sugar intake is a quick and easy way to make extra calories disappear. If you need to make your RealAge younger by losing weight or stopping weight gain, watching your sugar is a good place to start. Calories tend to be more concentrated in simple sugars, meaning that you consume more calories, usually nutrient-poor calories, per mouthful. Any calories that you don't use are stored as body fat.

What about honey and natural sugars? Unfortunately, these are not healthy substitutes for white sugar. The body breaks them down into the same molecule as white sugar, and they contain the same number of calories.

FIGURE 4.3 GET YOUNGER WITH FOOD.

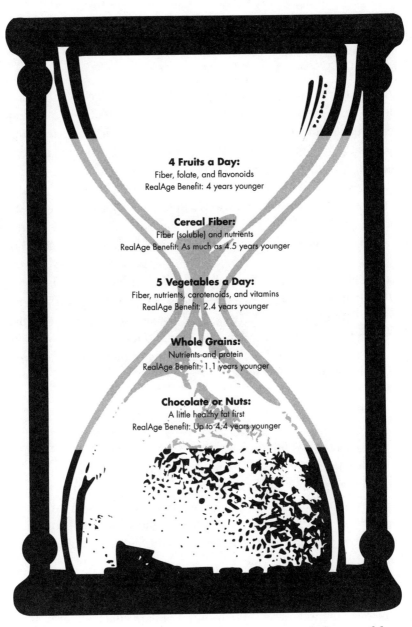

4 Fruits a Day:
Fiber, folate, and flavonoids
RealAge Benefit: 4 years younger

Cereal Fiber:
Fiber (soluble) and nutrients
RealAge Benefit: As much as 4.5 years younger

5 Vegetables a Day:
Fiber, nutrients, carotenoids, and vitamins
RealAge Benefit: 2.4 years younger

Whole Grains:
Nutrients and protein
RealAge Benefit: 1.1 years younger

Chocolate or Nuts:
A little healthy fat first
RealAge Benefit: Up to 4.4 years younger

Although the idea that eating too much sugar causes diabetes is false, many people find that a diet low in sugar helps keep their blood glucose levels more stable. Eating sugar in large doses tends to cause your blood sugar level to peak and then drop rapidly, sapping your energy. Simple sugars increase the amount of fat (triglycerides) in your blood, which also saps energy. Many people find that eating less sugar gives them more energy without the after-the-big-meal sleepiness.

Sweets and Sodas

Most sodas and fruit juice drinks contain lots of sugar and can wreak havoc on your blood sugar levels. Also, many beverages hide a great deal of sodium, so be sure to read the labels. Diet sodas are acceptable drink choices, but you should drink them in moderation. (We do not know for certain of any dangers of the currently used artificial sweeteners, but debate on saccharin and aspartame still exists.) Although diet sodas don't age you, they don't make you younger, either. Since the sodium and phosphates in diet sodas cause calcium and potassium loss, you need to get extra amounts of these two minerals in your diet if you drink diet sodas (about 200 mg of each for every six 12-ounce cans you consume).

There are also some sweets that will not raise your blood sugar levels significantly, though most have moderate glycemic indices (see Chart 4.3). If you have to indulge, oatmeal cookies, Twix caramel cookie bars, peanut M&Ms, and Snickers bars have the lowest glycemic indices of the sweets we have evaluated.

Remember, a little fat first slows the emptying of the stomach and reduces the aging that simple sugars cause.

Chocolate

There's some good news for chocolate lovers. Researchers in the Netherlands have discovered that chocolate contains catechins, a type of antioxidant that helps protect cells from damage and, therefore, the body from disease. In fact, dark chocolate (the kind from cocoa, not combined with milk) contains four times more catechins than black tea contains. Milk chocolate isn't as good, because it contains more saturated fat and fewer catechins—about the same amount as black tea.

Although all these benefits may reduce the guilt you feel when enjoying that "true" chocolate candy bar—from cocoa, not milk chocolate—remember to eat chocolate in moderation. A half-ounce of dark chocolate prior to dinner provides the right amount of fat.

Get Younger with Food

Small changes in your diet can make big differences in your RealAge and energy level. Even eating the RealAge way after surgery or chemotherapy will give you more energy for that recovery. Remember the RealAge hourglass to choose foods that slow your aging process and make you younger (Figure 4.3). Take notes on the foods that you enjoy and that make you healthy. Grab them at the supermarket. Before you go out to lunch or dinner, plan ahead so you can make wise decisions. If you've gone the whole day without any vegetables, be sure to make them a big part of your next day's meals. Fruit, fish, and foods with fiber and flavonoids should fill your cart at the market. And don't forget: Have a little healthy fat first at every meal. That's eating the RealAge way. The way to being younger and more energetic. And, yes, it's that easy—and that magical!

REALAGE CAFÉ TIP 4.24

Genetic Engineering: Should We Worry?

The controversy over genetically engineered or modified food centers around three concerns:

1 Potentially dangerous products may be sold to unwary consumers.

Pros: Genetic modification goes all the way back to the first mating of two strains of corn. We have eaten genetically modified foods for many years without one confirmed case of consumer harm. The same safety record exists for genetically engineered food. It has been over 11 years since the FDA approved the first genetically engineered (by gene splicing) food product—an enzyme used in cheese-making. Even in occasional mishaps, there has been no absolute link between consumption of genetically modified foods and actual disease.

Cons: Pharmaceutical firms that produce genetically modified food argue that the new gene-splicing techniques they use are merely a more sophisticated extension of classic breeding techniques. However, with recombinant DNA technology, genes from unrelated species can be inserted into the genetic makeup of animals or plants. At present, we just don't have enough information about how these products may affect us for us to eat the products without concern. The recent recall of corn suitable for animal consumption that found its way into taco shells reminds us of how hard it is to control these substances.

(continued)

2 Genetically modified food may be dangerous to our environment and to future generations.

Pros: The modifications may be a great boon to our environment. The new foods enable us to reduce the use of chemical herbicides, fungicides, and pesticides. Yields are up, and the cost of foods is down, so we may have less pollution because of genetically modified food. An occasional problem, such as milkweed contamination and the death of monarch butterflies, is to be expected.

Cons: New food crops contain genes that are tolerant to herbicides and resistant to insects. New scientific studies show that these genes flow easily in the pollen of these crops to surrounding fields. We do not know what happens when weeds take up these genes and become tolerant to herbicides and resistant to insects. We do know that real environmental harm results.

3 If consumed, genetically modified foods may create allergic and toxic reactions.

Pros: Although allergic or toxic reactions due to genetic modifications are, in theory, possible, they have *never* been proven to occur. The future of genetically modified food is even more promising. A new type of rice engineered to have more flavonoids and vitamin C may prevent aging, scurvy, or prostate cancer in poor or susceptible patients.

Cons: We just do not have enough data, and the FDA is allowing release of this genetically modified food without enough animal testing. Why wait for toxic reactions to protect the safety of our water, animals, and children? We know the hazards may be undetected for years. Many countries in Europe have banned genetically modified foods for just this reason.

Our Impression: We do not have enough data to state that you should avoid genetically modified food. However, we do believe that all genetically modified food should be labeled, and consumers should be able to choose, both in markets and in restaurants. Congress should enact enough safeguards to ensure adequate testing in animals before products that involve genes from unrelated species are inserted into foods and released into our food chain. We also believe that the potential benefit (including reduction of contamination from synthetic chemical herbicides, fungicides, and pesticides) is great, but that more caution and greater care should be exercised before genetically modified foods are released into the food chain.

5

How the Right Supplements Can Keep You Young

And a Trick for Remembering Your Supplement ABCs

Now that you've learned more about the right food choices, you're probably wondering if you need to take vitamins. Almost certainly yes! Taking a vitamin supplement is no longer optional for optimal aging; but taking the right vitamin and mineral supplements and avoiding the wrong ones can be an easy way to make your RealAge significantly younger.

The questions people most often ask me on radio and TV shows, online, and in my own clinical practice are questions about vitamins, minerals, and supplements:

> What vitamins, minerals, and supplements have been shown to make people's RealAge younger?
> Do I need to take a multivitamin?
> If I need a multivitamin, why doesn't my doctor tell me to take one?
> Why doesn't the multivitamin I bought at the store contain what you say should be in multivitamins?
> Why don't you recommend "X" or "Y" supplement?

In this chapter, I answer these questions. I recommend that you get all the vitamins, minerals, and other nutrients, from food or supplements, that have been repeatedly shown to make people healthier. I also recommend that you avoid those substances that may accelerate aging.

What to Look for When Buying a Multivitamin

Dozens of choices of multivitamins exist. Keep in mind that the FDA does not regulate the manufacture of vitamins and minerals or claims made on their package labels as tightly as it regulates drugs. With drugs, the manufacturer must prove safety and effectiveness beforehand. With vitamins and minerals, the FDA must prove lack of safety after the vitamin, mineral, or food supplement has already been sold. Multivitamins—even those manufactured by the big companies—may not have the right combination of vitamins in the exact amount you need to make your RealAge as young as it can be. You need to be aware of what you're buying.

After you read this chapter, you'll know what we believe are the optimal amounts of vitamins to slow your rate of aging, that is, the RealAge Optimum (RAO) doses. When selecting a multivitamin, these are the steps to take:

- Select a multivitamin that contains the RAO doses of the nutrients that promote age reduction, as we discuss in this chapter.
- Try to find a multivitamin that divides its daily dose into two pills. For certain vitamins and minerals (for example, the water-soluble vitamin C and calcium), it's better to divide the daily dose and take the halves eight to twelve hours apart, or at least six hours apart.
- Make sure the pill dissolves. A "USP" (United States Pharmacopeia) on the label indicates that it does. Or drop the pill into warm water and see if it dissolves within an hour when gently stirred occasionally.
- Look for the easy-to-spot contaminants. For example, try not to get your calcium from dolomite, oyster shells, or bone meal, which may contain minute quantities of lead or other heavy metals that are toxic.
- If you are allergic to wheat or some other substance, make sure it isn't on the label. You do want a yeast-based selenium, so do not choose yeast-free for your multivitamin.
- Make sure the multivitamin agrees with you. Drink half a glass of warm water before taking it, and a half glass afterwards, usually at the start of a meal. The water helps the vitamin dissolve. Take your multivitamin with a little healthy fat. Your body needs the fat to absorb the fat-soluble vitamins. If, after a month, the multivitamin seems to be causing stomach upset, switch to another. This is a trial-and-error process, but one that works for most of my patients.
- Avoid specialty versions that add cost but not value. For example, organic vitamins, mineral chelates, and vitamins that have "ester C" have not been demonstrated to have a RealAge advantage. They can increase cost needlessly. A multivitamin that meets all the recommendations in this chapter shouldn't cost more than $30 for a month's supply.

Of course, food is the number one source of nutrients. If you're eating a balanced diet that includes fruits and vegetables, whole grains, lean meats, fish, and olive oil, you're probably giving your body most of what it needs to stay strong, energized, and free of disease. Even when you're eating the best food, individual genetic variations and soil variations make vitamin and mineral deficiencies possible. It's difficult to get every vitamin and mineral you need from your food every single day. For some vitamins, such as vitamin E, it's nearly impossible to get the right amount from your diet. A broad-spectrum multivitamin that meets USP (U.S. Pharmacopeia) requirements from a reputable U.S. manufacturer will provide most of the vitamins and minerals your meals may be missing. The right amounts of calcium and vitamin E just will not fit in the size of one tablet that most people will take. So readers who want such amounts usually have to obtain a multivitamin that is meant to be taken daily in divided doses (several pills) or buy separate supplements of calcium, vitamin E, and vitamin C. (I suggest a U.S. brand because, in some countries, the laws governing the sale of nutritional supplements are even more lax than those in the United States.) After you've read this chapter, check to see if your multivitamin is missing important ingredients or has too much of others.

Before you rush out and buy a basketful of vitamins, you might want answers to these questions:

What are vitamins and minerals? What can they do for your health?
Which multivitamin should you choose? What should, and shouldn't, be in it?
How much of each vitamin do you need? How much is too much?
How can you tell if you're vitamin deficient? Can you focus on specific
   foods to get specific vitamins and minerals?
When should you take your vitamins for optimal absorption?

What Are Vitamins and Minerals— and What Can They Do for Me?

Vitamins are organic substances (derived from living organisms) that are present in natural foods; sometimes they're produced within the body. Vitamins are essential, in minute quantities, to your health. These substances do not provide energy or serve as building blocks but are very important to metabolic processes. Minerals are also essential, in minute quantities, to your health, but, unlike vitamins, minerals are inorganic—they're composed of matter other than plant or animal.

Your body uses vitamins and minerals for many processes, including cell growth and tissue repair. The right balance of nutrients keeps your body functioning properly, helps retard or prevent aging, and boosts your energy levels. Vitamins and minerals can help ward off a variety of ailments, from the common cold to osteoarthritis and progressive joint disease. Taking a multivitamin is a convenient way of getting most of what you need. Another advantage of taking a multivitamin is that certain vitamins and minerals perform better, or are absorbed better, in the presence of another vitamin or mineral, and this mix occurs when you take a multivitamin. Examples of these kinds of pairs are vitamins C and E, and calcium and vitamin D. You should avoid taking iron and vitamin C together, because iron inhibits the absorption of vitamin C. Remembering to take a multivitamin almost every day will help make your RealAge younger.

The Best Amount to Take? The RealAge Optimum

You've probably heard of the recommended daily allowance (RDA), now called the reference dietary intake (RDI). This is the minimum amount of a vitamin or mineral that the U.S. Department of Agriculture (USDA) recommends an average person should consume every day. The USDA also lists a daily value (DV), which is the RDI based on a 2,000-calorie-a-day diet. The problem is that the DV is the minimum amount of a vitamin or mineral that 95 percent of the American population needs to avoid illness from vitamin deficiencies. For example, the DV for vitamin C—formerly 60 milligrams (mg), now 90 to 105 mg—is an amount that ensures all of us will avoid getting scurvy.

In contrast, the *RealAge Optimum* (RAO) is the dose you need to slow aging and enjoy the best health. The difference between the DV or RDI and the RAO is the difference between treading water and having fun swimming. You may survive either way, but your quality of life in the water will be better if you know how to swim. To determine the RAO value for each nutrient, the RealAge scientific team analyzed hundreds of research articles on the effects of various doses of vitamins and minerals on health and aging.

Is More Better?

Although you don't want to be deficient in nutrients, taking more than the optimal amount for good health may not be a wise idea. Megadosing—taking large doses—of certain vitamins is potentially dangerous. The fat-soluble vitamins (vitamins A, D, E, and K) pose a particular threat. They are not easily eliminated from your body and are stored, instead, in body fat. When you megadose supplements, nutrients stored in body fat can reach toxic levels over time. These levels can then alter the production of proteins or other processes, or result in abnormal formation of bone or kidney stones that cause you to age or become ill. This danger is particularly high if you megadose minerals, since many remain in the body for a long, long time. If you get most of your nutrition from food and make up the rest through a balanced program of supplements, you won't need to worry about toxicity from accumulated excesses.

What You Need in Your Multivitamin

What exactly are the ingredients in a desirable multivitamin, and how do they make you younger? In the rest of this chapter we highlight the most important vitamins and minerals in your multivitamin and how they work for you.

The Water-Soluble Vitamins: Heart Helpers and Arterial Anti-Agers

Vitamins B and C are just a few of the water soluble-vitamins, but they seem very important, at greater than the DV or RDA amount, for slowing or even reversing aging. Being water soluble, they are flushed from your system relatively quickly. Because they are eliminated rapidly, they pose a low risk of toxicity; for the same reason, you must make sure you get adequate amounts relatively often (twice a day for vitamin C).

One thing these water-soluble vitamins have in common is that they all reduce cardiovascular aging in some way—something from which we can all benefit, no matter what our RealAge goals.

One reason some B vitamins play a major role in cardiovascular health is that they decrease the amount of homocysteine in the blood. Homocysteine is a normal product of protein metabolism that builds up in the blood. This can be a problem, because high levels of homocysteine are even worse for you than high levels of bad cholesterol. Although theories exist, we do not know exactly how homocysteine damages your arteries, but it does. Elevated homocysteine levels can triple your risk of heart attack, stroke, memory loss, impotence, and decay in the quality of orgasm. At least one-third of people who have cerebrovascular or cardiovascular disease—the precursors to strokes and heart attacks—have high homocysteine levels and thus unnecessary aging. Also, for some unknown reason, homocysteine levels increase as you age.

Although you could ask your doctor to determine your homocysteine levels, you can take precautions easily and painlessly by taking B vitamins. Vitamins B_6, B_9 (also known as folate, folic acid, and folicin), and B_{12} all work to lower homocysteine levels. With adequate amounts of these key nutrients, you can slow arterial aging.

Vitamin B_6

Aside from reducing homocysteine levels, vitamin B_6 helps break down fats, carbohydrates, and proteins so they are absorbed more easily. It is also essential for the formation of red blood cells, the production of antibodies, and normal neurological function.

AM I DEFICIENT? The common symptoms of an extreme vitamin B_6 deficiency are a sore mouth and tongue. Other symptoms are nausea, vomiting, dizziness, and mental confusion. A vitamin B_6 deficiency also increases the risk of depression.

WHAT'S THE RAO? Chart 5.1 shows the RealAge benefit of getting the right amount of vitamin B_6. If you get at least 3.7 mg of B_6 a day from food and supplements, you can make your RealAge more than 1 year younger. I play it safe and aim for 4 mg a day.

WHICH FOODS CONTAIN VITAMIN B_6?

Chicken, roasted light meat, no skin, 5 oz	0.8 mg
Banana, one medium	0.7 mg
Tomato paste, 1/2 cup	0.5 mg
Sunflower seeds, 1/4 cup	0.4 mg
Turkey, light meat, two thin slices	0.4 mg
Ground beef, 3 oz	0.4 mg
Crab meat, 1/2 cup	0.3 mg
Artichokes, one large	0.3 mg
Sweet potatoes, 1/5 cup	0.3 mg
Pork, one medium chop or slice of loin	0.3 mg
Tuna, sole, sardines, cod, or haddock, 3 oz	0.2–0.4 mg

Folate (Vitamin B_9)

Although folate (or folic acid or folicin—they're all the same nutrient) also reduces homocysteine levels and is a powerful ally in your fight against arterial

CHART 5.1

The RealAge Effect of Your Daily Intake of Vitamin B$_6$

	Less than 1.2 mg	1.2–1.5 mg	1.51–2.2 mg	2.21–3.7 mg	RealAge Optimum: More than 3.7 mg
Calendar Age			RealAge		
			MEN		
35	35.9	35.1	35	34.3	34.2
55	56	55.2	55	54.2	54.1
70	71.1	70.2	70	69.1	69
			WOMEN		
35	35.7	35	35	34.6	34.5
55	55.8	55.1	55	54.5	54.3
70	71.2	70.2	70	69	68.9

CHART 5.2

The RealAge Effect of Your Daily Intake of Folate

	100–200 mcg	200–400 mcg	400–700 mcg	RealAge Optimum: More than 700 mcg
Calendar Age		REALAGE		
		MEN		
35	35.3	35	34.7	34.6
55	55.5	55	54.3	54.2
70	70.6	70	69.4	69.2
		WOMEN		
35	35.3	35	34.7	34.6
55	55.5	55	54.5	54.3
70	70.5	70	69.4	69.3

aging, it has other benefits as well. It's essential for such cellular processes as the production of red blood cells and genetic material. Since rapid cell division depletes the supply of folate, people who have cancer, burns, or skin diseases, and pregnant women may need a higher intake of the vitamin to maintain normal levels. This vitamin is especially important for potentially pregnant women, since permanent nervous system defects can occur in newborns if the mother is deficient during early pregnancy.

AM I DEFICIENT? People who have an extreme folate deficiency may have anemia, a swollen tongue, gastrointestinal problems, and diarrhea. In two large studies, more than 65 percent of people over age 60 and more than 30 percent of all people tested deficient for folate.

WHAT'S THE RAO? Aim to get a total of about 700 micrograms (mcg) of folate a day. Since the average diet usually contains approximately 300 mcg, choose a multivitamin that has about 400 mcg of folate. Folate toxicity is rare, so you don't need to worry about getting a little more than the RAO each day. Getting the RAO of 700 mcg of folate a day can make your RealAge 0.8 years younger (see Chart 5.2).

WHICH FOODS CONTAIN FOLATE?

Asparagus, 1/2 cup	190 mcg
Artichokes, one large	150 mcg
Brussels sprouts, four large	130 mcg
Black-eyed peas, 1/2 cup	100 mcg
Sunflower seeds, 1/4 cup	80 mcg
Apples, one medium	75 mcg
Lima beans, fresh or frozen, 1/2 cup	75 mcg
Soybeans, 1/2 cup	70 mcg
Avocado, half	60 mcg
Spinach, fresh or frozen, 1/2 cup	60 mcg
Broccoli, fresh or frozen, 1/2 cup	50 mcg
Banana, one medium	45 mcg
Oranges, one medium	40 mcg

Most pastas, breads, cereals, fruit juices, and grains produced in the United States are fortified with about 25 mcg of folate per serving. Check the label to be sure. Most labels express folate content as a percentage of the DV, and the DV is 400 mcg. We know folate is safe up to about 2,000 mcg a day.

> ⧗ RealAge Café Tip 5.2
> ## Cabbage Killer
>
> Although some vegetables (for example, tomatoes) deliver more health benefits when they're cooked, cabbage is an exception. Cabbage contains a number of anti-cancer chemicals, but boiling it probably decreases their benefits. Research has shown that cooking cabbage removes about half its nutrients. Two compounds in particular—indole-3-carbinol and sulforaphane—make cabbage an especially potent cancer fighter. One cup of cabbage also has 250 milligrams of potassium and 83 micrograms of folate.
>
> When you can, enjoy cabbage in its raw form—in a salad, as coleslaw, or as a topping for tacos. Also use it in your stir-fry dishes. This cruciferous veggie keeps for ten days in a refrigerator crisper, so it's easy to have on hand.

Vitamin B_{12} (Cobalamin)

Vitamin B_{12} is the third vitamin that lowers homocysteine. This nutrient also aids many growth and repair functions of your body, including the production of red blood cells, nerves, and genetic material. Vitamin B_{12} is found almost exclusively in animal products, so vegetarians who do not take vitamin supplements may be especially susceptible to a deficiency.

AM I DEFICIENT? Symptoms of an extreme B_{12} deficiency are a sore tongue, fatigue, tingling, weight loss, and back pain. Severe and lasting deficiency results in pernicious anemia, a condition that has the potential for fatal paralysis.

WHAT'S THE RAO? Your body does not need much B_{12}—just 25 mcg per day from food and supplements. (The DV is 8 to 12 mcg, depending on age.) Since much more than that amount can be tolerated, and since some people have trouble absorbing B_{12} (for example, those with decreased stomach function), I recommend getting at least 800 mcg a day. To get this amount, you almost always need a supplement.

WHICH FOODS CONTAIN VITAMIN B_{12}?

Salmon, 1/2 cup	5.8–7.6 mcg
Tuna, 1/2 cup	2.2–3.0 mcg
Roast or hamburger, 3 oz	1.5–2.2 mcg
Lamb, chop, leg, or shoulder, 3 oz	1.4–2.0 mcg
Enriched bran or wheat flakes, 1 oz	1.5 mcg

Sole, haddock, 3.5 oz	1.2–1.4 mcg
Pancakes from mix, one 4″	1.3 mcg
Cod, fish sticks, swordfish, 3.5 oz	0.9–1.1 mcg
Yogurt, 8 oz	0.8–1.3 mcg
Milk, 1 cup	0.8–1.0 mcg
Macaroni and cheese, 1 cup	0.8 mcg
Egg, one large	0.6 mcg, mostly in the yolk

Vitamin C

Although vitamin C has long been associated with health, only recently has it been studied carefully by medical scientists. Vitamin C reduces arterial aging by functioning as an antioxidant. It helps keep blood vessels healthy by preventing fatty plaque buildup on blood vessel walls. It does this by helping to convert cholesterol to a substance that is not incorporated into plaque. Because it is water soluble, vitamin C enters the cells freely, where it attaches to free radicals (reactive chemical compounds) and prevents them from damaging DNA (genetic material). That's why vitamin C and vitamin E work as a combo: Vitamin E is fat soluble and attaches to free radicals in the fat-soluble parts of cells.

Vitamin C helps in other ways as well. It works to maintain a healthy matrix in blood vessel walls. It aids in the metabolism of proteins, boosts the immune system, promotes healing, and builds collagen in the skin. (Collagen keeps your skin elastic and makes you look younger.) Vitamin C also helps repair joint injuries, because of its effects on cartilage and collagen.

How you take your vitamin C may be as important as the vitamin itself. First, you should take your vitamin C with vitamin E, another antioxidant. The two work together to provide optimal age-reduction. It is also important to divide your vitamin C doses throughout the day.

Since vitamin C is water soluble, excess is flushed out of your system throughout the day. Therefore, this is one vitamin you may need to take as a supplement, in addition to your multivitamin, unless your daily multivitamin can be taken in two doses. Taking doses of vitamin C eight or twelve hours apart will help you keep a good level of the vitamin in your blood. Another option is to choose a multivitamin that you're supposed to take in several doses throughout the day. The label would say, for example, "serving size 2 tablets" or "serving size 1 tablet twice daily." In fact, formulating a vitamin with the correct amount of 1,200 mg a day of calcium and 1,200 mg of vitamin C makes the tablet too big, so it is convenient to have more than one of the same pill that combine to provide the 1,200 mg of these two Cs (vitamin C and calcium).

AM I DEFICIENT? A minor vitamin C deficiency decreases energy levels in athletes and even the rest of us. An extreme deficiency can produce loss of energy, painful joints, swollen and/or bleeding gums, and anemia. Vitamin C is further depleted if you smoke, use oral contraceptives, or take aspirin or tetracycline (an antibiotic) on a regular basis. Surprisingly, in one study in Arizona, vitamin C was found to be deficient or depleted in more than 36 percent of 494 people.

WHAT'S THE RAO? For maximum age reduction, take 1,200 mg of vitamin C a day, or 400 mg three times a day. By doing this, you can make your RealAge as much as 1.6 years younger (see Chart 5.3). Although vitamin C does not prevent colds, increasing your vitamin C intake to 4,000 mg a day (with an extra glass of water for each 1,000 mg taken) at the onset of a cold may decrease the severity and duration of symptoms (but, for some people, also causes diarrhea).

WHICH FOODS CONTAIN VITAMIN C?

Red bell peppers, one medium	150 mg
Orange juice, 1 cup	125 mg
Green bell peppers, 1/2 cup	95 mg
Papaya, half	85 mg
Strawberries, 1 cup	85 mg
Orange, one medium	70 mg
Cantaloupe, 1 cup	65 mg
Brussels sprouts, four large	60 mg
Mangos, 1 cup	45 mg
Broccoli, fresh or frozen, 1/2 cup	41 mg
Honeydew melon or watermelon, 1 cup	40–45 mg

 REALAGE CAFÉ TIP 5.3
Cheery News about Cherries

If you love chomping on cherries, check this out: This favorite summertime fruit packs a powerful combination of anti-aging antioxidants. Cherries not only contain the antioxidant quercetin, but also are loaded with anthocyanins and cyanidin. These two chemicals have anti-inflammatory effects and prevent cell damage from free radicals. What's more, cherries have heaps of vitamins C and E and a plentiful supply of potassium. If your taste buds prefer slightly sour tastes, try tart cherries; you'll pick up even more vitamins and great flavor.

RealAge Benefit: Getting the right amount of antioxidants and vitamins C and E in your diet or supplements can make your RealAge more than 3 years younger.

CHART 5.3

The RealAge Benefit of Getting the RealAge Optimum (RAO) Doses of Vitamins C and E Every Day

MEN

Vitamin C

At age 55: 1.4 years younger

At age 70: 1.6 years younger

Vitamin E

Age 55: 1.3 years younger

Age 70: 1.4 years younger

WOMEN

Vitamin C

Age 55: 1.1 years younger

Age 70: 1.3 years younger

Vitamin E

Age 55: 0.8 years younger

Age 70: 1.1 years younger

THE DAILY DOSE AT THE RAO LEVEL

Vitamin C

600 mg or more as a supplement, plus five servings of fruits and vegetables, to total 1,200 mg a day, in divided doses, separated by at least six hours (usually not to exceed 2,000 mg a day). Some people take 4,000 mg with four extra glasses of water when they start to feel a cold or flu coming on, to shorten the symptoms. Some data indicates that side effects of vitamin C start to occur when you routinely take more than 2,000 mg a day. Although the data are not clear yet as to the safe quantity, most evidence indicates that it's safe for the average person to take as much as 2,000 mg a day with no more than 600 mg taken in any six-hour period.

Vitamin E

400 IU

Note: Every time new data are published, the RealAge team recalculates the effect on RealAge. That is why the effects of vitamins C and E on RealAge are less in this book than in *RealAge: Are You as Young as You Can Be?* The direction of the benefits has not changed, but the size of the benefits has been reduced.

The Fat-Soluble Vitamins

The next group of vitamins, the fat-soluble vitamins, includes vitamins E, A, and D. Vitamin K is also a fat-soluble vitamin, but you do not need to supplement your diet with this nutrient as long as you get plenty of leafy green vegetables. The fat-soluble vitamins are usually found in such fatty foods as meat, eggs, dairy products, and fish; in green or yellow vegetables; and in vegetable oil. Since they are fat soluble, they need to be in the presence of fat to be absorbed by your gastrointestinal system, and they are stored in the fat tissue of your body. Fat-soluble vitamins are eliminated from the body at a slower pace and can reach toxic levels more easily than other vitamins.

Although toxicity can be a problem for those who megadose on fat-soluble vitamins, it is extremely rare to reach toxic levels with food alone, so you don't have to worry about the vitamins in the food that you're eating. In fact, even though fat-soluble vitamins are depleted slowly, many people develop deficiencies of vitamins D and E.

Vitamin E

Vitamin E is a fat-soluble vitamin that works with vitamin C, a water-soluble vitamin, as an antioxidant. These two nutrients complement one another because they act in different areas of the cell. Vitamin E concentrates in the cell membrane, which consists of fats. There it protects against oxidant-induced aging in the membrane. Vitamin C, on the other hand, enters the water-rich parts of the interior of the cell to collect free radicals lurking inside the cell. Together, these antioxidants keep your cells healthy inside and out.

Vitamin E gets right to work on artery walls. It helps keep the lousy (LDL) cholesterol in your blood from attaching to your artery walls. This lowers the risk of a heart attack by up to 40 percent in women and up to 35 percent in men. One important study in Great Britain found that vitamin E reduced the risk of heart attack by as much as 75 percent in people who already had arterial disease. Vitamin E also works as a mild blood thinner, making clots less likely to form. These anti-arterial aging effects of vitamin E confer the RealAge benefit.

Some studies have also shown that vitamin E helps protect against certain types of cancer, including prostate and lung cancer. The antioxidant properties of vitamin E may boost the immune system. Although the connection between cancer and vitamin E has not yet been confirmed, the results so far are promising. Thus, vitamin E may lower your RealAge even more than calculated in this book; we don't have enough data to say for sure.

Finally, vitamin E is good for your eyes. Preliminary research shows that this nutrient may help prevent macular degeneration and cataracts, two common eye diseases.

AM I DEFICIENT? In terms of the RDI or DV, very few adults in the developed world are deficient in vitamin E. On the other hand, virtually everyone who doesn't take a supplement with vitamin E will not be getting the RAO.

WHAT'S THE RAO? For maximum age reduction, you should take 400 international units (IU) of vitamin E a day. Because it's fat soluble, your body stores this nutrient until needed. One dose per day is all you need. Supplementation is necessary, since it's almost impossible to get enough vitamin E from food.

So, which is better, natural or synthetic? Vitamin E is the name given to a family of fat-soluble compounds called tocopherols, which come in several forms—alpha, beta, delta, and gamma. Synthetic vitamin E is usually alpha tocopherol, the form that confers many of the important benefits attributed to vitamin E. However, the other forms of tocopherol provide benefits, too, and natural vitamin E ("mixed natural tocopherols") contains all four forms. One study on animals found that natural vitamin E may be more effective in promoting a young RealAge. As of now, no data from humans indicates that natural vitamin E is preferable to synthetic vitamin E.

See Chart 5.3 for the RealAge effect of getting the RAO daily dose of vitamin E. Also, take your vitamin E with vitamin C. By taking your vitamin E and 1,200 mg of vitamin C a day, you can make your RealAge 3 years younger.

WHICH FOODS CONTAIN VITAMIN E? Vitamin E is found in high amounts in vegetable oils, beans, eggs, nuts, and avocados. Other foods that contain vitamin E include:

Almonds, 1 oz	6.7 IU
Hazelnuts, 1 oz	6.7 IU
Sweet potato, one medium	5.9 IU
Safflower oil, 1 tblsp	4.6 IU
Peanut butter, 1 tblsp	3.0 IU
Avocado, one medium	2.3 IU
Mango, one medium	2.3 IU
Corn oil, 1 tblsp	1.9 IU
Asparagus, four spears	1.1 IU
Apple, one medium	0.8 IU

Vitamin A

Vitamin A is another popular antioxidant. It's derived from beta-carotene, the substance that gives the yellow or orange color to fruits and vegetables. Vitamin A supplements have become a big industry, with Americans spending millions each year on this vitamin alone. Recent research has not proven vitamin A to be any sort of wonder drug. In fact, regularly taking too much vitamin A (more than 8,000 IU per day) can be quite dangerous.

Despite the warnings, vitamin A is an important nutrient. It has a number of functions, including the maintenance of healthy vision (especially night vision) and healthy teeth and gums, and improving the strength of hair, skin, nerves, and mucous membranes. Vitamin A also aids in immune and reproductive functions.

AM I DEFICIENT? An extreme vitamin A deficiency manifests as vision problems, tooth and gum diseases, skin changes, and an increased susceptibility to infection. Most Americans are not at risk of vitamin A deficiency.

WHAT'S THE RAO? In choosing a multivitamin, pick one that contains no more than 8,000 IU of vitamin A. Also, find one that contains vitamin A in the form of beta-carotene, which is less likely to be toxic than other forms of vitamin A. (Beta-carotene is converted to vitamin A only when your body needs vitamin A.)

The risk of toxicity from vitamin A supplements is high. At high doses, vitamin A turns from antioxidant to pro-oxidant, promoting free-radical damage rather than binding and neutralizing free radicals. High doses of vitamin A may also inhibit the metabolism of toxic compounds to nontoxic compounds. One 1993 study showed that people who took vitamin A supplements (beyond their multivitamins) had a higher risk of lung cancer, atherosclerosis, and, if they smoked, stroke. Chronic vitamin A toxicity causes headache, nausea, diarrhea, depression, liver damage, and even bone loss. Even though ingesting beta-carotene (a carotenoid), the precursor to vitamin A, is generally safer, toxicity from even carotenoids has occurred on rare occasions. Consumption of large amounts of beta-carotene can also produce a harmless yellow-orange discoloration of the skin.

If you want the protection of a vitamin antioxidant, it's better to rely on vitamins C and E rather than large doses of vitamin A. Most of all, get your vitamin A by eating a lot of fruits and vegetables.

WHICH FOODS CONTAIN VITAMIN A? The best source of vitamin A is food. Moreover, you don't have to worry about getting too much vitamin A from food. Breakfast cereal is a good source of vitamin A, as are egg yolks (though I'm not advocating that you eat yolks). Other sources include:

Pumpkin, canned, 1 cup	2,800 IU
Sweet potato, baked or boiled, half medium	2,200 IU
Cantaloupe, 1 cup	510 IU
Carrots, raw, one medium	300 IU
Spinach, fresh, frozen, or boiled, 1/2 cup	250 IU
Mango, 1 cup	215 IU
Swordfish, broiled, 3 oz	200 IU
Enriched bran or wheat flakes, 1 oz	125 IU
Winter squash, baked or boiled, one medium	115 IU
Red pepper, one medium	110 IU

Vitamin D

One of the most important vitamins in your age reduction plan may be vitamin D. The many benefits of this nutrient are just beginning to be understood. It is well known that vitamin D works with calcium to strengthen your bones. Recent research shows that vitamin D may also reduce your risk of certain types of cancers. No one knows how vitamin D works as an anticarcinogen, but studies have produced promising results.

For now, vitamin D is known to be a powerful ally in the battle to keep bones and joints working at their peak. First, it aids absorption of calcium. So, take your vitamin D when you take your calcium. Second, vitamin D may also help prevent osteoarthritis, the most common form of arthritis. Osteoarthritis, which affects more than 10 percent of people over age sixty-five, is a painful, debilitating disease that often restricts physical activity and the enjoyment of life and, in this way, makes you feel older and leads to further aging.

> Several studies have shown that taking calcium, vitamin C,
> and particularly vitamin D can delay the progression
> of and perhaps even prevent osteoarthritis.

In one large study, people who had high levels of vitamin D had less joint deterioration and fewer painful bone spurs, two common conditions in arthritis. Those who had low levels of vitamin D were three times as likely to suffer from rapid progression of arthritis.

AM I DEFICIENT? Despite all of these potential benefits, as many as 40 percent of Americans may be deficient in vitamin D. You may not even notice a mild deficiency of vitamin D, except as less than perfectly formed bones or arthritis. Severe deficiency can result in muscle weakness, tooth decay, osteoporosis, or severe bone deformities.

WHAT'S THE RAO? There are two ways to get vitamin D: from your food and from sunlight. The safest way is to get an adequate amount from food and supplements. Fish and shellfish contain vitamin D, and the vitamin is added to milk (but usually not milk products) and cereals to fortify them. Even so, most people don't get enough vitamin D from food alone. As you age, your body is less able to use sunlight to make active vitamin D, so older adults need to take more as a supplement. To get adequate amounts of vitamin D, take 400 IU a day as a supplement if you're under age seventy, and take 600 IU a day as a supplement if you're over age seventy.

Getting ten to twenty minutes of sun exposure a day without sunscreen (don't go out at peak sun time) is another way of getting your vitamin D. This amount of sunlight turns inactive vitamin D in your skin into active vitamin D, the same amount contained in four 8-ounce glasses of fortified milk. In reality, many people are not able to get ten to twenty minutes of sunlight that has enough energy to convert the inactive form of vitamin D to the active form. This deficiency is especially relevant in the northern climates. In fact, north of St. Louis, you cannot get enough energy from the sun between October and April to convert the inactive form of the vitamin to its active form. Whether the sun shines or not, err on the safe side and get your daily dose of vitamin D from foods or supplements.

Finally, don't forget your calcium! Getting 400 IU of vitamin D and 1,200 mg of calcium per day can make your RealAge as much as 1.3 years younger (see Chart 5.4).

WHICH FOODS CONTAIN VITAMIN D? Good sources are eggs, fatty fish, fortified milk, and fortified breakfast cereals. Some products list their vitamin D content in micrograms, so, for conversion's sake, remember that 1 mcg equals 40 IU.

Atlantic mackerel, 112 g (about 3 oz)	400 IU
Evaporated milk, 1 qt	100 IU
Milk, low-fat, fortified, 1 cup (not milk products)	100 IU*
Margarine (not recommended), 1 tblsp	60 IU
Atlantic cod, 115 g (about 3 oz)	50 IU

*The dairy, not the cow, adds vitamin D to milk; thus, products made from milk products such as cheese usually do not have much vitamin D. Soy milk often has the same amount of vitamin D added to it as dairy milk has. Check the label.

Granola, 1/4 cup	50 IU
Raisin bran, 1/2 cup	50 IU
Corn flakes, 1 cup	40 IU
Egg, one large	26 IU

The Minerals

Minerals help build bone and connective tissue and play an important role in cell signaling. Certain minerals, such as calcium, are key supplements. For many other minerals, you already get enough in the food you eat.

CHART 5.4
The RealAge Effect of Your Daily Intake of Calcium and Vitamin D

Calcium	Less than 200 mg	200–600 mg	600–1,000 mg	1,000–1,200 mg	More than 1,200 mg
Vitamin D	Less than 200 IU	200–400 IU	400–2,000 IU	400–2,000 IU	400–2,000 IU
Calendar Age			RealAge		
			MEN		
35	35.1	35.1	35.0	34.9	34.8
55	55.4	55.2	55.0	54.8	54.7
70	70.6	70.5	70.0	69.7	69.5
			WOMEN		
35	35.2	35.1	35.0	34.7	34.6
55	55.5	55.2	55.0	54.6	54.6
70	70.7	70.5	70.0	69.3	69.4

Note: If your calcium and vitamin D doses aren't in the same column, look at the column that contains the lower of your two values. Because there is little data on the number of deaths (from all causes) related to the depletion of calcium or vitamin D, these RealAge values probably underestimate the true aging effect of inadequate intake of calcium and vitamin D and the true RealAge benefit from the RAO doses of calcium and vitamin D.

Calcium

Men, women, runners, body builders, no matter what your age and fitness level, you need calcium to keep bones strong and to help prevent such diseases as osteoporosis and arthritis. The benefits of calcium go well beyond your bones. This nutrient is an all-star, helping many of your body's systems function and stay in shape. For example, calcium reduces premenstrual symptoms. It's also important for transmitting nerve impulses and regulating mood and blood pressure. In a recent study, men who took 1,000 mg of calcium a day had a 12 percent reduction in blood pressure. These results are controversial, because other studies didn't produce the same results. Nevertheless, calcium is essential in many ways, so the potential benefit of reduced blood pressure is just the beginning.

Calcium comes in a variety of forms, and many people are concerned about choosing the best source. Although there are slight differences in absorption, any kind of supplement will do—even over-the-counter antacids or the candy that contains calcium. I do advise against taking calcium supplements made from bone meal, oyster shells, or dolomite. These forms may contain minute quantities of lead or other heavy metals that can be toxic.

> **To get the full benefits of calcium, you need to skimp on salt and get your daily dose of vitamin D. Without sufficient vitamin D, your body won't absorb the calcium well. As mentioned, you need 600 IU of vitamin D a day if you're over age seventy, and 400 IU a day if you're under age seventy.**

If you consume a limited number of calories (for example, if you're on a weight loss plan), do a lot of physical activity that makes you sweat, or drink a lot of soft drinks, you may want to be doubly sure you're getting enough calcium from your diet. People who regularly restrict their caloric intake usually cut back on dairy products. Also, perspiring and drinking soft drinks increase calcium loss through the skin and urine, respectively.

AM I DEFICIENT? A lack of calcium may result in muscle cramps, spasms, osteoporosis, and, some say, premenstrual cramps and high blood pressure.

WHAT'S THE RAO? If you opt for supplements, find one that comes in 500- to 600-mg doses, because your body can absorb only that much at a time. Take one with breakfast and one with dinner; most people need 1,000 to 1,200 mg of calcium daily. Don't take iron or fiber supplements with your calcium, since both interfere with the absorption of calcium. You can make your RealAge as much as 1.3 years younger by taking 1,200 mg of calcium, along with 400 IU of vitamin D, every day from food or supplements. Most multivitamins don't have a lot of calcium, because it would make the pill too large. So, you'd need to take 400 mg of calcium three times a day. Chart 5.4 shows the RealAge effects of various daily doses of calcium and vitamin D.

WHICH FOODS CONTAIN CALCIUM?

Yogurt, plain, low-fat, 8 oz	415 mg
Parmesan cheese, 1 oz	390 mg
Macaroni and cheese, 1 cup	360 mg
Eggnog, 1 cup	330 mg
Soymilk, 1 cup	300 mg
Milk, 1 cup	290 mg
Swiss cheese, 1 oz	270 mg
Pink salmon, canned, 1/2 cup	215 mg
Kale, 1/4 lb	205 mg
Cheddar cheese, 1 oz	205 mg
Spinach, 1 cup	180 mg
Tofu, one cube $2 \times 3 \times 1''$	155 mg
Ice cream, 1 cup (not recommended)	150–180 mg

 REALAGE CAFÉ TIP 5.4

Kale and Hearty

If you're trying to add more greens to your diet, give kale a taste test. This bunch of curly green, white, and purple leaves is a type of cabbage. Like other cruciferous vegetables, kale contains natural plant chemicals that, research suggests, may stimulate enzymes that detoxify carcinogens and in this way help prevent a variety of cancers. Kale also contains (per ¼ pound) 60 micrograms of folate, 380 milligrams (mg) of potassium, and about 200 mg of calcium. Both potassium and calcium regulate blood pressure and therefore reduce arterial aging and the risk of stroke.

Potassium

You may not have heard much about potassium, but it's an essential nutrient and an important anti-ager. This mineral packs a punch against arterial aging and one of its consequences, aging of the brain (cognitive aging). Strokes are a major cause of cognitive aging, but you can minimize your risk by increasing your intake of potassium in food. Under no circumstances should you take a supplement of potassium unless guided by a physician; supplementing with potassium is an extremely dangerous thing to do. Under certain circumstances, taking potassium in pill form can cause an accumulation of potassium that can produce fatal irregular heart rhythms. If you are considering taking the pill form of potassium, you should have your potassium concentrations and kidney function monitored by a doctor.

Potassium reduces the risk of having a stroke in several ways. It reduces blood pressure, stabilizes arterial plaques, and decreases the oxidation of lipids (fats). In one study, people who ate foods with little potassium were over three times more likely to have a stroke due to arterial aging than were those who ate considerably more potassium.

Potassium is also involved in the transmission of nerve impulses and the maintenance of normal heart function. This nutrient even helps in the metabolism of carbohydrates and proteins.

AM I DEFICIENT? Probably not. If you are not taking diuretics (water pills), potassium deficiency is actually quite rare; less than half of the population gets the optimal amount, however. Just make sure you're getting enough potassium from food.

WHAT'S THE RAO? There is no DV value for potassium, but I recommend getting at least 3,000 mg a day *from food.* You probably get about half that each day if you eat a balanced diet. By focusing on potassium-rich foods (four servings of fruits and five servings of vegetables a day), you can increase your daily intake to the recommended dose of 3,000 mg. Three bananas provide more than 1,300 mg. Getting your recommended amount of potassium makes your RealAge 0.6 years younger.

WHICH FOODS CONTAIN POTASSIUM?

Tomato paste, 1/2 cup	1,340 mg
Dried peaches, five halves	785 mg
Baked potato, one large	780 mg
Sole, salmon, sardines, cod, 4 oz	585–720 mg
Watermelon, cantaloupe, honeydew, 1 cup	460–560 mg
Dried apricots, three to four medium	480 mg
Steamed scallops, 3 1/2 oz	455 mg
Bananas, one medium	450 mg

Grapefruit juice, 1 cup	405 mg
Yogurt, 8 oz	400–530 mg
Chestnuts, 100 g (about 3 1/2 oz)	380 mg
Milk, 1 cup	370–450 mg
Artichokes, one large	360 mg

Magnesium

Magnesium is essential for many basic cellular processes. It is required for energy metabolism and is involved in muscle contraction, normal heart function, absorption of calcium, and transmission of nerve impulses.

The benefits of magnesium are clear. A ten-year study of people at high risk of arterial aging showed that those who ate a magnesium-rich diet had less than half the cardiovascular-related complications as those on low-magnesium diets. You should benefit from a dose of magnesium that is one-third that of calcium.

AM I DEFICIENT? Unfortunately, magnesium deficiency is increasingly common. Experts estimate that up to 40 percent of Americans get less than 70 percent of the DV for magnesium. It turns out that life in the modern world is to blame. Stress, sugar, alcohol, and phosphates (commonly found in soft drinks) all deplete the body's store of magnesium. Exercise can also contribute to the deficiency, because we lose magnesium through perspiration. To make matters worse, magnesium deficiency produces few symptoms. Without adequate magnesium, your muscles and heart may act "tired," and your arteries age faster.

WHAT'S THE RAO? Magnesium is an important mineral. Women should get 400 mg, and men at least 333 mg per day from food or supplements. Getting this amount will make your RealAge as much as 0.9 years younger. With a balanced diet, you may not need to supplement, but if you're worried that you're not getting enough magnesium, take 400 mg in a multivitamin daily. You should consult your physician about your magnesium intake if you're pregnant or lactating, have kidney disease or diabetes, are on a low-calorie diet, or are taking digitalis preparations or diuretics (water pills). If you're in one of these groups, you need to be extra careful to get enough magnesium.

WHICH FOODS CONTAIN MAGNESIUM? Magnesium is found in whole grain breads and cereals. Other foods containing magnesium include:

Tofu, 120 g	130 mg
Soybeans, 1/2 cup	80 mg

Cashews, 1 oz	80 mg
Tomato paste, 1/2 cup	75 mg
Salmon, one steak (4 oz)	60 mg
Spinach, 1/2 cup	60 mg
Oatmeal, 1 cup	55 mg
Peanuts, 1 oz (thirty nuts)	50 mg
Potatoes, baked or sweet, one large	45 mg
Fortified cereals (bran or wheat), 1 oz	40–50 mg
Shrimp, 3 oz	40–45 mg
Brown rice, 2/3 cup	40 mg

What You *Don't* Need in a Supplement

Now you know what you need in your multivitamin. What about what you don't need? Many supplements purport to be wonder drugs, but when they're tested appropriately, they fail to show results. You are probably getting plenty of sodium, iron, zinc, chromium, potassium, and vitamin K from food, so there's no need to have them in your supplement as well.

Sodium (Salt)

Although sodium is an essential nutrient, it's one mineral you don't have to add to your diet. Sodium is abundant in the average Westernized diet. By most accounts, people get too much sodium from the foods they eat. Although you need only 116 mg of sodium a day, the average American consumes a whopping 4,000 mg each day.

Many people think that if they just don't add salt to their food, their sodium intake will be at a healthy level. Unfortunately, 75 percent of the salt in our diets is hidden in the processed foods we eat. Soy sauce, canned soups, and frozen foods are loaded with excess salt.

Don't get me wrong; sodium is necessary. It's required for transmission of nerve impulses, regulation of blood pressure, and metabolism of carbohydrates and protein. But for most people, high consumption of salt can lead to high blood pressure. In the most famous study on sodium intake, the InterSalt study, researchers evaluated sodium consumption in over ten thousand people and found that it definitely correlated with blood pressure. The more salt people consumed, the higher their blood pressure. This elevated blood pressure led to an accelerated rate of arterial aging. These changes in blood pressure caused by sodium were small but important: In a few people—those with salt-sensitive high blood pressure—salt caused dramatic increases in blood pressure.

For years, physicians prescribed low-salt diets to people with high blood pressure. However, since the advent of effective drugs that lower blood pressure, these diets have become less common. Nevertheless, the combination of a lower-salt diet, exercise, and weight control is still an important way to avoid high blood pressure.

Sodium can also be bad news for your bones. When sodium is excreted through urine or sweat, it takes a bit of calcium with it. This becomes a problem for the bones of the average American, who takes in far more sodium than the recommended 2,400 mg a day. To offset this effect, you could start reading all the food labels, counting up all the milligrams of salt, and limiting your salt intake, *or* you could increase your *calcium* consumption to about 1,500 mg a day. The second strategy is probably the simpler of the two.

How can you reduce your sodium intake? Because much of the sodium we consume is hidden, it helps to avoid fast foods and processed and preserved foods. In general, canned, prepared, and fast foods contain the highest levels of sodium. Fresh fruits and vegetables and fresh meats and poultry contain little sodium.

COULD I BECOME DEFICIENT? Although sodium deficiency is rare, certain conditions can deplete sodium stores. Illnesses (such as diarrhea and kidney disease), medications (diuretics), and heavy perspiration can produce a temporary sodium loss. In extreme instances, sodium loss can produce an electrolyte imbalance, which can cause fatigue, loss of appetite, thirst, vomiting, and severe muscle cramping.

WHAT'S THE RAO? Experts agree you should not ingest more than 2,400 mg of sodium a day. For optimal health, however, aim to keep your sodium intake below 1,600 mg a day. This can make your RealAge younger by as much as 3 years.

WHICH FOODS CONTAIN THE MOST SODIUM?

Soy sauce, 2 tblsp	2,665 mg
Dill pickles, one large	1,930 mg
Chili con carne with beans, canned, 1 cup	1,355 mg
Frozen dinners, one 11-oz meal	1,075–1,225 mg
Sausages, three small	560–720 mg
Pretzels, ten	480 mg

Green olives, five large	465 mg
Cheese pizza, one slice	455–490 mg
Canned soups, 1 cup	400–1,810 mg

REALAGE CAFÉ TIP 5.5

Salt Shakedown

If you're health conscious, you may want to keep red pepper flakes or lemon pepper in your saltshaker instead of salt. Or you may cook with garlic or chilies.

Even if you don't add salt to your food, you may be getting too much. Perhaps two-and-a-half times too much! That's because sodium usually sneaks into packaged and restaurant foods where you'd least expect it. It's not just the obvious chips, pretzels, and pizza. Diet soda, canned vegetables, and cereal also contain hidden salt. With hidden salt lurking in almost every food, is it even possible to cut back and protect yourself from hypertension and arterial aging?

Absolutely. Just being aware of hidden salt helps. For example, an innocent-looking low-fat tuna fish sandwich on whole wheat bread can pack 922 milligrams (mg) of sodium. That's more than half of what you should get a day—1,600 mg—to stay as young as you can be. The trick is to take a little more time reading the nutrition labels. For instance, different brands of tuna fish and bread contain different amounts of sodium. All else being equal, choose the one with the least sodium. Also, pick fresh fruits and vegetables over canned, and fresh meats and poultry over processed. If you want to stock up, freeze food in baggies yourself. And watch those frozen dinners. Even the low-fat ones can be full of salt, so check the labels before you check out.

By whittling down the sodium in your diet, you'll protect yourself from high blood pressure and lower your risk of cardiovascular disease, heart attack, stroke, memory loss, impotence, decay in the quality of orgasm, and even wrinkling of the skin. So, for a younger RealAge, put a great-tasting herb in your saltshakers.

Iron

Iron is another mineral you probably don't need to supplement in your diet. Premenopausal women, children, and occasionally vegetarians are the most likely to be iron deficient. If you're beyond adolescence and have not been diagnosed as being iron deficient, you should be more concerned about getting too much iron. Most of us get plenty of iron from the food we eat. It's in meats, fish, poultry, eggs, whole grains, beans, spinach, and fortified breads and breakfast cereals. Some experts have criticized U.S. food manufacturers for adding too much iron to breads and cereals. There is reason for concern—iron overload can be life-threatening and can make your RealAge older.

IRON OVERLOAD. Iron is stored in the body for long periods. Over time, excess iron ingestion can lead to toxic levels of the mineral. Early signs of iron overload are abdominal pain, fatigue, and loss of sex drive. Later symptoms include liver enlargement, diabetes, arthritis, and, in severe cases, abnormal heartbeats and heart failure.

Even a slightly elevated level of iron can be harmful. Although the evidence is preliminary, it's cause for concern. There are two ways that excess iron can lead to accelerated aging. First, excess iron may harm the arteries. One theory is that iron oxidizes bad (LDL) cholesterol (causes it to combine with oxygen), and the resulting oxidized cholesterol accumulates in arterial plaques in the lining of vessel walls. One Finnish study supports this theory. It showed that the rate of heart attacks doubled when the concentration of iron in the blood was high. The risk quadrupled when this high iron level was coupled with a high level of bad cholesterol.

Again, this research is preliminary, but I don't think you should increase your risk of aging by taking iron supplements. Some data even suggest that donating blood regularly, and thus decreasing your iron, may result in a longer, healthier life. Giving blood also makes many people feel good (by doing good for others), so perhaps some of the RealAge benefit comes from that, regardless of the iron-reducing benefit from blood donation.

The second way that excess iron accelerates aging involves, once again, its role as an oxidant. Acting as an oxidant, iron may increase the quantity of free radicals in the body. These free radicals cause DNA damage that can lead to cancer. Another theory is that cancer cells, which proliferate quickly, require more iron, so that having excess iron may actually facilitate cancer cell growth. Although neither of these theories has been proven, research in the United States and Finland indicates that increased iron levels may lead to a higher risk of cancer. The bottom line is that you should not take a multivitamin containing iron unless you are iron deficient and are directed to do so by a physician.

With all this negative news about iron, you may be wondering what good it can do. Although you want to avoid iron overload, iron is still an essential mineral. One of its primary functions is to bind oxygen in red blood cells, for the delivery of oxygen to body tissues.

Is It Possible to Become Deficient? Without adequate amounts of iron, you may be fatigued, breathless, or unable to concentrate or have cold hands and extremities. If so, talk to your doctor. The amount of iron you get in your food should be enough to avoid a deficiency.

What's the RAO? The DV for iron has been established at 18 mg. We believe that the RAO for iron is whatever amount you get eating a balanced diet (of appropriate calories) that is rich in fruits, vegetables, and whole grains, *without supplementation.*

Which Foods Contain Iron?

Enriched bran flakes, 1 oz	18.0 mg
Enriched Cream of Wheat, 1 cup	9.0 mg
Oysters, six	7.2 mg
Clams, six	6.0 mg
Enriched wheat flakes, 3/4 cup	4.5 mg
Wheat bran, 1 oz	4.2 mg
Whole grain wheat flour, 1 cup	4.0 mg

Zinc

Zinc is a trace mineral vital to the synthesis of genetic material, that is, DNA and RNA. Therefore, zinc is especially important during times of rapid cell growth, for example, during healing processes, especially wounds in the skin.

Recently, zinc has received attention for its possible role in fighting colds. Zinc does not prevent colds, but it may shorten the duration of symptoms. One study found that zinc lozenges helped ease the symptoms of a cold, while another study did not.

Although further studies are needed before a definitive determination can be made, it appears that the effect of zinc on the duration and severity of cold symptoms is minor, less than the effect of vitamin C or even chicken soup.

Could I Become Deficient? Zinc deficiency is rare because most people get enough zinc from the foods they eat. When zinc deficiency does occur, the symptoms include depression, skin inflammation, and memory problems.

What's the RAO? For adults, the RAO for zinc is 12 mg per day from food or supplements, and you shouldn't get more than 30 mg a day. Try to find a multivitamin with less than 15 mg per day. Boosting your zinc above 30 mg a day may do more harm than good. Too much zinc can interfere with the actions of another mineral—copper—and may also impair your immune system. If you take 50 to 75 mg per day, the extra zinc may reduce your healthy (HDL) cholesterol levels and, in this way, increase arterial aging.

WHICH FOODS CONTAIN ZINC? It's unlikely you'll get more than 30 mg of zinc per day from your diet alone (unless you eat oysters daily), so eating foods that include zinc is a safe thing to do.

Oysters, six	25.0 mg
Enriched bran flakes, 1 oz	3.7 mg
Turkey, dark meat, four thin slices	3.5 mg
Baked ham, 3 oz	3.4 mg
Beef, 3 oz	3.1–5.0 mg
Lamb chops, one average	3.0 mg
Pork, one medium chop or slice of loin	2.2–2.3 mg
Black-eyed peas, 1/2 cup	2.0 mg
Shrimp, 3 oz	1.8 mg
Chicken, roasted light meat, 5 oz	1.7 mg
Yogurt, 8 oz	1.5–2.0 mg

Chromium

Chromium was once said to promote weight loss, prevent osteoporosis, alleviate depression, build muscle, and increase longevity. Unfortunately, research in the past decade has disproved most of these claims. Claims that chromium furthers weight loss are unsubstantiated. In fact, one study showed that chromium might even cause weight *gain* in overweight women. In addition, there's little evidence that chromium helps build muscle mass.

Nevertheless, chromium is an important mineral. It is involved in glucose metabolism and increases sensitivity to insulin. Chromium also aids in the anabolism (building up) of fatty acids and cholesterol and functions in the catabolism (breaking down) of proteins. Having adequate amounts of chromium helps regulate metabolic processes.

COULD I BECOME DEFICIENT? Chromium deficiency may lead to a buildup of fatty acids in the blood, elevated blood glucose levels, and even nerve degeneration. However, most people get more than enough chromium from their diet, so there's no need to supplement. In fact, large doses of chromium can cause high blood pressure, heart palpitations, and psychosis. Avoid potentially harmful supplementation and rely on your diet for adequate amounts of this mineral. Just about the only indication for possible chromium supplementation is diabetes. If you are diabetic, talk to your doctor before taking chromium.

WHAT'S THE RAO? The DV for chromium is 120 mcg, and the RAO is unknown.

WHICH FOODS CONTAIN CHROMIUM? Getting your chromium from foods is a safe thing to do. Chromium can be found in meats, whole grains, dairy products, wine, beer, and yeast.

Selenium

Since selenium is a trace mineral that has antioxidant properties, it has created quite a stir recently. Several preliminary studies indicate that selenium may protect the body from damage by free radicals and thus boost the immune system and reduce the risk of cancer.

A study recently published in the *Journal of the American Medical Association* found that among people who took 100 mcg of selenium twice a day there was a 50 percent reduction in cancer deaths. This was the second study to show such dramatic benefits. Other research has suggested that selenium boosts resistance to several viruses. The data are tantalizing but preliminary. At least five studies funded by the National Institutes of Health are now underway, so we should know soon whether the benefits of selenium outweigh the dangers of possible toxicity—and there *is* toxicity.

The good news is that most people get adequate amounts of selenium from their diet. Selenium is found largely in such plant foods as garlic, celery, and onions, which absorb the mineral from the soil. Because taking too much selenium can be toxic, it's best to get this mineral from food sources instead of supplements. Your diet is a safe source of selenium.

COULD I BECOME DEFICIENT? Selenium deficiency is rare but may be linked to certain conditions and diseases, including high blood pressure, cystic fibrosis, cancer, and atherosclerosis (hardening of the arteries).

WHAT'S THE RAO? The RAO for selenium is 200 mcg per day. If you take supplements, make it organic selenium supplements (from yeast), since the two studies found no anti-cancer effects with inorganic selenium.

WHICH FOODS CONTAIN SELENIUM? Aside from garlic, celery, and onions, you can find selenium in the following:

Tortilla chips, 1 oz	284 mcg
Brazil nuts, two	200 mcg
Pistachios, three	200 mcg
Corn chips, 1 oz	182 mcg
Tuna, 3 oz	99 mcg
Wheat bread, three slices	67 mcg
Salmon, 3 oz	64 mcg

Other Supplements

We discussed other supplements, such as melatonin, ginkgo, St. John's wort, SAM-e, DHEA, and garlic, in *RealAge: Are You as Young as You Can Be?* Except for garlic, none of these supplements seems to slow aging in or bene-fit people who don't have specific conditions. (Discussing remedies for very specific conditions is not the aim of this book.) The many other supplements on the market that are causing a stir have not yet been proven to have a defi-nite, significant effect on your rate of aging. Some look promising and appear to offer more benefits than risks, for example, saw palmetto for benign pro-static hypertrophy, glucosamine and chondroitin sulfate for arthritis, St. John's wort for depression, and garlic and perhaps ginkgo for arterial aging. I recommend that you avoid most others, because either too little is known and a bad effect is possible or the underlying science is shaky. You can get more information on these supplements in the first RealAge book and at www. RealAge.com.

Why Doesn't My Doctor Tell Me to Take a Multivitamin?

Medical schools have so much to teach that until recently most physicians received very little education on nutrition. The two of us combined received fewer than eight hours of education on nutrition in more than six thousand lecture hours in medical schools. We've had to study hard to make up for these deficits. Today, things are a little better, though; for example, at the University of Chicago, it's still only about twenty-eight hours of nutrition lectures in twenty-five hundred lecture hours.

In medical school, I was taught that if you ate a balanced diet, you obtained all the nutrients you needed—all your RDAs. However, having studied large groups of people and evaluated more than 3 million people who've taken the nutrition program at www.RealAge.com, we now know that fewer than 1 percent of people get the RAO amounts of essential nutrients, such as calcium, vitamin D, folate, and vitamin B_{12}. Furthermore, as many as 60 percent of supposedly well Americans do not get even the RDA or DV amounts of these nutrients. These results are new, however, and are just now starting to be taught in medical schools.

Although your doctor tries to stay current on the latest medical findings, recent findings that the level of nutrients in people's usual diet is low are very different from traditional teaching. As a result, some physicians have not yet incorporated these new data into their routine practice. Studies show that most physicians are so pressed for time that they seldom discuss standard preventive care measures, such as doing strength-building exercises, eating healthy fats, and taking daily vitamins, with their patients.

Take your nutritional printout from www.RealAge.com to your physician and ask questions. Also, compare your vitamins with the recommendations we offer at the end of this chapter.

Time Your Vitamins Correctly

To make your body's absorption of vitamins consistent, try to take them at about the same time every day. I take half of mine in the morning with my cereal or egg white omelet. As a visual reminder, I keep my bottle of multivitamins in the same cupboard as my cereals. I also keep a bottle of vitamins in a drawer at the office, in case I don't have breakfast at home or I forget to take them before I leave the house. If you are taking a multivitamin in several doses (read the label to see how many you should take a day), stagger them throughout the day. I take the second half of my vitamins at the start of dinner, right after I've had a little healthy fat. Generally, the best time to take a vitamin is with a meal, because the presence of water and a little fat helps you absorb the fat-soluble vitamins and avoid stomach upset.

Nutrient Deficiencies

With each of these nutrients, I have included information about the symptoms of deficiency. Did you see yourself in any of those profiles? If so, take a look at your supplements and see how much of the nutrient you're getting. You should also take a look at your diet. Getting your nutrients from food is the safest way to obtain what you need. Do not rush out and start taking massive doses of a nutrient. If dietary changes and a balanced supplement routine do not relieve your symptoms, you should discuss your concerns with your health care provider.

Still Not Convinced You Need a Multi?

What about those days when you're not making the best food choices? It's just too easy to find yourself eating food that isn't all that nutritious, especially when you're too busy to cook. If you lead a hectic lifestyle, are on a special low-calorie diet, or cannot eat certain foods, taking a multivitamin is an especially important way of filling in your nutritional gaps. If you look at the nutrient analyses of the bestseller diets we reviewed in Chapter 3, you will see that without supplements no diet—not even the RealAge Diet Plan—has the RAO amounts of vitamins C and E or calcium, and most fall short on folate. Even though it's not included in the analyses in that chapter, almost all of the bestseller diets also fall short on vitamin D. So do your RealAge a favor and add the protection of a good multi.

> One thing to remember is that many multivitamins contain iron and vitamin A. Unless you're on a particular diet, you probably get enough of both from your food, and too much of either can be toxic. So choose a multivitamin that does not contain iron and vitamin A or one that contains less than 10 mg of iron and less than 8,000 IU of vitamin A.

In fact, taking too much of almost any vitamin could be toxic. That's why it's best to steer away from megavitamins that contain an excess of your daily RAO.

Putting It Together: What Should My Multivitamin Contain to Hit the RAO?

When you shop for a multivitamin, the first thing to do is read the label. The multivitamin should have the usual DVs of the vitamins and minerals we've talked about. Then you need to supplement that amount, so that you reach the RAOs for each vitamin and mineral listed below. The vitamins are sequential from A through F. Then you have to remember four minerals (sorry, there's no shortcut). Just photocopy this list and take it with you when you go to buy your multi.[†]

A	More than 8,000 IU is too much
B_6	4 mg a day
B_{12}	800 mcg a day
C	400 mg × 3 (remember it's water soluble, so you need several doses over the day), or 1,200 mg a day
D	400 IU a day
E	400 IU a day
F (folate)	400 mcg a day (folic acid or folate, or folicin is sometimes listed as vitamin B_9)
Calcium	1,200 mg a day in divided doses
Magnesium	400 mg a day
Selenium	200 mcg a day
Potassium	Four fruits plus a normal diet should do it

Before you go, check your cupboard and evaluate what you already have. Check expiration dates. Throw away the vitamins that contain more than you need in a day. If you're worried about arterial aging, make sure you get the antioxidant vitamins E and C and the homocysteine-lowering vitamin, folate. If you're concerned about osteoporosis, arthritis, or immune aging, pay careful attention to your calcium and vitamin D intake.

[†]Readers of *RealAge: Are You as Young as You Can Be?* expressed an interest in having a multivitamin that provided the RAO doses. As a result, RealAge, Inc., encouraged at least one manufacturer to produce such multivitamins. I do not personally receive income from such activity. However, I do own equity in RealAge, Inc., which hopes to receive income or royalties from such multivitamins.

6

You *Can* Change Your Eating Habits

Eleven Strategies That Make Healthful Eating Easier and More Enjoyable

How's your attitude? The most important factor in being able to adopt a healthy diet is a positive attitude. Do you see changing your food choices as a chore or an adventure? Eating the *RealAge* way isn't about denying yourself the foods you love. Rather, it's an opportunity to explore new foods, recipes, and taste sensations. You'll have more foods to love, better health, and a RealAge that's as much as 14 years younger.

Sometimes it seems a hard task to change your eating habits. People frequently ask me how they can make healthy eating a permanent part of the RealAge lifestyle. Having a positive attitude makes it a lot easier. You can do it—I've seen many people do it who formerly were fixtures at the vending machines. You can make changing your habits a great, joyful adventure. Here are my top eleven strategies for making healthful eating easy and, most important, *enjoyable*:

1 Make eating, and the place you eat, special, and eat only in those one or two special places.
2 Plan menus and learn to cook.
3 Be a smart shopper.
4 Read the labels.

5   Make substitutions.
6   Add variety to your diet.
7   Eat a little fat—the right kind—first.
8   Keep your portions energy-giving, not energy-sapping. Stop as soon as you first feel you might be getting full.
9   Don't eat absentmindedly.
10 Be a savvy snacker.
11 Drink lots of water.

Strategy 1: Make Eating, and the Place You Eat, Special

Make eating a special, enjoyable experience. At first I didn't realize how valuable this strategy could be. Now I think it's essential. Adopting this attitude makes eating just plain fun. In fact, all the other strategies, though important, come after it.

> **My most successful patients (and their families) have a special place in their home that is the only place for eating. Not eating anyplace else—not the TV room, not standing up, not out of the refrigerator—is their rule.**

To make that place special, decorate it beautifully. Make it a great spot. Give it energy. For example, choose bright, colorful plates and accessories that cheer you up and bring a smile to your face.

And no reading or watching television while you're eating! Mealtime should be a time to enjoy our friends and family, and an opportunity to give thanks for the happy parts of our lives. Savor the smells and sensations of the food, the visual delights of the food, the special dinnerware and decor of the place where you eat, and the stimulating company of your eating companions.

Even if you're eating alone, pick a great spot, and make eating special. Enjoy the colors on your plate; savor the flavors you've created. If at all possible, *sit down when you eat.* Try not to eat while standing at the kitchen counter or sitting on the sofa or at the computer.

Eating in the car can get you a big waistline. You may save time, but for what? And it's hard to savor the experience of eating while avoiding road rage. If you crave food while in the car, keep a bag of crunchy veggies on the front seat.

When you relish the food you eat, you won't eat too much. We eat more food than we need, because we eat too quickly. We don't savor the colors and tastes sufficiently. The satisfaction and sense of fullness that come from having enough food don't register in the brain until twenty minutes after you begin eating. If you eat quickly, you probably won't realize that your body's needs have been satisfied until you've eaten way too much. Give your body enough time to process the signal that it's been fed. If you slow your pace, your hunger will be satisfied in a healthier way.

Since it may be the most important energizing strategy, it bears repeating:

- Make the place you eat special.
- Eat only in a special place at home or at work.
- Eat only when your food is on a special plate.
- Never eat standing up or in a car (drinking water or similar beverages in a car is fine, of course).

Strategy 2: Plan Menus and Learn to Cook

Menu planning is a skill that safeguards against impulsive choices that can sabotage your health goals. And, it can be a fun part of eating. Enlisting the help of your children—for example, asking them to choose between two healthy choices—empowers them. Also, asking family members what tastes, flavors, smells, and colors they most enjoy can yield surprises and make dining together, and even cooking together, even more fun. When you plan your menus, you also:

- Save time by making each trip to the store more productive.
- Make your RealAge younger by electing choices that are nutrient rich.
- Guarantee variety, preventing feelings of deprivation.
- Enjoy healthy snacks that are always on hand.
- Save time by preparing extra portions of food for future use.

Another benefit of menu planning is that within one daily menu plan, you can maximize benefit to all family members simply by increasing or decreasing the number of servings from food groups. For example, teenage boys require more calories than most other living creatures; this requirement is easily satisfied with extra servings of whole grain breads, pasta, or even vegetables or fruit smoothies. Boys and girls in their teens require more calcium, as do pregnant and nursing women. Planned snacks of yogurt, low-fat milk, or low-fat cheese or broccoli spears are ideal sources of calcium.

REALAGE CAFÉ TIP 6.1
Yogurt Is a Good Source of Calcium

Ever wonder what's the best source of calcium? It's yogurt. You need only eat three servings of nonfat yogurt a day to get the recommended 1,200 milligrams (mg) of calcium. Each serving of yogurt has a little over 400 mg of calcium, whereas a glass of milk or soy milk has just about 300 mg.

Use your food journal (see Strategy 9) to help you design your menu. If you've been eating the same kinds of food over and over, your journal will show it. Plan your meals so you try something new at least one day a week. And if you don't do the cooking in your family, learn to cook. Learning to cook not only helps you appreciate the primary cook in your family, but also makes it possible for you to help vary food choices in the family. You can experiment with spices, smells, tastes, and colors you enjoy to make new meal creations. With children, this method is even better; they can rate the food you choose to cook, and you can rate what they create and cook. (You might need a different rating scale from the one we provide in Chapter 10.)

REALAGE CAFÉ TIP 6.2
Cranberry Thanks

Cranberries typically appear at the dinner table only once a year around holiday time, but you might want to consider making them more of a dietary staple. Cranberries are a rich source of ellagic acid, an antioxidant. Early research suggests that ellagic acid may even help prevent cancer cells from growing once genetic damage has occurred. Cranberries are also a great source of flavonoids, the antioxidants that are thought to help prevent arterial aging (and are associated with fewer heart attacks) and immune aging, making your RealAge younger.

To get the biggest bang from your berry, eat cranberry relishes made from uncooked cranberries. Cooking may destroy some of the valuable nutrients in the cranberry.

Strategy 3: Be a Smart Shopper

If you don't *buy* food that's bad for you, you won't *eat* food that's bad for you. That's attitude—pay only for food that's good for you. A few subtle changes in your shopping style can produce an amazing increase in the healthfulness of your diet. Before you put any item in your grocery cart, read the label. Find out what's first, second, third, and fourth in the list of ingredients. If any of the first four are a saturated fat, a partially hydrogenated vegetable oil, a simple sugar, a carbohydrate that is not whole grain, salt, or a meat, put the item back on the shelf, *fast*. If you're still tempted, ask yourself, "Why would I pay for or eat something that will make me older and sap my energy?"

REALAGE CAFÉ TIP 6.3
Read the Label, Cut the Fat

Here's an easy trick for cutting fat in your diet: Read the label. According to a recent study by the National Cancer Institute, people who read labels before buying food in the grocery store consume 6 percent less fat than people who don't. Reducing fat intake by even a small amount can reduce your risk of developing a variety of conditions, including unwanted weight gain, cardiovascular disease, and some forms of cancer.

The next time you shop, read the label and choose products that are low in saturated fats and trans fats, both of which are linked to an early onset of cardiovascular disease. Although trans fat isn't listed on the label, foods that contain partially hydrogenated oils contain trans fat. In contrast, foods that contain monounsaturated fats, such as olive oil, are actually good for you. When you look at the label, remember that similar products often contain very different amounts and types of fat.

RealAge Benefit: People who eat a low-fat diet (in which fat makes up about 25 percent of calories) and who, when they do eat fat, eat healthy unsaturated fats have a RealAge as much as 6 years younger than those who don't.

Try not to go grocery shopping when you're hungry. You'll spend more money and be more likely to make unwise food decisions. If your schedule is tight and you want to shop on your way home from work, take an ounce of nuts or a piece of fruit and a bottle of water with you; try to drink 8 ounces before you enter the store. These practices help stave off the hunger that can push you into making bad decisions.

What to Buy

One of my patients, Donna S., said it best: "The most healthful place to shop is primarily around the perimeter of the store." The perimeter contains the healthy basics: skim milk, fish, eggs, freshly baked whole grain breads, and fresh fruits and vegetables. Donna says that in addition to other strategies, spending most of her shopping time in the produce section has enabled her more easily to quit smoking and lose 23 pounds. Although John and I shop for produce almost three times a week, we've learned how to do it in less than twelve minutes. Also, if you shop for produce first, your cart will be fuller and you'll be less likely to add unnecessary, nutrient-poor foods to your purchases. A cart that's full of produce is a great visual reminder that will reinforce your commitment to healthy selections.

REALAGE CAFÉ TIP 6.4
Silly for Sea Vegetables

Bored with green salad? Try sea vegetables.

Many U.S. consumers know about sea vegetables only from Japanese restaurants. Sea vegetables include wakame (seaweed), komu dashi (kelp), and nori (often used for wrapping sushi). They are an excellent source of minerals, taste great, and can be added to soups and salads with little preparation time.

You might want to try some sea vegetables merely because they taste good and add variety to the diet. Also, if you don't eat much iodized salt, or if you're a woman with a history of benign breast lumps, you might want to try them. Sea vegetables are a good additional source of dietary iodine.

Don't forget the fresh seafood section. How much fish should you purchase? Although eating at least one serving of fish a week can make your RealAge younger, you get maximum benefit from three 4-ounce portions a week (a typical can of tuna counts as almost one-and-a half portions). After all, the benefits of eating just these few ounces of fish a week make your RealAge at least 1.1 years younger than if you ate no fish. In fact, eating fish at least three times a week may lower your risk of a heart attack by 50 percent.

Which fish makes your RealAge the youngest? I do not know. All we know is that eating fish prolongs your healthy life. Why or how it does so we aren't sure.

As I stated in the Introduction, the RealAge scientific team does not make statements that are not supported by data. The data we have indicate that fish—and not just fatty fish—make you younger. Although we really don't know if it's the fat, the protein, or some other nutrient in fish that's responsible for making us younger, fish slows arterial and immune aging.

A recent workshop at the National Institutes of Health
discussed five studies that indicate another possible benefit of
fish: a lower risk of some psychiatric diseases with consuming either
more fish or more oils that are typically found in fish, namely,
EPA and DHA (both are omega-3 polyunsaturated fats).

Even survival after a heart attack is better for people who eat more fish. Why? One reason may be that fish oils reduce the tendency of blood to clot. This is consistent with the fact that people who eat fish suffer fewer strokes, less memory loss, and less impotence. Not only that, but higher fish consumption is also associated with less cancer, perhaps because of the oils fish have or because of the content of selenium often found in saltwater fish. Selenium, in moderate (200 mcg) amounts in two studies (not enough for a RealAge effect yet), reduced cancer rates by up to 50 percent. In addition, I could speculate that fish oils reduce the body's inflammatory reactions, contributing not only to the lower risk of cancer but also to the pain relief reported by many arthritis sufferers. All I conclusively know is that eating three 4- to 5-ounce servings of fish a week makes your RealAge years younger.

Good choices of fish include haddock, mackerel, whitefish, tuna, scrod, salmon, anchovies, rainbow trout, sardines, cod, catfish, and pike. In fact, if you decide to have *any* fish for dinner tonight, you're making a good decision, as long as you use a low-fat cooking method such as broiling, baking, poaching, steaming, or grilling.

Before you leave the perimeter of the supermarket, stop by the dairy and egg section. The foods in this section contain such healthy nutrients as calcium and vitamin D, which retard or even reverse aging of the bones, muscles, and joints and slow aging of the immune system. Dairy or dairy-substitute products are particularly recommended if your diet has been high in meat proteins. (Soy milk and soy proteins might be even better choices.) Excessive meat proteins can leach calcium from your bones. Although dairy products are a good counterbalance for meat consumption, remember to use the low-fat versions and substitute, whenever possible, egg whites for whole eggs.

Now that you've been around the perimeter of the grocery store, venture into the middle aisles. The aisles stocked with uncooked beans, whole grains, and whole grain breads hold the most promise. Eating more whole grains makes your RealAge younger.

In addition to maintaining the health of your digestive system, a high-fiber diet helps you feel full longer (and thus cut back on unhealthy late-morning and afternoon snacking) and decreases arterial aging. One study of women in

Iowa reported that those who chose whole grains benefited by lower rates of IQ deterioration, memory loss, stroke, and heart disease.

The amount of complex carbohydrates you should choose for an optimal RealAge effect is unknown. We do know that simple sugars *age* you and that soluble fiber makes you younger. The amount of complex carbohydrate you should eat for the youngest RealAge is the amount that gives you the number of calories that maintains a healthy body weight for you. I know that depending on your height and metabolic rate (see Chart 1.1), you should eat somewhere between 1,200 and 2,500 calories a day to be at your optimal weight. I also believe that for the youngest RealAge, about 25 percent of those calories should come from fat—300 to 625 calories, or about 33 to 69 grams (g) of fat a day. I do not know if it makes a difference whether you choose complex carbohydrates or healthy protein for the rest of your calories.

However, when you choose carbohydrates, make them complex. Look for words like "whole grain" or "100 percent whole wheat" as the first ingredient on the product label. The words "healthy" and "multigrain" do not necessarily ensure a whole grain food. Remember to look for the following claim on the food package: "Diets rich in whole grain foods and other plant foods and low in total fat, saturated fat, and cholesterol may reduce the risk of heart disease and cancer." It lets you know the product contains at least 51 percent whole grains. Whole grain foods are a healthy eating decision because they are high in fiber and also contain antioxidant vitamins, minerals, and plant chemicals (phytochemicals) that help protect against disease.

What Not to Buy

Avoid the aisles that offer snack foods and convenience foods. You'll save time and money and feel better about your healthier purchases. These foods tend to be high in saturated and trans fat, calories, sodium, and chemical preservatives. If you venture down those aisles, be sure to read the labels. Even frozen foods that claim to be healthy alternatives and low in saturated fat or cholesterol may contain harmful, arterial-aging trans fats.

Some of my patients find it helpful to shop at only one grocery store. They know exactly which shelves and aisles contain healthy food products and, more important, which aisles to ignore. I subscribe to another point of view, that shopping at a few different stores may provide unforeseen benefits. For example, sampling produce and fish at different markets might lessen the buildup of hidden contaminants, give you a wider choice of healthy foods, and help you make your RealAge younger.

Strategy 4: Read the Labels

Food producers don't advertise the saturated or trans fat, sodium, or cholesterol in their products, so it's up to you to find out how the foods you buy
rank in nutritional value. Reading labels provides the information you need
to make good decisions every time you pay for food.

> For example, I once took a few minutes to compare the ingredients for
> four different brands of refried beans. One was high in partially
> hydrogenated oil, another contained lard, the third contained
> canola oil, and the fourth was oil free. All are refried beans,
> but with three very different levels of healthfulness.

What the Label Reveals

What's the easiest way to find out whether a food is high in saturated fat or
sodium?

First, look at the nutritional information on the label to determine the serving size and the amount of calories, cholesterol, total and saturated fat, and
sodium in each serving. The serving size helps you decide how much you
should be eating. For example, two products may have the same calories but
very, very different serving sizes.

Second, read the list of ingredients. Be on the lookout for saturated and
trans fats. These fats can show up as palm or coconut oil, hydrogenated (or
partially hydrogenated) vegetable oil, vegetable shortening, or whole milk
solids. Manufacturers are not yet required to break out the trans fat separately, so you'll have to calculate that yourself. Subtract the combined amount
of saturated, monounsaturated, and polyunsaturated fats from the total
amount of fat that the product contains. The resulting number tells you the
amount of trans fat. Use these numbers to distinguish age-reducing foods
from foods that make your arterial and immune systems older.

Be prepared to read the nutrition label critically. Prepackaged or convenience foods can be misleading. The number of fat grams and the percentage
of fat calories from total calories may be presented as "as-packaged" values,
which makes them appear artificially low.

> For example, a prepackaged box of rice pilaf lists the total fat as 1 g,
> with 0 g of saturated fat. However, those numbers apply only if you eat
> the rice uncooked, straight out of the box. If you prepare the rice as

directed—adding butter, chicken broth, and other ingredients—a single 1 cup serving delivers 9 g of total fat, most of it aging, saturated fat.

Also inspect the list of ingredients to find out what's most prevalent; the ingredients are listed from most prevalent to least prevalent. Some nutritionists recommend that you simply forego products that have so many ingredients they barely fit on the label. Similarly, some nutritionists avoid products containing artificial colors, artificial sweeteners, nitrites, sulfites, potassium bromate, and brominated flours. They also use as few products as possible that contain monosodium glutamate (MSG), aluminum, and the preservatives BHA, BHD, and TBHQ. I agree. Here's a handy tip:

If saturated and trans fats, simple sugars, salt, or meat products are in the first four ingredients of a product, make another choice.

Don't get discouraged. Not everything on the food label is negative or leads to aging. Take a look at the amount of calcium, dietary fiber, monounsaturated fat, whole grains, tomato products, vegetables, vitamins C, D, and E, and folate. Make sure your diet emphasizes these nutrients to reach their RealAge Optimum, the amount necessary to obtain the greatest age reduction.

The great thing about nutrition labels is that most of the time, they do the math. You don't need to perform complicated equations or learn scientific definitions to figure out how to meet your body's nutritional requirements. By using the information called "percentage of daily value (% DV)," you can judge the relative merits of specific products. The percentage of daily value also makes it easy for you to balance your diet. By taking a quick look at the % DV, you can monitor your intake of fat, cholesterol, and sodium and make

---

 REALAGE CAFÉ TIP 6.5
Trans Fat Trouble

Think all vegetable fats are the same? Think again. Hydrogenated and partially hydrogenated vegetable oils, both of which contain trans fats, may be the worst fats of all. When liquid vegetable oils are put through the process of hydrogenation to become solids—like margarine—they also become what are known as trans fats. Trans fats, found in hundreds of foods, increase artery-clogging LDL cholesterol even more than saturated fats.

Be warned: These trans fats are not itemized yet in the Nutrition Facts box, so check the ingredients list carefully. If you see the words "hydrogenated" or "partially hydrogenated," steer clear for the sake of your arteries and your heart.

adjustments accordingly. For example, if you consume something high in fat at breakfast, balance it out by consuming food with lower fat content the rest of the day. Or the next day. As long as you consume around 100 percent of your recommended daily allowance for total fat (about 25 percent of your total calories), you're making your RealAge younger.

The Skinny on "Reduced" Foods

A word about fat-free, low-fat, and reduced-fat products. Many of these *can* be good choices for reducing the amount of saturated and trans fats you bring into your body. Some of these products will be good for you and will form an integral part of eating the *RealAge* way. However, manufacturers need to reduce the regular amount of an ingredient by only 25 percent in order to use the word "reduced." So, reduced-fat processed meats and cheeses can still have a very high fat content, *and* the fat may be trans fat. Moreover, these "reduced" products can also be loaded with simple sugars. Refined and simple sugars age your arteries. Limit these to less than 10 percent of your total daily caloric intake.

Manufacturers often believe that for the sake of flavor, they must compensate for the lower amount of fat in "fat-free" and "low-fat" foods. As a result, they frequently add ingredients (usually, sugar) that actually boost the calorie content. Unaware of this, you may think that fat-free cookies and ice cream can be eaten without limit. Unfortunately, this substitution makes your RealAge even older, because you will consume many (usually more) empty calories.

Strategy 5: Make Substitutions

Small and easy substitutions in your diet can make incredibly important changes in your rate of aging. For example, substituting monounsaturated and polyunsaturated fats for saturated and trans fats can make your RealAge more than 3 years younger. But just because you're making changes in your diet doesn't mean you have to throw away your favorite cookbook! Learn how to make healthy substitutions in recipes that have always been unhealthy. When a recipe calls for butter, ask yourself, "Could I use something else? Could I swap olive oil for the butter? How about orange juice and ginger?" Garlic, ginger, vinegar, onions, and spicy ingredients more than compensate for saturated fat in a dish.

REALAGE CAFÉ TIP 6.6

The Auspicious Onion

When it comes to onions, don't be shy. Opt for more of these pungent beauties. They may be bad for your breath if eaten raw, but they're a boon to your body eaten any way. A study in the Netherlands showed a strong association between onion consumption and a reduced risk of stomach cancer. Onions contain high concentrations of quercetin, a flavonoid antioxidant that protects cells from free-radical damage. They also are thought to be rich in other nutrients that protect the heart and arteries. Low in calories, rich in nutrients, and great tasting—a RealAge treat.

Here's how to de-fat the traditional recipe for mashed potatoes, which uses milk and butter. First, roast a head of garlic. Roasting gives the garlic a mellow flavor and the consistency of butter. Then add the cloves when you're mashing the potatoes, plus a little broth to soften them. Horseradish is also a delicious add-in.

Fruit butters (such as apple butter) and whole fruit preserves (from apricot to Seville orange) contain no fats and are a good substitute for real butter when you need a spread for toast or muffins or for refined sugars in recipes.

Similarly, you can really cut the fat in your baked goods by substituting unsweetened applesauce or prune puree for oil, shortening, or butter. Applesauce is high in soluble fiber and adds moisture and texture to baked goods. It usually has a neutral effect on flavor and, best of all, helps you eliminate excess fat from your diet. A cup of oil contains 220 g of fat, whereas a cup of unsweetened applesauce contains none. Also, a cup of oil has 1,920 calories, and a cup of applesauce only 244. For most recipes, you can simply substitute applesauce for the same amount of oil. You can also replace just a portion of the oil with a substitute. Experiment to find the amount that suits your taste buds. Try other fruits, too, such as mashed bananas or pureed pumpkin, or even silken tofu, to create a delightfully different texture, color, and flavor.

If you're roasting a chicken or other meat, put it on a rack so all the fat drips away. To make a tasty sauce for everything from grilled chicken to roasted eggplant to penne pasta, enliven store-bought tomato sauce with a little good balsamic vinegar and simmer it with oregano and thyme. Baste your meats with fruit juice, not fatty drippings from the pan. Make sauces out of vegetable purees, and use good wine instead of cream or butter for deglazing the pan. Soups can be made creamy by thickening them with cooked potatoes or other pureed vegetables instead of cream.

Here are some quick substitutions that maximize the flavor and nutrients and minimize the saturated fats in recipes:

CHART 6.1

Easy Recipe Substitutions

IF A RECIPE CALLS FOR . . .	USE . . .
Whole egg	Two egg whites or the equivalent amount of egg substitute
Butter	Olive oil or a lesser amount of vegetable oil or canola oil
Whole milk	Skim milk
Light cream	Equal parts of 1 percent milk and evaporated skim milk or soy milk
Mayonnaise (made with partially hydrogenated vegetable oil)	Mayonnaise made with olive or canola oil, or a fat-free salad dressing with a touch of olive oil, or drained low-fat or nonfat yogurt
Sour cream	Nonfat yogurt; low-fat or nonfat sour cream

Strategy 6: Add Variety to Your Diet

Why is variety in your diet so important? Many people don't eat a balanced diet. Forty percent of Americans don't eat fruit daily, and 30 percent don't consume any dairy or soy products regularly. On average, Americans get less than half of the 25 to 30 g of fiber they need a day. Eating a diverse diet that is low in calories and high in nutrition decreases aging from arterial and immune dysfunction and makes your RealAge as much as 4 years younger. If you eat from all five food groups daily, your RealAge can be as much as 5 years younger than if you ate from only two. The five groups are whole grain breads and cereals; fruits; vegetables; dairy and dairy-substitute products; and meats, nuts, legumes, and other proteins (see Chapter 4).

REALAGE CAFÉ TIP 6.7
Mighty Mite

The grape tomato is the latest popular food found to be rich in lycopene, an antioxidant that has been linked to a lower incidence of cancers and heart disease. Originating in Taiwan, these delicacies are now available year round in the United States. Check your produce aisle.

It is also important not to choose just one thing from each food group but to eat diversely within each food group. For example, some vegetables contain lots of one nutrient and virtually none of another.

Try to eat four servings of fruit, five servings of vegetables, some whole grains, and some nuts or legumes every day. That mixture will provide you with the vitamins and fiber you need without the excess calories.

Are you having difficulty adding fruits or vegetables to your diet? Here are a few quick and easy ways to round out your diet:

- Put vegetables other than lettuce and tomato in sandwiches. Sprouts, sliced squash, red onions, peperoncini, cucumbers, and poblano and bell peppers are tasty additions.
- Keep sliced or baby carrots or blanched and chilled cauliflower or broccoli handy for quick snacks.
- Add sautéed onions, mushrooms, tomatoes, peppers, and fresh herbs to scrambled egg whites and egg white (cheeseless) omelets.
- Add corn and sliced vegetables (carrots, zucchini) to tomato sauce.
- Take one or two pieces of fruit with you when you leave home for the day.
- Fill a container with cut-up fruit (melon, berries, grapes, bananas, or all four) that you can eat at breakfast or as a snack, perhaps with low-fat or nonfat yogurt.
- Add fresh or dried fruit to cold or hot cereal.
- Add fruit to salads (raisins or grapes to carrot or mixed lettuce or mesclun salads, crushed pineapple to coleslaw, or sliced pears to wild rice or brown rice pilafs) and sprinkle dried fruit (cherries, raisins, and cranberries) on salads.
- Add fruit to entrées, for example, apples or apricots to baked five-spice tofu or pork, peaches or cranberries to roasted chicken, and mango or pineapple to stir-fry dishes or pizza.
- Serve grilled fruit on skewers with the main course or for dessert.

Strategy 7: Eat a Little Fat—the Right Kind—First

This is an important recommendation, especially if you're overweight or if you're young and trying to avoid arterial aging and its consequences: Eat less fat, eat the right kinds of fat, and eat fat at the right times. Remember, all fats contain a lot of calories, but avoiding "four-legged" (animal) fat, and having a little healthy fat first, makes your RealAge younger.

Is Fat Always Bad?

Overwhelming evidence shows that eating a diet high in saturated fats and trans fats provokes many serious health problems: aging of the immune and arterial systems and, consequently, cancer, infections, heart disease, stroke, memory loss, impotence, decay in the quality of orgasm, and even wrinkling of the skin. Although definitive studies are lacking, experts estimate that 10 to 70 percent of all cancers stem from eating too much saturated fat and trans fat and too few fruits and vegetables. Studies in many countries have shown that the more saturated (and probably trans) fat you eat, the greater the chance of rapid growth of prostate and breast cancers. Furthermore, a study published in the *Journal of the American Cancer Society* reported that women who ate more than 10 g of saturated fat a day had a 20 percent higher risk of ovarian cancer. Consuming red meat more than once a week has been linked to increased aging from colon cancer and heart disease, presumably because of the saturated fats in red meat.

It is just as clear, however, that monounsaturated and polyunsaturated fats will make your arteries younger. Furthermore, some studies have shown that too little fat in the diet can lead to nerve dysfunction, depression, a shortened life span, and even suicide. Clearly, fat is not always bad.

Eat Dessert First?

In the first RealAge book, I told the story of how I accidentally rediscovered what other researchers had shown before, the value of eating a little fat before a meal. One evening, during a father-and-daughter outing, my daughter, Jennifer, was famished. Sitting in the restaurant waiting for the menu, Jennifer could barely hold out until her entrée arrived. I suggested we share a dessert first, knowing we could get it quickly. I reasoned that a small amount of dessert would be a quick input of calories and fat that would buy time while we waited. After all, Mom had always said that dessert would "spoil your appetite," right? I hoped that, if done correctly, our appetite could be "spoiled" just a little bit, and in a good way.

As it turns out, that instinct was correct. Eating a little fat first, not necessarily dessert, is beneficial.

Why Should I Eat a Little Fat First?

For one thing, a small amount of fat slows digestion—more specifically, the emptying of stomach contents into the small intestine. This means that your

REALAGE CAFÉ TIP 6.8
Why Does Red Meat Age You?

One reason that red meat is associated with premature aging is that it is high in saturated fats, which are tied to the onset of cardiovascular disease, or arterial aging. However, people who eat diets rich in red meats appear to undergo other kinds of aging, too. They have higher incidences of colon, prostate, and breast cancer and other types of cancer as well. Although no one knows exactly why, new research provides some interesting clues.

When the amino acids and creatine contained in meats are exposed to high temperature, HCAs (heterocyclic amines) are produced. Well-done beef, pork, and even chicken contain high concentrations of HCAs, which cancer researchers believe may be carcinogenic. Although barbecuing appears to be the worst form of cooking, since the charring process provokes the production of HCAs, broiling, panfrying, and other forms of grilling also create HCAs. Steaming, poaching, boiling, and stewing appear to generate few HCAs because the temperature does not get especially high.

Does this mean you can't eat red meat? No, but to avoid the risk of aging from cancer related to cooking, you might consider some easy-to-adopt practices.

- Marinate meats. Marinating meats for even just one hour before cooking dramatically reduces the production of HCAs. Then don't make a sauce using pan drippings, since HCAs congregate in the sauce. Make a sauce from pureed roasted tomatoes or sautéed onions and mushrooms.
- To further avoid exposure to HCAs, eat less meat and avoid eating meat that is well done.
- Preheating meats before cooking them in the microwave can help prevent the formation of HCAs. (Be sure to throw away the excess juice before cooking.)
- Avoid eating lots of barbecued meats.

Besides producing HCAs, barbecuing can provoke the formation of other possible carcinogens. When fat from cooking meat drips on the hot coals, chemical substances called PAHs (polycyclic aromatic hydrocarbons) form, which can then be absorbed into the cooking food. Although it is unknown whether PAHs cause cancer in humans, animal studies show PAHs to be carcinogenic. If you do barbecue, use lean cuts of meat; marinate for an hour; avoid cooking directly over hot coals; use hardwood charcoals, which produce less heat (or use a gas grill set at a lower temperature); and avoid charring or blackening unmarinated meat.

---

stomach stays full for longer. As a result, you *feel* full, your appetite decreases, and you eat less.

Second, a little fat helps keep blood sugar levels stable. Because sugars are largely absorbed in the intestine, the fat-induced delay in the movement of food into the intestine means that sugars are absorbed more slowly. (Just six to twelve almonds or half a teaspoon of olive oil will slow digestion and decrease rapidity of absorption.) As a result, the level of sugar in the blood rises more slowly and doesn't peak as high. Evening out the peaks in the levels of sugar in the blood retards some of the aging that the arteries experience when blood sugar levels are high.

The third reason to eat a little fat first is that healthful fats help the body absorb fat-soluble vitamins such as A, D, E, and K and fat-soluble nutrients such as lycopene.

Fourth, healthy fats help improve your blood cholesterol levels. Although the exact mechanism is not known, monounsaturated fats reduce the amount of lousy (LDL) cholesterol in the blood. At the same time, people who include healthy fats in their diets are more likely to see an increase in their healthy (HDL) cholesterol levels.

What Kind of Fat Should I Eat?

The ideal fat to eat is monounsaturated or polyunsaturated fats, the fats most prominent in olive oil, avocados, nuts, and fish. All foods have a mixture of fats, but a major portion of the fat found in olive oil is age-reducing mono-unsaturated fat. Even the fat in dark chocolate (not milk chocolate) doesn't raise your cholesterol levels or contribute to aging, if eaten in moderation.

How Much Fat Should I Eat?

The right amount of fat is a dipping of olive oil (half a tablespoon or less), a tenth of a medium avocado, or a half ounce of nuts (four Brazil nuts, twelve almonds, nine cashews, six macadamias, eight pecan halves, or seven walnut halves, on average). You could even eat a half-ounce of dark chocolate (not milk chocolate). A little bit of healthy fat goes a long way toward making you younger.

Strategy 8: Keep Your Portions Energy-Giving, Not Energy-Sapping

Patrolling your portion sizes is a great way to watch calories and control your weight, particularly if you're overweight or at a higher risk of arterial aging due to abnormalities of fats in your blood (triglycerides and lousy cholesterol).

In our culture of "mega-meals" and "super-sizing," we can forget what an appropriate portion is. Don't consider the usual restaurant entrée as an acceptable meal size. Instead, use your fist as a measure of meal size. Because your stomach is roughly the size of your fist, eating meals larger than your fist can stretch your stomach beyond what's comfortable or healthy. Remember to eat a little fat first. Then pause before the rest of the meal. And remember, stop eating as soon as you first sense you might be getting full—before the full feeling hits. Here are some other ways to judge what a single portion is:

- A single serving of grain is 1 ounce. Typical coffee-house bagels are 4 ounces, and typical restaurant muffins are 3 to 6 ounces. Some bagels and muffins are more than 8 ounces each.
- A single serving of pasta is one-half cup cooked. Restaurant plates are often large enough to hold 4 to 8 cups of pasta. That's eight to sixteen servings!
- A single serving of meat is 3 ounces cooked. A good comparison is to look at the amount of tuna in a single-serving 3-ounce can. The 16-ounce steakhouse steak is almost five times the amount of red meat for optimal aging in a week!

To patrol your portions, have a game plan before you start your meal. If you do not plan to freeze some for a later day, try cooking only the amount that will be eaten. This not only provides a psychological edge that reduces the temptation to get second helpings, but also minimizes waste. Look at the food on your plate.

Make your food the most sensuous, tasty, and colorful composition possible. Fight the feeling that you have to eat everything. When you're no longer hungry, leave the rest of the food on your plate. If you feel as if you are wasting food—and many of us do—be sure to take the food home with you.

Dear Dr. Mike:
What do you say to people who don't want to waste food but think it's tacky to take food home, or are embarrassed, particularly in good restaurants?

TT
Orlando, Florida

Dear TT:
It's never tacky to be healthy! Terrific restaurants expect you to take something home and often have special ways of packaging the take-home items. (One chef told me she is flattered by such requests.) Some

people say you can judge the quality of the restaurant by the quality of the take-home packaging and the degree to which they make you feel welcome taking home extra portions. Taking the extra home for tomorrow is RealAge smart.

Dr. Mike

Strategy 9: Don't Eat Absentmindedly

All too often, eating is an unconscious act. We lift the fork, swallow absent-mindedly, and lift the fork again. Sometimes we overeat, because we just aren't paying attention. We're bored, nervous, or busy. Often, we're not even hungry. Instead, eat mindfully. Be actively conscious of what you're eating and why. Use all of your senses to enjoy the color, texture, smell, and flavor of your food. Not only will you enjoy your food more, but you'll also slow your rate of consumption. There are several easy things you can do to eat less absentmindedly.

Having trouble taking your time? Make sure to finish one bite before you begin another. One trick is to put your fork down between bites. One of my patients adds time to his meal by taking a break between his salad and his entrée. If you eat with others, you can also slow your rate of eating by really listening and participating in the conversation. One of my single patients reads a newspaper between portions of the meal (but does not eat while reading).

Identify Your Eating Triggers

Become aware of the thoughts, feelings, and events that trigger eating and overeating. Identifying *your* cues for eating and overeating is easy:

- Notice the impulse to eat.
- Write down what happened right before and after the impulse.
- Record these events for a week.
- Look for patterns.

For example, suppose that overeating occurs after you have an argument with your spouse. Observe and record your behavior. Another eating episode may follow a conflict with your teenager. Observe and record the event. With consistent record-keeping, you will recognize *your* pattern of unhealthy eating. If angry interactions with your family trigger your eating episodes, then anger is the eating trigger. Once you've identified your eating triggers—which can include solitude, depression, frustration, celebration, nervousness, an upset stomach, constipation, and many other conditions—the possibilities for responding in a different way are unlimited! You could, for example, go for a walk, do breathing exercises, or take a bubble bath instead of responding with aging eating habits. Once you have identified your eating triggers and responded healthfully, you will actively make your RealAge younger.

Ask Yourself If You're Really Hungry

When you reach for something to eat, ask yourself, "Am I really hungry?" Imagine eating a carrot or a slice of cucumber or any other healthy food you like. Does that sound satisfying? If not, your appetite is probably the result of nervous tension, boredom, timing, or time of day: Maybe it's break time, and the vending machines are calling you. Also, thirst can sometimes masquerade as hunger. Drink a glass of water, which can curb your appetite and snacking. If you get the urge to eat when you're really not hungry, do something else. Go for a walk, do a chore, phone a friend, or jog in place. Do anything that will give you the time to assess whether the source of hunger is a true need for food or something else.

Eat Regularly

Many people believe they'll lose weight if they starve themselves all day, only to stuff themselves at dinnertime. This habit can adversely affect your body metabolism. When we eat only infrequently, it triggers a "starvation response." Our body worries that it's not going to get enough food and slows our metabolic rate so we won't starve to death. Then, every calorie we eat—be it protein, carbohydrate, or fat—is more likely to be stored as fat ("for future use in case we don't get any more food for a while"). That's why you're better off not going long periods without food. If your goal is to lose weight, skipping a meal can actually hinder your efforts.

Don't Skip Breakfast

Is breakfast really so important? Absolutely! If you're trying to lose excess weight, eating breakfast is a great way to do so. Research has shown that people who eat breakfast have a lower overall food intake than those who skip breakfast. Even if you're happy with your weight, breakfast makes your RealAge more than 1.1 years younger. We don't know exactly why. Is it because most people get at least half their daily vitamin intake at breakfast? Is it the fiber in cereals? Or is it because you're starting the day off with family and social support? For whatever reason, eating a healthy breakfast starts the day off right and makes your RealAge younger.

Studies that reported an age-reducing benefit from breakfast were conducted in the era of hot cereal and before the era of fast food, of egg-, cheese-, and bacon-filled biscuits and donuts. These latter make your RealAge older, whereas oatmeal, omelets made from egg whites and vegetables, and whole grain breads plus fruit make you younger. The sugar and other refined carbohydrates in today's pop-up food items and fast foods produce a spike in blood glucose that gives you a quick boost. You'll soon feel sluggish, however. The saturated and trans fats found in these kinds of foods are absorbed into the bloodstream and alter the normal functioning of blood vessels. As a result, blood vessels are not able to respond to energy demands as they should. The muscles get less energy, and that makes you feel tired. Eating saturated and trans fats at breakfast means a lack of energy at mid-morning or earlier. If you make delicious healthy choices, breakfast can give you energy and make your RealAge younger.

 REALAGE CAFÉ TIP 6.9
Be Sugar Smart

If you're trying to cut down on the amount of sugar in your diet, be aware that sugar comes in many guises. Just because you don't see the word "sugar" in the ingredients list doesn't mean the food is sugar free. Sugar comes in many forms, and most of their names end in "ose"—sucrose, dextrose, lactose, maltose, fructose, and glucose. Sugar also masquerades as honey, molasses, and syrup (as in malt and corn syrup), all of which can be very high in calories (see RealAge Cafe Tip 1.5).

Keep a Journal

Keep a diary of what you eat and when you eat. Don't be too judgmental about what you're writing in your journal, because you want an honest recording of the calories you're consuming. Note that you tend to skip breakfast and eat a late-morning cookie and a big lunch to compensate, if those are the facts. Your journal will show when you're most likely to snack and the foods you snack on. Also, you can check your journal to make sure you are getting enough of each food group (see Chapter 4).

Using the information in your journal, you can make simple, life-affirming choices for yourself. For example, Doris M. knows she likes to snack when her favorite TV show, *The Practice*, comes on, so she has bowls of soy nuts and cut carrots nearby.

Ageproof Your Environment

One last tip to help you savor healthy eating: After you've retrained your palate to relish healthy food choices, don't ruin that training by making unhealthy choices too available. Take a look at your refrigerator and pantry. Do you still have prepackaged foods that increase arterial age? Get rid of the items that make you age faster than necessary. Throw them out or give them to a charitable organization. (To lessen temptation until you can give them away, try not to store them in a place where they're too visible.)

Go through your recipe file and remove recipes that require a lot of butter, cream, and other fats. (If these recipes are treasured memories, put them in a scrapbook that's not kept in the kitchen.) Or, cross out aging ingredients and write in healthy substitutions, for example, two egg whites for one whole egg. Replace high-fat recipes with recipes that make you feel better, both physically and emotionally. If you have a collection of take-out menus or cookbooks, toss the ones that contain predominately unhealthy foods. Keep the menus that feature some healthy selections.

Finally, surround yourself with family members and friends who are upbeat and encouraging; they will strengthen your resolve and help you succeed. Ask your friends and family to help you by offering you only healthy snacks and taking walks with you. A true friend will not try to undermine your efforts.

Strategy 10: Be a Savvy Snacker

Instead of snacking out of the vending machine or doughnut box, consider breaking your usual three healthy meals into six smaller ones that you consume throughout the day. A University of Toronto study found that people who ate this way had significantly lower blood cholesterol levels and a lower risk of heart disease and arterial aging than people who ate the same amount of food in three sittings.

However, it's difficult to resist snacking. Work environments tempt many of us to add between-meal snacks. Be prepared with healthy alternatives to the high-calorie treats you may be offered at work. Make vegetables or fruit, even following six nuts or a half ounce of dark chocolate, your new snack food. I keep bags of precut baby carrots and other vegetables in the refrigerator, fruit in a bowl, and veggie burgers in the freezer. When I'm looking around for something to munch on, I start there. Cucumbers, celery, peppers, radishes, and even mushrooms all make great snacks. Even when snacking, remember that a little monounsaturated fat is needed for the absorption of fat-soluble nutrients.

Strategy 11: Drink Lots of Water

Because your body is 60 percent water, you need at least eight glasses of fluids a day to keep it running optimally. Water serves many functions in the body:

- It flushes out waste.
- It transports nutrients to all body tissues.
- It regulates body temperature.
- It's necessary for every chemical reaction in the body.
- It helps maintain the body's acid–alkaline balance.

If you're not drinking enough water on a daily basis, you may experience headaches, tiredness, and dry skin. If you become severely dehydrated—because of illness, extremely high temperatures, or intense exercise—your circulatory and vascular systems will suffer. If you're exercising or the weather is hot, drink extra water to keep yourself properly hydrated.

It may be helpful to know that you can get water from eating as well as drinking. The body uses water whether it's from beverages or solid foods. Fruits and vegetables supply the most water. The produce that provides the most water includes watermelon, oranges, grapes, apples, cucumbers, iceberg lettuce, and tomatoes. But drinking water itself (after a little fat) makes you feel full faster and provides extra energy.

I hope these strategies are as useful to you as they are to me. Whenever I shop, I start with a tour of the perimeter of the market. And although I have presented the strategies in sequential order, from food planning through shopping, eating, and snacking, the first strategy, eating only in a special place, has been particularly useful for me.

Use these eleven strategies, and you'll soon be much closer to reaching your RealAge goals. And, as a RealAge devotee told me, "You'll love the way you're eating—eating only sensuous food and savoring it, whether eating in or eating out."

7

What about When I Eat Out?

Be the CEO!

When you eat out, lots of factors can make your food choices less than perfect. You might think that if you're paying a lot for food, it should be something you really want. Sometimes, especially after a hard day or when you're on vacation, you feel you deserve an indulgent food fix, and you tell yourself it's just this once. Fellow diners may influence you to order food that's not especially healthy. Finally—and this is perhaps the most dangerous to your RealAge—you could be somewhere that doesn't seem to serve healthful foods—a restaurant, grocery store, or fast-food drive-in.

If you ate out only once a year, these issues wouldn't be a problem, but we're eating out more and more often. So the restaurant experience should be very much a part of your RealAge Diet Plan. You should enjoy your food, be satisfied, *and* do your body some good. Why pay for food that will make you older? The key is to be the CEO (chief executive officer) every time you pay for food.

You might think most CEOs achieved their success by cunning politics or individual brilliance, but many studies say such people became leaders by being questioners and listeners—"Can you get me the finance report?" "Can you see if marketing has that done yet?" "What do you [Mr. or Mrs. Customer] want or need?"—and then making informed "gut" decisions.

It is in this way that you can be the CEO when you eat out and be RealAge smart. If you ask your server, "Can you ask the chef if he or she could prepare my dish with marinara sauce?," the answer is usually "Yes!" And that's the key to eating out successfully: First, ask questions about your food, *and* then ask if they can make it your way.

Whether you're in an American, French, Italian, Latin American, or Mexican restaurant, or on a boat, plane, or train or simply stuck on a long car trip, you can use the RealAge Diet Plan. It's much easier and more fun than you might think, and the food tastes great!

First, don't deprive yourself. If the occasion is a special one (see Chapter 8), order exactly what you want. But no matter how delicious it is, don't make the mistake of trying to eat everything on your plate, or you'll likely regret it later. Restaurants tend to serve overly large meals: One plate can contain 2,500 or more calories, more than you need for the entire day! Take half of it home or split the meal with a friend.

Eating out used to be a special occasion, but today it's almost an everyday occasion. The good news is that almost all restaurants now offer something that is not only healthy but also delicious. Hundreds of people who read *RealAge: Are You as Young as You Can Be?* or took the RealAge test at www.RealAge.com have written to me. They have asked many, many questions about eating out in restaurants. Here are some of them and the strategies that will keep your RealAge young without requiring that you give up on flavor and enjoyment.

Dear Dr. Mike: I've been eating healthfully at home, and I feel terrific. My weakness is restaurant food. Sometimes, even when I think I'm ordering something good for me, it arrives in a dish of fattening white sauce. Help!
—Nancy P., St. Louis

Ordering in a restaurant is tough, especially if you haven't been to the restaurant before or you're trying a new dish. In most restaurants, the servers are trained to know about what goes on in the kitchen. Most have been quizzed on the ingredients, how the food is prepared, and what the options are. The first thing to do is to be the CEO and *ask.* Simply asking the server about the details will probably give you all the facts you need. He or she will probably describe the features most important for you to avoid, for example, entrees "seared in butter" or "covered in a creamy white garlic sauce."

I've found that cooks at restaurants want to give you exactly what you want. They want your business next week, too, and that means making you happy today.

The number one strategy is: Don't be shy when it comes to asking questions and specifying your needs.

Here are some basic strategies for getting what you want. Plain-colored foods are usually not filled with good-for-you nutrients. That goes triple for white sauces, which are most often made of cream or butter and therefore full of saturated fats. So ask for the sauce on the side, instead of on top of or under your meal. That way, you can just dip your fork (not your spoon) into the sauce on your way to the rest of the food. This strategy also helps control how much you eat.

Do the same thing with other sauces and salad dressings. Some salads arrive already tossed with *a lot* of dressing. Ask for your salad dressing on the side, and dip your fork before each bite. You'll be surprised at the amount that's left over. You can also ask for low-fat salad dressings. Sometimes even a vinaigrette salad dressing contains egg yolks and cheese that drive up the calorie and fat count.

When ordering your beverage, consider seltzer with lime, club soda, iced tea, sparkling water, plain water, or even calorie-free diet soda. (The amount of phosphates in a diet soda is usually not so great as to pose a hazard; as discussed in Chapter 5, if you drink a six-pack of diet soda a day, you need about 200 milligrams more of calcium a day in diet or supplements.)

When the bread comes, be sure to drink a full glass of water before you dig in, so you won't eat too much. Try skipping the butter and asking for olive oil, instead. The unsaturated fats in the olive oil are good for your arteries and will slow your digestion, so you'll feel full longer. And the olive oil is chock-full of world-class flavor.

If you'd like to order poultry, ask whether it is oiled before it is grilled, whether butter or other fat is injected into it, and whether a lot of butter is used in preparing it (if so, order it differently or choose something else). When your selection arrives, make sure the skin has been removed or remove it yourself.

If the portions are large, cut everything in half and put it to the side. You're much less likely to eat everything you're served if you've designated half as tomorrow's lunch.

Consider having a dinner of side dishes instead of an entree. If you're with a group of people who enjoy tasting a little of everything, order a dinner of favorite appetizers: The portions are usually reasonable, and the flavors great. You can always order more if you're still hungry. Chances are you won't be.

Taking the RealAge Diet Plan into Restaurants

French Restaurants

At fancy French restaurants, expect smaller portions. This portion size may be the key to the "French paradox" of rich food and fewer heart attacks. The

French consume fewer calories than Americans. Although you may be disappointed when you get your dish, you'll be surprised how full you are at the end of the meal. To avoid arterial aging from the saturated fat in traditional French food, and to make your RealAge younger, here's what you might order at a French restaurant:

- Salad with dressing on the side (French vinaigrette or olive oil and vinegar)
- Salade niçoise (a salad with tuna and olives)
- Endive or watercress salad
- Baguettes or French bread (one or two slices) with olive oil, not butter
- Bouillabaisse (fish stew)
- Steamed mussels
- Steamed or sautéed vegetables, including broccoli, spinach, kale, onions, and green beans
- Anything "en papillote"—in this method of cooking, a filet of chicken or fish is steamed in its own natural juices in lightly oiled parchment paper and topped with a little butter and vegetables (ask for it with olive oil instead of the butter).
- Pot-au-feu—a boiled dinner, such as poultry poached in white wine, herbs, or stock
- Poached fish
- Anything "coulis," which means that the food (usually tomatoes, carrots, red peppers, or other vegetable seasoned with herbs or just salt and pepper) has been reduced by means of brief cooking
- Lightly sautéed seafood
- Chicken in wine sauce
- "Nouvelle" dishes made with "light" sauces
- Fresh fruit and meringue

Here are the French foods that, if eaten often, will make your RealAge older:

- Pâtés and foie gras (fattened liver, usually duck or goose)
- Quiche (a custard pie that contains vegetables, fish, meats, and/or cheese)
- Au gratin (cheese) dishes
- Duck or goose
- Heavy cream sauces, such as hollandaise, béchamel, and béarnaise
- Fondue
- Crepes

- Brioches, croissants, éclairs, and other pastries
- Anything "confit" (cooked and preserved in its own fat)

Italian Restaurants

If you find yourself at an Italian restaurant, you're in luck. Many of the dishes have a red sauce (marinara) or pesto base, both of which make your RealAge younger. You don't have to ask for these on the side. You know about tomato products and lycopene. Olive oil is also a big plus at Italian restaurants, usually comprising the base for pesto and garlic dishes.

Marsala sauce, made from marsala wine and chicken or vegetable stock, is also a good choice in an Italian restaurant. Some chefs "finish" the sauce with oil, butter, or cream, so be sure to be the CEO and, when ordering, ask the wait staff, "Is cream or butter used to finish the marsala sauce?" If so, politely ask, "Could you ask the chef if that could be omitted from my dish?" Remember, if the waiter works to help you stay young, consider rewarding him or her more generously than usual.

If you can't stop yourself from ordering the fettuccine Alfredo (a butter, cream, and cheese pasta dish), ask for the sauce on the side. Then dip your fork into it on its way to the pasta. Perhaps you could also order a bowl of chunky, heart-warming, age-reducing minestrone soup, brimming with pasta and vegetables, to eat before the meal. This low-fat soup will fill you so you won't overeat when the pasta arrives.

Look for these RealAge diet choices on the menu at an Italian restaurant:

- Vegetable antipasto plates
- Salads with dressings on the side (vinaigrette, olive oil and vinegar, balsamic vinegar)
- Caprese salad and tomato and low-fat mozzarella with a little olive oil on the side (again, dip the fork into the dressing before each bite)
- Minestrone and bean soups
- Steamed or sautéed vegetables, like broccoli, spinach, kale, and zucchini
- Grilled vegetables with vinaigrette sauce or "light" olive oil
- Pizza with low-fat cheese, or just a little or no cheese, topped with vegetables
- Pasta with vegetables (primavera) with tomato sauce or very little olive oil
- Boneless, skinless chicken breast with tomato or tomato-mushroom sauce
- Seafood (shrimp, mussels, clams) sautéed, in "light" wine sauce
- Chicken, seafood, or veal steamed or grilled, topped with marinara sauce

- Chicken cacciatore (tomatoes and olives)
- Eggplant pomodoro (tomato sauce)
- Fresh-fruit dessert
- Italian ices
- Cappuccino made with skim milk

Here are Italian foods that, if eaten often, will make your RealAge older:

- Caesar salad or other salads with creamy dressings
- Anything "Alfredo" (cream, butter, and cheese)
- Fritto (fried) appetizers, including fried eggplant, mozzarella, and calamari (squid)
- Buttered garlic bread
- Pizzas with Italian sausage, pancetta (bacon), or prosciutto (ham)

REALAGE CAFÉ TIP 7.1

Make Mine Mediterranean

In the 1950s, scientists noticed that heart disease was far more prevalent in northern Europe than in southern Europe. The highest rates were in Finland, and the lowest were in southern Italy and Crete.

More recently, large European studies have shown that a diet of olive oil, fish, whole grain pasta, fruit, vegetables, and legumes (a "Mediterranean diet") helps prevent heart disease, a second heart attack, and stroke. A French study agrees. Half of 605 patients who had had a heart attack were put on a standard low-fat, low-cholesterol diet recommended by the American Heart Association. The other half were put on a diet similar to that on Crete, a Greek island in the Mediterranean: little or no red meat, no butter or cream, olive oil as the main fat, canola oil, fruit, vegetables, beans, cereals, whole grain breads, and alcohol (mostly red wine). After twenty-seven months, there were 70 percent fewer deaths and heart attacks in the group eating the Mediterranean diet. The researchers attributed much of this benefit to the substitution of olive oil and canola oil for the typical salad and cooking oils.

The lower levels of saturated fatty acids found in the Mediterranean diet mean lower levels of lousy (LDL) cholesterol. This form of cholesterol ages the arteries and promotes heart disease, atherosclerosis, stroke, and impotence. The Mediterranean diet is also rich in antioxidant vitamins (C and E) and folic acid. In addition to helping prevent birth defects, folic acid reduces levels of homocysteine, an amino acid that ages the arteries.

- Meat-centered antipasto plates
- Veal, chicken, or fish in cream sauce
- Breaded, fried, Parmesan-style dishes
- Pastas, such as tortellini, ravioli, cannelloni, and manicotti, that are not made with whole grains or are made with heavy, full-fat cheeses
- Lasagnas that are made with full-fat cheeses
- Sauces such as Bolognese (which contains beef) and carbonara (which contains eggs, bacon or ham, and cheese), or those made with sausage or white clams and cream (clam sauce is often oil and vinegar and not cream—be the CEO)
- Veal scallopini and other breaded and pan-fried veal dishes
- Spumoni (ice cream)
- Cannoli (a fried pastry containing ricotta cheese)

 REALAGE CAFÉ TIP 7.2
A Well-Oiled Diet

As if its superb taste weren't enough, there are many other reasons to celebrate olive oil. This heart-friendly fat reduces the level of lousy (LDL) cholesterol and usually boosts the level of healthy (HDL) cholesterol. Olive oil is also a natural storehouse of vitamins A, D, E, and K.

On the grocery shelf, go for the extra-virgin olive oil. It has a higher concentration of what we think are cancer-fighting antioxidants: omega-3 fatty acids and squalene. Squalene is a compound that may help prevent colon cancer. "Extra virgin" means the acidity is less than 1 percent; the oil came from the first pressing of olives, and the olives were cold-pressed, a process that preserves the nutrients and keeps the oil flavorful. The darker the color, the deeper the flavor.

Go easy on portions, though: Olive oil packs 9 calories per gram, or about 125 calories per tablespoon.

One way delightfully to enhance the flavor of olive oil is to infuse it with a fresh herb or spice. Add a sprig of your favorite herb to a small bath of oil and warm the mixture until the aroma touches your nose, that is, to a temperature of not quite 160°F (just below a simmer). Then store the oil in a dark, cool place for about a week before draining it into a cruet.

Mexican Restaurants

A traditional Mexican restaurant offers meals that are high in fiber and complex carbohydrates and low in animal protein. As with Italian food, you'll also find a wide range of red sauces and salsas that contain many nutrients. Most

Mexican restaurants offer some age-reducing options—try the sauces and salsas with cut vegetables or corn tortillas, not the oil-soaked chips that will age your arteries.

Not only that, but just half a cup of whole pinto or black beans has more than 7 of the 25+ grams (g) of fiber you need each day. Moreover, the fiber is soluble. That means it reverses arterial aging by reducing bad cholesterol, assuming the beans haven't been cooked in lard, a saturated fat from solid pork drippings. Remember to be the CEO and ask questions.

Here are ways to make dining at a Mexican restaurant a RealAge experience:

- For starters, order warm, fresh corn tortillas instead of the crispy chips that are packed with saturated and trans fat. Corn tortillas are healthier than flour tortillas, because they have less fat and calories, are made of whole grains, and have no synthetic chemicals.
- Eat lots of salsa. No need to worry about salsa and toppings like pico de gallo or picante sauce. They're virtually free of calories, and the lycopene in salsa is a great age reducer. Unlike French sauces, most Mexican sauces are made of vegetables—tomatoes, onions, chilies—and nuts.
- Chili or black bean soup makes a good appetizer or even an entree, but because melted or shredded cheese and sour cream are standard garnishes for such dishes in Mexican restaurants, *ask for all garnishes on the side.* Guacamole seasoned with lime and a dash of salt, on the other hand, provides some healthy zest; avocado is rich in monounsaturated fat. But just a little, since avocado has a ton of calories.
- Gazpacho, a cold tomato soup with vegetables, and tomatillo-based salsas and soups are loaded with antioxidants and are truly delicious.
- Two other RealAge choices are ceviche and mole. Both are low in fat and high in omega-3 fatty acids, and seem to reduce blood pressure and fight heart attacks by stemming the buildup of arterial-aging plaque. Ceviche is fish marinated in lime juice and sometimes onions and herbs. Small amounts of mole, a blend of chiles, tomatoes, nuts, and sometimes chocolate that accompanies the main dish, actually makes your RealAge younger. The nuts contain healthy fats, and by eating a smidgen of mole first, you'll feel full sooner.
- Steer clear of the taco shell in a taco salad and beef or pork fajitas topped with sour cream and cheese. Vegetable, chicken, and seafood fajitas that don't contain extra fat are fine. Also avoid chimichangas (fried burritos), chorizo (a Mexican sausage), and carnitas (pork cooked in lard).

- On special occasions, there's flan, a popular Mexican dessert. A half cup of this caramel custard, which we like with tangerines and blueberries, has about 200 calories.
- Enjoy a margarita, beer, or wine with dinner.

When you're craving Mexican food, here are your best bets:

- Salads with salsa or lime as dressing
- Soups and stews
- Black bean soup
- Corn tortillas
- Whole beans
- Refried beans cooked without lard
- Chili made with beans
- Brown rice
- Jicama ("Mexican potato")
- Gazpacho (cold tomato soup)
- Ceviche (fish "cooked" by means of an acidic marinade)
- Grilled chicken or fish
- Arroz con pollo (chicken with rice; request brown rice)
- Chicken, shrimp, or vegetable fajitas prepared with little oil
- Tacos al carbon with chicken (soft tacos; request corn tortillas)
- Chicken enchiladas (request no cheese)
- Camarones (sautéed shrimp)
- Fruit (guava, papaya, mango, soursop, berries, melon) and fruit ices
- Flan (baked custard)

Here are some Mexican foods that are sure to make your RealAge older if you choose them too often:

- Tortilla chips
- Nachos
- Taco salads topped with cheese and sour cream in a crispy taco shell
- Chalupas (fried tortillas) or tostadas
- Chile rellenos (stuffed peppers)
- Quesadillas
- Chimichangas (fried burritos)
- Beef or cheese enchiladas
- Ground beef or pork dishes

- Tacos (fried)
- Tamales made with lard
- Heavy cheese and cheese sauces
- Sour cream
- Refried beans cooked with lard
- Churros (deep-fried sticks of dough) or sweet bread

Asian Restaurants

If the choice of the day is Asian food, your body could be happy with you. Few diets are healthier than Asian diets, thanks to all those fresh, quickly cooked, crunchy vegetables and whole grain rice, green tea, fish, and protein-rich soy products (soybeans, sauces, and assorted varieties of tofu). And chopsticks slow the pace of eating.

Of course, lumping Japanese, Chinese, Thai, and other Asian food together is a little misleading. Each country has its own distinctive preferences and flavors, not to mention regional variations. But Asia is different from the rest of the world, in that so much of its cuisine is so healthy and uniformly delicious. It's no coincidence the Chinese rank just behind the Japanese in terms of having low rates of aging-related ailments such as heart disease, obesity, colon cancer, and diabetes. Their diets are similar.

Asian meals are mostly plant based: lots of vegetables, maybe noodles (be a CEO and ask whether yours have been dried in lard, as they are in many take-out meals), and small portions of whole grain rice. When cooked, long grain rice is fluffier than short grain rice. Brown rice is even better, since it's unrefined, meaning the B vitamins and fiber haven't been removed along with the hull and bran. More important, Asian meals are usually low in saturated and trans fats, because seafood is the main source of protein. And seafood contains those essential, heart-friendly, anti-aging fatty acids called omega-3s. As we said earlier, it may be the particularly healthy form of protein in fish that gives fish some or most of its anti-aging benefit. Also, a favorite Japanese beverage is green tea, which studies show is associated with lower rates of cancer.

Like the Japanese diet, the Chinese diet is heavy on vegetables, noodles, and grain. However, the Chinese dishes kung pao chicken and orange crispy beef are high in saturated fat. The Center for Science in the Public Interest (CSPI) uncovered some startling facts in 1997, when it analyzed the nutritional content of fifteen popular dishes from twenty mid-priced Chinese restaurants around the United States. It found that a 2.5-cup portion of kung pao chicken contained 38 g of fat, equal to *two* quarter-pounders at a fast-food outlet. Two cups of orange crispy beef packed more than 800 calories, about the same as two large orders of French fries.

So, if a dish is "batter-dipped," "sweet and sour," or "deep-fried," you know it will make your RealAge older. Another cue is "in a sauce," since most Chinese sauces contain aging oil. Try to go for stir-fried and steamed dishes.

> One of my favorites, and a great source of monounsaturated fats,
> is sesame noodles in peanut sauce with extra sesame seeds,
> fresh scallions, and dried chilies. But remember to ask whether the
> noodles have been dried in lard (saturated fat). If your food
> server doesn't know the answer, choose another dish.

When you're in a Chinese restaurant, choose the following to make your RealAge younger:

- Chicken won ton soup (almost all won ton soup is pork; there is so little meat one does not have to worry!)
- Hot and sour soup
- Steamed dumplings and other steamed dim sum
- Fresh spring rolls (the egg rolls found in regular neighborhood Chinese restaurants are almost always fried); you could also ask for the steamed dumplings
- Steamed rice or plain boiled noodles
- Spicy green beans or eggplant
- Vegetarian delight
- Chicken chop suey
- Drunken chicken
- Moo shu vegetable or shrimp
- Shrimp or chicken with broccoli, snow peas, mushrooms, or other vegetables (stir-fried with little oil)
- Shrimp with tomato sauce
- Boiled, steamed, or stir-fried vegetables
- Tofu (not fried)
- Whole steamed fish
- Sauces such as black bean, hoisin, oyster, plum, and sweet and sour (which is low in fat but high in sugar, so request a light portion)
- Litchis (a fruit)
- Fortune cookie (it has only 30 calories)—but some are made with partially hydrogenated fats

The Chinese foods that, when eaten often, will make your RealAge older are:

- All foods described as "fried" or "crispy"
- Salty soups
- Fried egg rolls or spring rolls
- Too much soy sauce (request low-sodium soy sauce and use in moderation)
- Monosodium glutamate (MSG), another form of sodium
- Peking duck
- Egg dishes, such as egg fu yung, which is just eggs but is often fried and served with a heavy gravy
- Sweet and sour dishes (most are deep-fried)
- Pickled foods
- Chow mein topped with fried noodles
- Spareribs

Vegetables are key age reducers because they contain a wealth of fiber, vitamins, and phytochemicals, substances that may protect against aging of the immune system and its consequence, cancer. No one can complain about too little variety when it comes to Chinese vegetables: There's everything from water chestnuts and bok choy to bamboo shoots and bean sprouts.

At Japanese restaurants, the first task is translating words such as *donburi, oshinko,* and *sunomono* so you know what you're ordering.

When you sit down at a Japanese food restaurant, you might, first thing, order some edamame (soybeans) and dip them in black bean, hoisin, or plum sauce. Then order foods that will make your RealAge younger:

- Sea vegetables
- Any nonfried, cooked fish dish
- Green tea

Two RealAge drawbacks in Japanese cuisine are deep-fried dishes, such as tempura, and smoked and pickled foods and other foods cured with salt. Many studies have shown an association between salt-cured foods and gastrointestinal cancer. In fact, Japan has the highest rate of stomach cancer in the world. Americans aren't guilt free in this department; many have a passion for such foods as dill pickles, which are high in preservatives, sodium, and nitrites.

CHART 7.1

The RealAge Guide to Japanese Food

Dish	Translation	Eating This Will Make Your RealAge:
Agemono	Deep-fried (for example, tempura)	older
Donburi	Boiled rice topped with meat, fish, eggs, and/or vegetables, and broth	older (with beef and egg)
Edamame	Fresh (boiled) soybeans	younger
Pickled ginger	Pickled young ginger root	younger
Ikebana	Steamed vegetable and seafood dumpling	younger
Ikura	Salmon caviar	unknown
Kamaboko	Boiled fish paste	younger
Kani-su	Snow crab and cucumber in vinegar sauce	younger
Miso soup	Clear soup made from fermented soybeans	younger
Nabe or nabemono	Lobster or other shellfish plus vegetables in miso and fish stock, cooked in a pot	younger
Negina	Chicken or beef rolled up with scallion	older
Ohitashi	Boiled spinach with fish stock	younger
Oshinko	Pickled Chinese cabbage	younger
Salmon naruto	Salmon wrapped in radish, seaweed, or cucumber	much younger
Sashimi	Raw, sliced fish served with rice	unknown
Shabu-shabu	A simmered beef (usually) dish	older
Soba	Noodles made from grain (like buckwheat, wheat flour)	younger (if not lard dried)
Sukiayaki	Stir-fried dishes	probably younger
Sunomono	Shrimp, octopus, mackerel, snow crab, and shellfish in vinegar sauce	younger
Sushi	Vinegary rice dish with fish and vegetables	younger

(continued)

Dish	Translation	Eating This Will Make Your RealAge:
Tempura	Anything deep-fried	older
Teriyaki sauce (chicken, fish, or shrimp)	A blend of soy sauce, mirin, sake, and sugar	younger
Tofu/tofu salad	Soybean curd	younger
Tsukudani	Food boiled down in soy sauce	younger
Wasabi	Green horseradish	younger
Yakimono	Usually, marinated meat grilled, broiled, or pan-fried	older
Yakitori	A type of yakimono dish, usually chicken	unknown

REALAGE CAFÉ TIP 7.3

Soy Joy

Discover the joy of soy, a great source of protein without the saturated fats in meat. Soy contains chemicals called phytoestrogens, which have the remarkable ability to mimic estrogen, the female sex hormone. Phytoestrogens are claimed to alleviate the effects of menopause in some tissues and to stifle certain cancers in others. Cell, animal, and human studies suggest that phytoestrogens help prevent cancer, heart disease, osteoporosis, and the symptoms of menopause, but the data are not clear enough to give soy a RealAge effect as of yet.

Here are some of the many forms of soy:

- Soy sauce
- Soy milk
- Tofu (bean curd)
- Tempeh (cultured soybean cake)
- Miso soup (soy soup)
- Soy flour
- Whole soybeans
- Soybean oil
- Textured soy protein
- Soy protein concentrates
- Imitation soy-based bacon bits
- Soy flakes
- Soy grits
- Soy nuts

Dear Dr. Mike: On the first Sunday of almost every month, we take the kids to a family restaurant for dinner. They always choose the greasy foods. If we try to influence them, the whole event becomes stressful for all of us. I don't want to give up our family outing, but I don't want to instill bad restaurant habits, either. Any suggestions?—Jan in Topeka

Dear Jan: Don't give up on your outings just yet. Having a special night out with your family can make your RealAge younger in several ways. No worries about what to shop for, what to cook, and whose turn it is to wash the dishes! Besides relieving stress, your night out can also strengthen the family bonds, which also makes your RealAge younger. And a family restaurant that has healthful food choices, a relaxed atmosphere, complimentary crayons, and white paper tablecloths is ideal for dining out with kids.

When you order food with good health in mind, you become a RealAge model for your children. Researchers at Harvard Medical School showed that parents probably have more influence than they think by just being a "food choice" model, without having to prohibit anything. Studying the eating habits of sixteen thousand children, the researchers found that those who ate dinner with their families ate more fruits and vegetables and less fried foods, saturated fats, and trans fats than those who rarely ate with their families. They also ate more fiber.

On the other hand, if your outing is more stressful than enjoyable, you could be making your RealAge older. If your kids are throwing tantrums, maybe it's best to leave the restaurant and try again next month. Or maybe it's best to simply wait until they're older. After a stressful day at work, or any other time, dining out should be a pressure release, not a pressure cooker.—Dr. Mike

If your children are older, maybe you can give them choices. If they have some say about what they're eating, it will be more fun for them and you may have less complaining. If they choose the least healthful food, so be it. Remember, it's only once a month that you're dining out, so they won't be doing their health much harm. In the meantime, make sure you're eating healthy at home. Who knows, maybe they'll tire of the same old thing and try some of your suggestions. Or try the dessert first (split three or four ways) followed by a healthy soup.

Congratulations on taking an active interest in your children's eating habits. Many people believe that healthy eating isn't an issue for youngsters. Unfortunately, children are prone to arterial aging, too. Moreover, obesity rates among youth are skyrocketing, with possibly dire consequences down the road. Not only are overweight kids more likely to be inactive, they're more

CHART 7.2
Dessert by the Numbers

8-oz servings (1 cup)			
Dessert	Total Fat (g)	Calories (kcal)	Protein (g)
Low-fat plain yogurt	3.5	145	12
Regular plain yogurt	7.5	180	8
Low-fat frozen yogurt, vanilla (Dreyer's)	1.5	100	2
Regular frozen yogurt, vanilla	8.1	228	5.8
Regular vanilla ice cream	14	270	5

likely to be overweight as adults. And being overweight will put them at greater risk of arterial aging and its consequences—heart disease, stroke, impotence—as well as diabetes and aging of the immune system (cancer, infections, and other ailments)—when they grow up.

All is not gloom and doom, however. More and more family restaurants are catering to health-conscious patrons—for example, Bennigan's "Health Club" entrees, the Olive Garden's "Garden Fare," Applebee's "Low-Fat and Fabulous" menu, and Friday's "More Good Stuff." Also, some restaurants list the calories and nutrients in their dishes. Remember to make each choice nutrient rich, calorie poor, and world-class delicious. And you can teach your children how to be CEOs, too.

Healthy fare at family restaurants these days includes broiled chicken and fish entrees, vegetable platters, baked potatoes, lentil stew, bean soup, marinara sauce, and side orders of broccoli and grilled mushrooms—and, of course, salad with the dressing on the side. Here are other ways to make the family restaurant outing a RealAge experience:

- Create your own healthy meal by ordering two or three appetizers for everyone to enjoy. Skip those that are fried (mushroom caps, mozzarella sticks) and anything described as "crispy" or "crunchy."
- Consider ordering half portions of entrees.
- Decline the oh-so-soft white dinner rolls, which contain saturated fat or trans fat, and ask for real bread, bread sticks, or whole grain crackers.
- Stick with olive oil and reduced-fat salad dressings.

- Add grapes, tangerines, or other fresh fruit to your salad. Avoid the croutons (they're full of trans fat), bacon bits, shredded cheese, and eggs.
- Detour around the pasta salad; it will bust your calorie budget. Or, take a small, fist-sized portion and consider that your limit for saturated fat in the meal.
- Go light on the grated cheese (Parmesan) you sprinkle on your food.
- Hold the butter, sour cream, and cheese on the baked potato. Ask for salsa, ketchup, or an order of broccoli instead.
- Substitute lime juice and red pepper flakes for butter as a topping for broiled fish.
- Choose steamed, roasted, or grilled vegetables, rather than the creamed variety, as side dishes. Or make two vegetables and an appetizer your main meal.
- Give your kids choices: "You can have the dessert or French fries, but not both." "If you want a Coke instead of milk, juice, or water, then you have to have grilled chicken instead of a hamburger."
- Order a dessert for your whole family to share, before the meal, and let it be a choice rotated week to week among family members.

 REALAGE CAFÉ TIP 7.4
Like Father, Like Son

As many as two out of every ten youngsters between the ages of five and eighteen may be very obese (weighing 40 percent more than they should for their age, sex, and height). One-fourth to one-half of this group will probably be fat in adulthood, too.

The biggest risk factors for obesity in childhood are:

- A parent who is overweight
- An inactive lifestyle
- Residence in the Northeast (children in the Northeast are more likely to be overweight than those in the West, South, or Midwest)

Dear Dr. Mike: My friends are a "Let's-hang-out-in-bars-and-coffee-shops" kind of crowd, and we always have fun together. The trouble is, I find that I'm never really eating a meal, just picking at whatever they order for the table— for example, Buffalo wings or fried potato skins. It tastes good at first, but then leaves me feeling heavy and sluggish. If I don't eat it, they tease me and I end up starving and miserable. What can I do?—PJ in Chicago

Dear PJ: I see your dilemma. Coffee shops and bars don't often give you many healthy alternatives when it comes to food. So, maybe it's best to go to coffee shops for coffee and to the bar for a beverage, with no intention of eating anything. Fill up on soup and whole wheat crackers before you go, and then you won't be lying when you say you're not hungry. Also, if the bar is part of a restaurant, you might be able to order something more nutritious and satisfying from the regular menu. Ask the host or bartender. And, eating a *few* nuts, even bar nuts, is a healthy habit.—Dr. Mike

Coffee shops are a great place to meet friends and a great way to make your RealAge younger. Coffee itself doesn't hurt, either. It is low calorie and has no effect on your RealAge one way or the other. In fact, researchers recently demonstrated that caffeine can help alleviate both tension headaches and migraine headaches and may prevent Parkinson's disease.

REALAGE CAFÉ TIP 7.5
Tea-ing Off at Coffee Shops

Ready for a hole-in-one? A single cup of black or green tea a day may be beneficial. It was recently reported to cut your risk of heart attack nearly in half! Moreover, drinking tea on a daily basis makes the aging bones of women *five years younger*. It also reduces the risk of bone fractures (the biggest cause is osteoporosis, low density of minerals in the bone).

A study of approximately twelve hundred women between sixty-five and seventy-six years of age suggests (but doesn't prove) the benefits of drinking tea. Researchers at Cambridge University in England found that the average bone-mineral density was 5 percent higher in women who drank at least one cup of tea every day. According to the researchers, that figure translates to a 10 to 15 percent lower risk of bone fractures.

Herbal teas are safe in moderate amounts. However, you should choose them for their aroma and flavor, not their alleged medicinal benefits. Long-term studies have yet to prove or disprove such claims, so there's no known RealAge effect, yet.

Drink the coffee but avoid the unhealthy add-ons: sugar, flavored syrup, cream, whole milk, cream substitute (usually from partially hydrogenated vegetable oil), and whipped cream. If the coffee is prepared for you, be sure you know exactly what's in it. Be a CEO! For example, a café latte has more milk—and therefore more calories—than a cappuccino. If you'd like some dairy with your coffee, try skim milk.

Bars, too, are a great place for camaraderie. Of course, overindulging on alcohol won't do your RealAge any good. In fact, over time, it will put you at risk of such ailments as respiratory arrest and liver disease and will increase the likelihood of driving accidents. So, if you're drinking, drink in moderation and *never drink and drive.* "Moderate" means one or two drinks a day for men and one drink a day for women. One drink is 5 ounces of wine, 12 ounces of beer, or 1.5 ounces of spirits.

Which form of alcohol is best? The alcohol in all drinks is the same, so, on that front, all drinks are equal, and slow arterial aging. In terms of nutrients, however, red wine could be even better than other types of alcohol, since red grapes contain more resveratrol, a powerful antioxidant that may help reduce

---

CHART 7.3

The RealAge Benefit of Alcohol

MEN

Drinking one alcoholic drink a day

At age 35:	0.9 years younger
At age 55:	1.7 years younger
At age 70:	2.3 years younger

Drinking three to six alcoholic drinks a day

At age 35:	0.1–1.4 years older
At age 55:	0.2–5 years older
At age 70:	0.3–7.6 years older

WOMEN

Drinking one alcoholic drink a day

At age 35:	Probably none, since the benefits for women do not usually occur until after menopause.
At age 55:	1.8 years younger
At age 70:	2.2 years younger

Drinking three to six alcoholic drinks a day

At age 35:	0.1–1.4 years older
At age 55:	0.2–5 years older
At age 70:	0.3–7.6 years older

Note: For those without a personal or family history of alcohol or drug abuse.

your risk of cancer. According to researchers at the University of Illinois in Chicago, the University of Missouri, and others, this organic molecule lowers the risk of cancer in laboratory animals. Resveratrol is being tested (funded by part of the National Institutes of Health) in at least three studies in humans, so by 2005 or so, we should know whether the benefits of resveratrol are as great for humans as they are for test animals.

Then, again, if you're a beer drinker, take heart. New research shows you may get benefits from drinking beer, as well. A study in the Netherlands found that people who drank beer with dinner for several weeks had lower levels of homocysteine than did people who drank wine or gin. High levels of homocysteine are associated with aging of the arteries and the early onset of heart and vascular disease. So beer and wine make you younger by at least two processes.

Remember to eat before you drink, especially something that contains a little fat, like nuts. Also, drink water with your alcohol. You will feel fuller and drink more slowly, and the water will help to counteract the dehydrating effect of alcohol, so you won't wake up the next morning with a dry mouth.

REALAGE CAFÉ TIP 7.6
Water with Wine

Have you ever drunk too much wine and awakened the next day with "cotton mouth"? Your thirst is a symptom of the dehydration that alcohol may cause. Alcohol curbs the production of antidiuretic hormone (ADH), which is secreted by the pituitary gland. Normally, as a conservation measure, ADH allows tubules in the kidneys to pass water back to the body. However, when alcohol suppresses ADH, the tubules are less permeable to water, so water flows out of the body as urine. Rather than conserve water, you lose it and thus feel dehydrated.

Dear Dr. Mike: I travel a lot. My RealAge test results suggest that I eat more dark green vegetables and less saturated fats to make my RealAge younger. However, I'm always in an airport food court or in a rented car at a fast food joint. How can I possibly eat right?—Kirsten, Denver

Dear Kirsten: More and more people are finding themselves on the go, including me. Two slices of Domino's twelve-inch classic pizza with extra cheese, Italian sausage, and black olives have 492 calories and 20 g of fat. Depressing. Even if I order something that I think is good for me—grilled chicken sandwich without mayo, a banana, and a large diet Coke—I do the math and realize that this quick lunch has 450 calories and 6 g of fat. Still, that's a lot better than having fries (approximately 300 calories and 27 g of fat) instead of the banana. Small substitutions that are easy (the banana for the fries) and are made consistently make big differences in your energy and RealAge. You'll feel and be vital for a much longer time if you substitute a banana for fries every time you can.

You can eat fairly well when you're on the move, if you know what to order. For one thing, don't "supersize" anything unless it's water or a diet drink. Ask for extra lettuce and tomato on your grilled chicken sandwich, and always hold the mayo. Remember, even fast food restaurants want you to be a CEO and "have it your way."—Dr. Mike

---

 REALAGE CAFÉ TIP 7.7
Steering a Healthy Course

All of us have found ourselves at a roadside joint with few food choices. Here are tips for avoiding that predicament:

- Before setting out, get the names and locations of the better restaurants along your route.
- Pick restaurants that offer the most choice.
- Be a CEO every time: Ask questions about the food, and then ask if the chef or cook could prepare it a certain way. I've seen over fifteen hundred meals ordered this way, and all but one made the diner's RealAge younger.
- Eat foods that are most similar to those you eat at home.
- Don't overlook the salad bars at supermarkets.
- Prepare food, such as turkey sandwiches and carrot sticks, and set out appropriate portions before the journey.
- Bring along easy-to-eat fruit (pears, apples, bananas, grapes, and boxes of raisins).
- Keep food fresh in plastic bags, and carry a frozen bottle of water to keep them cool (and for drinking). Wrap sandwich ingredients separately so bread doesn't become soggy.
- Carry a soft cooler loaded with RealAge goodies.

Once you board the plane, eating right takes a little forethought. Either stash something in your carry-on—granola bars, a turkey sandwich, and a banana work well on a short flight—or call ahead and specify your needs. Most airlines offer a variety of food choices to passengers who make a request. Remember to be the CEO twenty-four hours in advance. "Can I have a low-calorie vegetarian or fish plate, please?" is my usual request. And it's usually delicious!

What are your options in the air? Here's just a small sample:

- Low-calorie food
- Low-cholesterol food
- Low-sodium food
- Fresh fruit bowl
- Heart-healthy platter
- Vegetarian meal, with or without dairy products or eggs
- Seafood platter
- Diabetic meal
- Gluten-free meal
- Kosher food
- Hindu food
- Muslim food
- Peanut-free meal

Another RealAge trick is to drink as much water as possible en route. It not only reduces your appetite by filling your stomach but also fights the dehydration caused by low-humidity air in the cabin.

RealAge Café Tip 7.8
Airport Fuel

Healthy food selections are taking off at airports. When the American Dietetic Association studied the choices at twenty-eight major airports in 1997, it found big improvements since a similar survey three years earlier.

For example, all of the airports sold fresh fruit and fruit juices, and many sold low-fat or nonfat yogurt, pretzels, and bagels. Less common were salad bars (39 percent of airports), nonfat milk (40 percent), and low-fat muffins (15 percent). San Francisco International and Philadelphia International offered "make-your-own" whole grain pasta meals, and Chicago's O'Hare International prepared custom sandwiches.

By the way, those long hikes between gates at O'Hare may be a pain, but they're also a RealAge bonus. The American Dietetic Association estimates that travelers walking from Terminal 1 to Terminal 3 burn about 150 calories.

Dear Dr. Mike: I'm going on vacation soon, and I'm worried that I'm going to slip back into unhealthy habits. If I restrict calories a couple weeks before I take off, can I eat more freely and without guilt when I get there?—John C., San Francisco

Dear John: Unfortunately, severely restricting your caloric intake now so you can eat macadamia nut ice cream in Hawaii every day next week is not a good idea. Here's why.

First, when you stop eating, your body thinks, "Uh-oh, I'm not getting fed. I'd better slow down to conserve energy." So calories aren't burned, they're stored. This "starvation response" is a survival mechanism that harkens back to primitive days when humans beings could live longer if their metabolism slowed in response to lean pickings. Second, a week of saltines and cabbage soup is enough to make anyone feel deprived. That sets the stage for overindulgence on vacation, and the resulting weight gain and discomfort. You'll waste a lot of effort, too: You've trained your palate to love healthy food. Eating food that ages you will retrain your palate, and you'll be on a diet yo-yo again. So, consistency is an important—perhaps the most important—part of the RealAge Diet way.

There *is* something you can do before your trip. To avoid the starvation response and to plan wisely for indulgences ahead, cut back on calories by small amounts before you leave. You can easily eliminate sugar and salty snacks before you go.

Much more important, once you're on vacation, be sure to keep up all those good eating habits you've already faithfully adopted. For example, continue eating for flavor.

Perhaps the best vacation perk is having time for physical activity, be it casual strolls on the beach, tennis, swimming, or pumping iron. So, if you do want to consume a few extra calories on vacation, think of fun ways to burn them off while you're there.

If you really want to sink into healthy eating and pampering, perhaps it's not too late to consider a spa. Most spas serve lots of fresh fish, salad, fruit, and vegetables; and hydromassage is a fabulous way to rejuvenate yourself and reduce stress.—Dr. Mike

Dear Dr. Mike: For many reasons, my mom and I recently became vegetarians. We'd already had a cruise planned for next year, but now I'm worried we won't get the protein we need during those two weeks on board. Should we cancel the trip?—Timmy S., Pensacola, Florida

Dear Timmy: Absolutely not. The time with your mom is important, and there's no reason you shouldn't be able to get everything you need on a cruise. In fact, cruise lines, like airlines, supply all kinds of special foods, be they low-cholesterol, low-sodium, diabetic, or kosher. If you need the ship to stock tofu and soy milk for you, give the company a call a few weeks ahead of time and

REALAGE CAFÉ TIP 7.9
Calories on a Ship

All hands on deck. Here's how many calories you can burn on a cruise in thirty minutes of exercise:

Exercise	You Weigh 110 lb	You Weigh 185 lb
Aerobics (low impact)	145 calories	244 calories
Tennis	185	311
Snorkeling	132	222
Swimming	158	266
Stationary bike (vigorous)	277	466
Weight lifting	79	133
Rowing machine (moderate)	185	311
Stair-step machine	158	266
Running (ten minutes/mile)	264	444

According to a 1996 report in the *New England Journal of Medicine,* the average person burns about 700 calories an hour during a "somewhat hard" workout on a treadmill.

request it. Most cruise lines will be happy to accommodate you. After all, they want you back.—Dr. Mike

The problem most of us run into on cruises, however, isn't that there won't be enough choices for you to eat, but there will be too many! One thing that sets cruises apart from many other vacations is food. And more food. And still more food. But menus are changing, and more and more frequently you're able to choose among nutrient-rich, calorie-poor options, including vegetarian meals and healthfully cooked seafood. "I haven't been on a cruise in the last two years that hasn't had a healthy spa selection on the menu," reports Lesley Abravanel, managing editor of *Porthole/The Cruise Magazine* in Fort Lauderdale, Florida. "The menus are designed for people who want to stay healthy and not gain fifty pounds on vacation."

Remember, there are good and bad choices. That rule applies whether you're in Dallas on business or in Tahiti on vacation, or at the eatery across town or the bistro down the block. Ask your server about how the food is prepared, first. Then, be the CEO and ask if your meal can be prepared the way you want it. You'll enjoy the food more, and you'll be years younger for your efforts.

8

Distinguish Which Occasions Are Really Special, and Then Distinguish Yourself

A few times a year, occasions arise that are truly special: your birthday, Thanksgiving, your anniversary. These events are almost always celebrated with food—rich, incredibly buttery homemade or gourmet food. If it's a true celebration, it's almost impossible not to dive into the delicacies around you. And why shouldn't you? Sharing your happiness over a delicious meal or special food is a fabulous and cherished part of life.

The problem is that rich, buttery gourmet foods have become available all the time, and for many people special occasions are no longer once-in-a-while events. So, if you're one of those people who find themselves attending lots of parties, you have a decision to make. From a RealAge standpoint, you need to decide how many events are worth the downside of eating all those aging, nutrient-poor foods.

On one hand, you want to be satisfied both physically and emotionally when you leave the party. On the other hand, you don't want to end a month of back-to-back celebrations ten pounds heavier and four years older than when you started. You need to decide what kinds of occasions are truly special to you, so you can then let yourself be carried away with an indulgent reward.

It's Not What You Eat, But How Much You Eat

Once you begin to make a habit of eating the *RealAge* way, you might find that your food strategies are automatically good ones. You might share your birthday cake with someone near you, or taste your uncle's home-baked, newly arrived apple pie and then discreetly stash it in the kitchen. You might take smaller portions of everything on the table and leave space on the plate between each food. This controls your portion sizes and lets you taste everything without overdosing. You might drink a large glass of water at a restaurant before you order, so your appetite doesn't get the best of you.

For me, I choose to eat food that isn't part of my RealAge lifestyle only when I'm celebrating something especially personal—an anniversary or an achievement I've been striving toward for months. If the celebration is a family gathering or someone else's personal achievement, I eat only the things I want and only until I feel I'm about to be full. Then I'm content to just sip and stir my coffee.

You might have different criteria for designating which occasions are special enough to stray from your RealAge goals. Just remember, a special occasion should be a rare event. Try limiting yourself to four a year. Choosing which four requires a little looking into the future. One friend picks Thanksgiving, Christmas, Easter Sunday, and Mother's Day, while another friend picks Super Bowl Sunday, the NBA finals deciding game, the Fourth of July, and his own birthday. Any more than four, and it's too easy to break the good habits you've created for yourself.

You're probably thinking, "That's easier said than done." You're right. At first, it's hard to break the habit of overindulging at every celebration. A few months down the road, once you've been sticking to your plan for a while, you'll probably look back and wonder how you ever lived otherwise. In fact, you might even feel that eating the *RealAge* way isn't denying yourself at all— it's exactly what you want to do! Until then, here are some good strategies for managing those special occasions that are most challenging for our RealAge goals—the holidays, parties, catered events, business dinners, picnics, tailgate parties, and more.

The Holiday Marathon

Although the "holiday season" usually refers to the five weeks between Thanksgiving and New Year's Day, it really starts earlier, at Halloween, when all that candy suddenly shows up in your house and workplace. The secret to staying young through the holidays isn't so much *what* you eat as *how much* you eat. Continuing to eat even though you're full, no matter what the reason, is a choice that adds years to your RealAge.

Whether you're playing host or visiting family and friends, the holidays mean a change to your routine. A big change. Even though the room may be filled with laughter, you're under pressure to arrive on time, entertain, and make sure that your guests are fed and the children are cared for. You're distracted. There's just so much going on, so much to think about, and so much to do. It's easy to eat without thinking about it—to eat while you're cooking and to snack while you're chatting. All of these are subconscious eating habits.

During the holidays, you might keep a small notebook with you at all times. Write down *everything* you eat. This keeps you from eating subconsciously or absentmindedly. Also, recording everything you eat deters snacking. It's sometimes too much trouble to eat if you have to write it down every time.

A study published in *Health Psychology* takes a look at the habit of recording one's food. Researchers studied thirty-eight men and women who had been watching their weight for about fifty weeks and had lost an average of 21 pounds before the holidays. During the weeks between Thanksgiving and New Year's, the 25 percent who most consistently recorded every bite of food lost an average of 7 pounds, whereas the other 75 percent regained an average of 3 pounds.

Once you realize what the pressures are, it's much easier to gain control. Yes, there's lots of food around, but that doesn't mean you have to eat it. Eat only world-class food. Try to stick to the RealAge lifestyle you've developed as much as possible. It's difficult when the party isn't at your own home, and you should give yourself permission to vary a little. For the most part, if you stick to the eleven RealAge strategies discussed in Chapter 6, you should find yourself surviving the holidays with a stable weight and a lot of pride in yourself.

One strategy for keeping yourself focused on your RealAge lifestyle is to really listen to the people around you. You can't eat fast if you're engaged in a good conversation. After all, talking to other guests is the main purpose of these social events, right? You can even engage in more personal or devoted one-on-one conversation by taking a walk with someone. Less food and no interruptions can make such a walk really special.

By planning ahead, you can enjoy nutrient-rich, calorie-poor foods during the holidays without stinting on pleasure. For example, if you're worried that the empty calories at an upcoming bash will age you, bring along a dish that you've made yourself, ensuring that you'll have something healthful to eat. Take a shrimp cocktail, dressed with tomato, mango, papaya, or pineapple salsa. It's an excellent starter and doesn't have any saturated fat. You can also take a preemptive strike at hunger by eating at home before the party. This way you don't arrive famished, ready to devour everything in sight.

Another helpful practice is exercising before the party, or taking a brisk walk or bike ride after the meal and before dessert. Exercise not only burns some of those extra calories but also reduces the stress that comes with end-of-the-year festivities. But don't use these strategies to allow yourself a lot of "special occasions." Stick to four for the year.

Substitutions are a great strategy. Think pumpkin pie instead of pecan during the holidays. There are 229 calories and 10 grams (g) of fat in the average slice of pumpkin pie and as many as 450 calories and 20 g of fat in a slice of pecan pie. Pecans themselves aren't to blame. In limited amounts, they're RealAge-friendly, but all the other ingredients in traditional pecan pie aren't nutrient rich and calorie poor. If you love pecan pie, you might take one that's been adapted to make your RealAge younger. Or, instead of pecan pie, try another crowd-pleaser: dark chocolate (not milk chocolate). Since either choice will be high in calories, practice moderation.

Roasted sweet potatoes mashed with roasted garlic and sweetened with a touch of orange juice make a great alternative to mashed white potatoes, which usually contain butter and cream. You might also consider bringing your own eggnog—4 ounces of the traditional eggnog packs 335 calories and 16 g of saturated fat. A RealAge alternative is soynog, which has only 1 percent fat but also the rich flavors of vanilla and nutmeg. Look for it in your dairy beverage case.

Another good beverage choice is mulled wine or straight red or white wine; a four-ounce glass contains just 90 calories and is brimming with flavonoids (red wine has more flavonoids than white wine). Moderate quantities of red wine may slow aging of both your arterial and immune systems.

Of course, even the best holiday eating plans can go right down the drain if your companions insist you take seconds. In some families, taking seconds is the only way to really praise the cook. One of our friends wrote the following:

Mike: Absolutely the truth! My aunts and mom get really hurt if I don't eat more. It's not worth it to me to refuse seconds; it hurts their feelings too much. Better to get itsy portions, go back for seconds, and make a big deal about "YUM, YUM, YUM." This is really difficult (itsy portions), because their food is drop-dead delicious.

These situations call for polite but firm responses. You could say, "It was so good, but I'll burst if I eat another bite." Our friend responded:

Mike: This comment would have NO effect whatsoever on a determined aunt or mother. So I say, "Thanks, but I've already had two servings and want to be sure to save room for dessert." Then take dessert, eat a little, and leave the rest. I also like the idea I gave you about taking really small second helpings. It lessens the amount of chatter about food.

Or you could say, "I can't take those leftovers home—they'll spoil while I'm away skiing next week."

Our friend's response:

Mike: A pretty good save, but sometimes it's better just to take the leftovers home and dump them. Your excuse is a little too limited. It should be so broad you can use it automatically, without looking like you're lying. For example, skiing is too specific, too easy to catch as a lie. Devise something generic, like this: "I'll be out most nights this week and the food will spoil. I'd hate to waste such delicious food. Why don't you freeze what you can for my next visit?" Or, as Sukie Miller said, "Take the food home and give it to someone on the street or drop it off at a homeless shelter. You can't say no when people offer you food—not family. You'd be cursed if you turned down family."

 REALAGE CAFÉ TIP 8.1

A Fancy for Flavonoids

Think of flavonoids as the safety patrol for your cardiovascular system. Flavonoids relax smooth muscle in the cardiovascular system and thus lower blood pressure. Flavonoids also prevent the oxidation of lousy (LDL) cholesterol that otherwise could build up as plaque in the arteries.

Here are some sources of flavonoids:

- Vegetables: tomatoes, broccoli, green peppers, onions
- The edible pulp of fruits: grapes, apples, citrus, apricots, cherries, berries
- Green tea
- Herbs: yarrow, hawthorn, milk thistle, gingko, bilberry

Since the French eat lots of saturated fat and drink lots of red wine but have lower rates of coronary heart disease than Americans, researchers suspect that the flavonoids in red wine provide a shield against aging of the arteries and immune system. With the exception of champagne, flavonoids are much less plentiful in white wine, as the skin, leaves, stems, and seeds of grapes are separated from the juice immediately after the grapes are crushed. See Chart 4.5 to calculate how many flavonoids you consume in an average day.

Though the holidays may be the most hazardous bump on the RealAge road to youth, they certainly aren't the only one. Catered parties can put the skids on good eating habits at any time of the year. The key to survival at catered events, as you'll see, consists of three words: plan, plan, plan.

REALAGE CAFÉ TIP 8.2

Holiday Dos and Don'ts

Dos

- Do eat a meal before the party.
- Do perform physical activity before or walk with guests as part of the party.
- Do bring your favorite RealAge recipe to the festivities.
- Do use a small plate and leave space between foods.
- Do eat a little healthy fat first, before your meal.
- Do listen to your stomach. Stop eating when you're almost full.
- Do engage in more conversation (and less eating).
- Do keep a daily journal of how much you eat and how much physical activity you get between Thanksgiving and New Year's Day.
- Do modify recipes to make them low in saturated fats. If you're the host, test your recipes before the party to make sure they're so good you'd order them in a restaurant. Find a caterer who will make recipes that make your RealAge younger and will let you taste them well before the party. RealAge foods can, and should, taste great.
- Do be selective. Eat foods that are nutrient rich—fruits, vegetables, legumes, and nuts.
- Do drink a moderate amount of wine with dinner, as well as water.
- Do go light on desserts.
- Do use nonstick cooking spray on pots and pans.

Don'ts

- Don't try to lose weight. You'll simply frustrate yourself.
- Don't skip meals in anticipation of the feast.
- Don't let friends and relatives pressure you into eating foods that age you or make you too full.
- Don't hover near the appetizers or buffet table.
- Don't volunteer for serving hors d'oeuvres.
- Don't eat gravy, rich sauces, or fried foods.
- Don't return for seconds.
- Don't leave the party with leftovers. If you're the host, see if you can tactfully and appreciatively send leftovers home with whoever brought the dish, or with other departing guests.
- Don't place cookie jars and candy dishes around the house or office.

REALAGE CAFÉ TIP 8.3
About That Turkey

All turkeys are not created equal. Here are tips we edited from *Prevention* magazine about buying and preparing a RealAge-friendly holiday bird:

- Avoid "self-basting" turkeys; usually these have been injected with butter or other high-fat additives.
- Add aromatics, herbs, and spices under the skin. Even if you remove the skin after baking, the meat will have a fuller flavor.
- Baste with a saturated- and trans-fat-free broth or fruit juice rather than drippings.
- Leave the turkey skin, which is the fattiest part of the bird, on the cutting board.
- Prepare dressing without giblets, using broth instead of drippings to moisten it. Make sure to bake the stuffing outside the turkey, so the dressing won't absorb fat, and so the stuffing gets to the right temperature.
- Prepare gravy by separating the fat from the pan juices and thickening the juices with pureed vegetables and cornstarch instead of flour and fat. Use soy or skim milk instead of cream.

REALAGE CAFÉ TIP 8.4
A+ for Applesauce

There is a simple, delicious way to trim unhealthy fat from holiday baked goods: Substitute unsweetened apple sauce or another fruit puree for at least half the oil, butter, or shortening in a recipe. Fruit purees (apple, plum, pumpkin, and prune) contain fiber that traps moisture in cakes, muffins, and breads. Purees also make baked items tasty and moist.

Lightly flavored recipes that call for lemon, blueberry, or oatmeal are especially good for swapping unsweetened applesauce for part of the fat. In chocolate recipes, pureed prunes can offer a delightfully dense, fudgy texture when substituted for half of the chocolate.

Catering to Appetites

As a catered event approaches, recall all the things you did right during the holidays to make them a RealAge victory, and then apply them here. About an hour before the big Thanksgiving meal, you had a light snack with some healthy fat or fiber (or both) and a big glass of water (or better yet a bowl of light soup) so you wouldn't be famished. Also, you probably exercised earlier in the day. You sidestepped the hors d'oeuvres, or at least kept them to a minimum. You selected your dinner foods carefully, after considering all the options and choosing only ones you really wanted to eat. You made sure none of the portions on your small plate touched each other.

Here are more strategies for catered events:

- Enlist a partner to lead you away from unhealthy food if you can't do it yourself.
- Always keep one hand free. Don't keep both hands full of food or drink, because you'll consume more. This tip is perhaps the most valuable one for me. In the one hand I use, I alternate food with two other choices: a glass of wine with a glass of ice water with lemon or lime.
- Immerse yourself in conversation. Focusing on words and people instead of food and drink can trim calories dramatically.
- Chew food slowly and put your knife and fork down between bites. Stretching out a meal reduces the likelihood of a calorie overdose.
- Take a bite of the cheesecake your host absolutely insisted you try, then discreetly (and quickly) put the rest in the trash can or dirty dish tray. Even better, split one dessert three or four ways—you'll be doing at least three friends a favor, too!

At wedding receptions, there's another fun activity that, along with the 2-mile run or the weights you lifted earlier in the day, sweats off calories right away. It's dancing! In one study, researchers determined that individual dancers covered nearly five miles in one evening out on the floor. In thirty minutes, a person who weighs 150 pounds can burn 255 calories doing the polka, 200 calories square dancing, or 120 calories waltzing. Although you usually can't have your cake and eat it, too, wedding cake and dancing may be the exception when it comes to compensating for extra calories.

There might even be healthy alternatives to wedding cake or the dessert table: an orange compote with Cointreau (orange liqueur) or a fresh fig and honey galette (a kind of dessert pizza).

Decide before you get to the event which item is going to be your favorite. Is it the cake? Ribs? Bread (you can even ask for olive oil at most catered events)? Whatever it is, it's okay to eat some, as long as it is only some, and you choose wisely the rest of the time. If you choose bread, maybe you'll skip the potatoes and definitely the butter. Did you choose the cake? You might compensate by selecting a grilled or poached item for your main course at dinner. Tell your friends you're saving room for what you really love. The fruits and vegetables you eat will be a RealAge plus, of course.

Catering on Home Turf

Hosting an event can be a ton of work, but it's also very rewarding. The trick is finding the right caterer. To do so, you have to ask questions. Seek referrals from people who are also concerned about healthful eating. Then start calling. If a caterer is not able to provide what you need or tries to sell you something you don't want, just politely say you'll consider what they've offered.

Good caterers will do everything possible to accommodate special orders. After all, they want your repeat business and referrals. Of course, even the most accommodating and resourceful caterers face some limitations. You might request some fruits and vegetables that are not in season or some items that are not their specialty or that they can't find. That's why it's best to shop around. If a caterer is creative, energetic, eager to please, and knows how to shop, you'll probably find yourself with a delicious *and* healthy meal.

Most caterers can produce a variety of dishes that are low in saturated and trans fat, from salads and vegetable soups to lean cuts of meat that gain flavor in wet or dry marinades. Remember to ask questions and take charge; for example, "Can you make it without butter?" Of course, whether your guests number four or four hundred, you can't satisfy everyone's tastes. You can ask guests to RSVP with any special dietary restrictions, which aren't the same as culinary preferences. Since many people are concerned about arterial aging and high blood pressure, you'll want to provide plenty of healthy choices so no one feels left out. It's probably wise to have the caterer salt food lightly and season it deliciously with garlic, mustards, and other herbs and spices.

I'm a great fan of this next tip. A surefire way to make sure your party food is healthful and delicious is to arrange a tasting at least one week before the big event. Many caterers are willing to bring samples to your house. You and a few friends can taste and rate every food on a scale of 0 to 10 (see the RealAge tasting scale, in Chart 10.2). If an offering doesn't score an 8, don't serve it. It's also your chance, as the one in charge, to ask the caterer to tweak some of the recipes. This makes your meal not just another get-together, but a really memorable special occasion. Don't be shy: Taste two or three times as many foods as you plan to serve. That way, your guests will have a variety of delicious and healthful choices. But, remember, it's a *tasting*, not nine meals—take tiny portions to taste!

Eating with Your Colleagues

Whether you're a lawyer, agent, or consultant who wines and dines clients, or a teacher, computer engineer, or office assistant who lunches with colleagues, you're probably going to find yourself, on occasion, eating with people whom you need to impress, sway, or simply get along with.

Sometimes, when you're eating with your peers, it can be more difficult to eat the RealAge way. You might be self-conscious about asking your server a number of questions about the food and its preparation or making a special request regarding your meal. Sometimes, especially at work get-togethers, your colleagues may even pressure you into eating unhealthful foods or more than you really want. What do you do?

Food choices are personal issues. Period. You have to eat what's best for you, whether your dining partner is Bill Gates or the Bill next door. That said, consider how the RealAge approach to eating at restaurants might just bolster your image with a potential business partner. By taking charge when it's time to order, you're showing confidence and initiative. By asking intelligent questions, you're showing curiosity and attention to detail. By politely posing questions to the server, you're showing grace and an ability to enlist others in accomplishing a goal. All of these are admirable traits in any business world.

That's not to say that dining with a future client, your boss, or your peers will always be easy; some social situations are just plain awkward. But there are things you can do to turn the tide in your favor. One is to let your boss or client set the tone by ordering first. This does not mean, of course, that you should order the same thing. Who knows? Maybe she or he shares your desire for healthy food and will put an immediate end to your worries.

After the meal, your colleague may suggest dessert, even though you feel comfortably full and even a bite would put you over the edge. In these situations, you might encourage your dinner partner to order whatever he or she wants, then perhaps order fruit or coffee or tea for yourself. The challenge is to keep control of your choices.

Let's face it. These occasions aren't about food; they're about mutually beneficial relationships. The first task is to maintain that bond with your guest across the table, and the second is to satisfy your RealAge appetite with delicious choices. Choices *you* make.

Outdoor Parties and Picnics

Some people claim tailgate parties make the best setting for outdoor eating. Other people don't need the game as an excuse to get all their friends together for backyard barbecues. At any outdoor eating event, you have a multitude of RealAge choices. If there's a grill, my favorites are veggie, soy, or turkey burgers with whole wheat buns, sliced onions, and tomatoes. Prepared-in-advance chicken kabobs with mushrooms, onions, and cherry tomatoes are also easy, colorful, and tasty. If there isn't a grill, bring along hummus sandwiches made with pita bread or whole wheat bread, tomatoes, lettuce, and cheese. Yogurt-dill dip and carrot, jicama, and celery sticks are great substitutes for other picnic snack items like heavy sour cream dips and potato chips.

 RealAge Café Tip 8.5
Heavenly Hummus

Heart-friendly hummus, a classic Middle Eastern dish, is a mashed concoction of chickpeas (also known as garbanzo beans), lemon juice, garlic, olive oil, and tahini (sesame paste). Hummus has a rich, earthy flavor and is high in soluble fiber. It's served with pita bread, which is flat, hollow, and round, whole or cut into triangles for dipping. There are many different recipes, including some that substitute soybeans or chana dal (a yellow dried legume) for garbanzos. Try some yourself, and then experiment a little. Roast the garlic, for example, before adding it to the blender. Add a little lemon zest, plus the lemon juice. Add a tablespoonful of yogurt for smoothness and a little more tang. Squiggle basil-infused olive oil on top. Go hummus!

Another wonderful idea is to bring smoked salmon, some whole grain breads, and some seasonal fruits. Or bring a few ears of organic corn still in the husk (soaked in water for just a few minutes) to toss on the grill and eat first. The fiber will help fill you up so that you'll eat less, and the sweetness of the corn will make you thankful that you did. Remember to enjoy a few nuts first to make you feel and be fuller, and to decrease the sugar level that sweet corn could cause.

At many of these casual outdoor events, you're feeling relaxed and there's so much food around, it's easy to snack all afternoon. Here are some tips to help you eat less:

- Eat something nutrient rich and calorie poor before you attend the game or picnic. This could be something that has a little fat, for example, six

nuts, a little whole wheat bread dipped in a little olive oil, a small wedge of tortilla, avocado, and tomatoes, or two whole pieces of fruit.
- Keep track of what you eat.
- Munch on fruits and vegetables instead of chips.

Regarding the alcohol that is typically available at these events, it's probably best if you bring your own choice in great enough quantities for the whole group. Bring a fine wine or beer you'll truly savor. Also, who says your drink has to be alcoholic? Thirst-quenching alternatives include freshly squeezed juices, sparkling apple cider or grape juice, sparkling or mineral water, seltzer, or club soda. And remember the tip of having food or drink in only one hand at a time.

At a potluck, use a recipe from Chapter 11. And remember you can be in charge and make your RealAge younger deliciously, even at special occasions. The choice of four special occasions and planning how to distinguish yourself are yours to make.

REALAGE CAFÉ TIP 8.6
Alcohol: Friend or Foe?

Many recent studies have tried to gauge the health effects of different quantities and types of alcohol. For those who aren't at risk of alcohol or drug abuse, the results indicate that moderate amounts of alcohol (two drinks a day for men and one drink a day for women) reduce the aging of arteries. The type of alcohol may not be as important as the amount.

Researchers at Harvard studied more than twenty-two thousand men ages forty to eighty-four for nearly eleven years. The risk of dying was 28 percent less for those who had two to four drinks a week, and 21 percent less for those who had five or six drinks a week. Although heavy drinkers were no more likely to die from heart disease than others, their risk of death from cancer was double.

The Northern Manhattan Stroke Study found that people who had up to two drinks a day pared their risk of stroke by 45 percent when compared with nondrinkers. However, more than five drinks a day tripled the risk of stroke. Some studies have shown that alcohol reduces the level of lousy (LDL) cholesterol in the blood and boosts the level of healthy (HDL) cholesterol in the blood. Although this may not be the reason for the benefit, a little alcohol will make your RealAge younger.

9

You Can Reach Your Goals Faster!

Through the Door, or Turning Heads Once Again

You've just learned how to eat the RealAge way at home. You have even learned how to be the CEO at every restaurant and to make your RealAge younger when you eat out, even on special occasions. My patients who've adopted RealAge eating habits frequently ask, "How can I achieve my goals faster?" When we change our lifestyle, we want to see the effects as soon as possible. It's difficult to wait for benefits that take months of effort; we need immediate gratification. There's good news. Nothing beats physical activity for slowing and reversing aging, and for making you feel, look, and be younger *quickly.*

Within days, even hours, exercise provides important age-reducing bene-fits. Physical activity improves your attitude, self-image, and ability to manage stress, anxiety, and depression. Not only will you *feel* as if you have more energy, you *will* have more energy. Benefits that come quickly include increased stamina, flexibility, and metabolism; healthier arterial and immune systems; and better sleep patterns. Best of all, you'll probably find yourself reaching for more healthful RealAge foods to make your workouts more youth promoting.

Even when you believe in the benefits of exercise, it can be a challenge to start and stay motivated. It's especially tough if you have time constraints or physical problems. Nevertheless, it is possible to slide a ten- or twenty-minute activity into the busiest schedules. For example, if you have one-on-one meet-ings anytime during the day, make some of them walking meetings. You won't be interrupted by phone calls or e-mail, and you'll enjoy the energy that physical activity gives. No matter what your situation, do some physical activity every day (or almost every day) and enjoy yourself. You can always find something that's fun for *you*.

The RealAge Café: Real-Life Success Stories

Although everyone wants to be successful in an exercise program, success means different things to different people. The following two stories illustrate these differences, but both are success stories: Carol and Janice have each made their RealAges over 10 years younger. How each started and the goals they set illustrate the range of goals you might have, and how exercise can help you make eating the RealAge way more fun.

Carol's Story

For Carol, just entering the club meant success. At 5'3" and 185 pounds, Carol was fifty-one years old and overweight. Her sister, two years older, who had a similar physique, had developed breast cancer. Abetted by her great gourmet cooking ability, Carol had been overweight for at least twenty-five years. She wanted to avoid breast cancer and not to feel sluggish. She had become an empty-nester when her daughter graduated from high school. Now, without the goal of getting her daughter to school, she felt she needed more motivation than ever to get going every day. The sluggishness she had often felt in late afternoons was starting to creep into the mornings. She was (and is) a successful public relations consultant and needed stamina for her work. To lose weight, Carol decided to go on the Atkins diet, as modified in Chapter 3 of this book to be more RealAge healthful. She also decided to see if she could make her RealAge younger and feel more energetic by doing physical activity for the first time in over thirty years.

Carol felt she needed the environment of a health club to help her start. She wrote that a RealAge goal was just to enter the health club three times a week. That's right—for her, simply going into the health club was a measure of success. At first, Carol's goal was a little disappointing to me, until I realized what a truly great start this was for her. It was something she had never done before. In the past, she had always worried she wouldn't be one of the beautiful bodies in the health club. When she arrived, however, she saw a wide range of body types and realized hers was just one point on the continuum. To reward herself for meeting her RealAge goal of entering the club six times in two weeks, she bought herself a new outfit.

After her first visit, Carol started to wander around a little bit, walking from one area to another. She then started walking for twenty minutes at a time. That soon became thirty minutes. Then she started lifting weights, too. She hired a trainer to teach her the right regimen for her ten-minutes-a-day, three-days-a-week commitment to weight lifting. So, she started with walking, then added resistance exercise (weight lifting, for her), and now she's even doing some stamina exercise. She has indeed been successful: She met her goal; set newer, higher goals; and rewarded herself with some new clothes. Just putting on those clothes made her feel more energetic and more likely to exercise.

Janice's Story

For Janice, the goal was different. She wanted to "turn heads once again." She wanted to get in good enough shape so that people would tell her she was beautiful, and she could believe them. When Janice came to see me, she asked, "That's all there is? Just these small lifestyle changes and I'll be twelve to sixteen years younger? I can do that." And she did.

Janice had been a 5'4", 123-pound head-turner. Then, in her last two years of college and throughout her career, she gradually gained weight. Not much at any one time, just a few pounds here and there. When she turned forty-eight, she realized she was quite a few pounds (40+) over her ideal weight. She bought the first RealAge book and then she came to see me to find out if living younger was really as easy as it seemed. She wanted a plan for life—not a quick fix.

She began with strength-building exercises, just thirty minutes a week. Then she took her workouts a little further; she hired a trainer for one session on the weekend and worked out twice a week lifting weights with her son. She then started walking on a treadmill at a six-degree incline at the rate of 2.5 miles an hour. Over the next several months, she built up to 3.5 miles per hour for thirty minutes at the same incline. Once she was confident in her routine, Janice was ready to tackle her eating habits. She wanted to know what to eat, how to eat, and when. She adopted the RealAge eating plan slowly, easily, and with just small changes.

Within a year and a half, Janice was back to her ideal weight, even with the increased muscle mass. In fact, she had redesigned her body as she gained muscle and lost fat. She had regained much of her youthful physique. Of course, some people have a more difficult time changing their habits, especially habits that have been in place over several years.

Although Janice had some difficult moments, she didn't give up. Once her new lifestyle was in place, staying with it just got easier and easier. When I saw her next, I could see that her new lifestyle had given her a more youthful glow, a ready smile, and an energetic bounce to her step. She had met her goal and was turning heads once again.

What's Your Goal?

When it comes to goals, most people are somewhere between Carol and Janice. Some want to feel healthier; some, to cross the threshold of the health club or exercise room; and some, to feel like Superman or Superwoman. The aim should be to choose a goal that is achievable for *you* and that will make your RealAge younger.

Healthy eating and physical activity go hand in hand toward making your RealAge significantly younger. Daily exercise will reinforce your healthier eating choices and accelerate your progress. To make exercise a part of your life, you've got to look forward to it. Make it fun. If you try a certain kind of physical activity and don't like it, don't give up on exercise: Try another activity. As with your food choices, you should find ways to enjoy exercise or your resolve will not last.

The Benefits of Exercise

Exercise is more than just a way to look and feel better. It's a choice you make in order to become significantly younger. For men who are fifty-five years old and participate regularly in a balanced exercise program, the RealAge benefit is more than 8 years younger. For women, the benefit can be even greater, as many as 9 years younger. Instead of viewing exercise as a chore that eats up your free time, remember that you're adding some very positive things to your life—good health and a stronger, more capable body. Those of us who can choose to walk, to increase the stamina of our heart and lungs, or to lift weights have options that some others do not. When you exercise, you're adding more years in which you can enjoy a full range of physical motion.

If you don't make exercise a part of your life, you may be depriving yourself of activities later in life—walking on the beach, playing on the floor with your grandchildren, spending the day at the fair or the mall, or even throwing a ball at a picnic. With ailments that may arise from a sedentary lifestyle, including obesity and joint problems, many middle-aged people have a difficult time even standing quickly after a movie. Comparatively, you'll be a virtual teenager just three years after you start your physical activity program. Physical activity gives you more time; it not only lengthens your life but also makes it more enjoyable. Here's how.

Exercise and Weight Management

Exercise can be the most enjoyable part of a weight management program. Most often, if you want to lose weight, you're going to have to reduce the number of calories you eat. However, if you try to lose weight only by eating less, your metabolism may slow down. Exercise, on the other hand, increases your body's metabolic rate. You'll lose weight faster if you're physically active.

Obesity affects one of every five men and one of every three women. Also, more of us (including our children) are obese than ever before. What is obesity? For a man, it's a body fat composition of 25 percent or more; for a woman, it's a body fat composition of 30 percent or more. That means if a man weighs 160 pounds, more than 40 pounds would be fat. Or, if a woman weighs 150 pounds, more than 45 pounds would be fat. Another way of looking at it is that obesity is a body mass index of 30 or more (see Chart 9.1).

If you are able to keep active and avoid high blood pressure, being overweight—even to the point of obesity—makes only a small direct contribution to aging of the arteries and immune system, and to diabetes and osteoarthritis. That's why being overweight has only a small effect on RealAge (see Charts 9.1 and 9.2). But if being overweight causes lack of physical activity, it can contribute significantly to aging of the arteries and immune system.

A leading scientific researcher in this field joined the Cooper Clinic, planning to be like Dr. Cooper and in the process get in shape, lose weight, get taller (!), and regain his hair. Although he has become fit, he's still obese. Nevertheless, his RealAge stays young, because he exercises consistently and well and has avoided the consequences of obesity—high blood pressure, diabetes, arthritis, high levels of bad cholesterol, and heart disease. Physical activity also decreases your risk of at least four other diseases that occur more frequently in the obese: gall bladder disease and colon, prostate, and breast cancer.

Losing weight—and keeping it off—is no easy task if you try to do it without changing food choices. Instead of going on a tempting, but temporary, fad diet, however, it's best to change your eating and exercise behaviors. This means that you need to retrain your palate (see Chapter 10), retrain your eye,

CHART 9.1

What Is Your Body Mass Index?

	Body Mass Index (kg/m²)													
	19	20	21	22	23	24	25	26	27	28	29	30	35	40
Height (inches)	Body Weight in Pounds													
58	91	96	100	105	110	115	119	124	129	134	138	143	167	191
59	94	99	104	109	114	119	124	128	133	138	143	148	173	198
60	97	102	107	112	118	123	128	133	138	143	148	153	179	204
61	100	106	111	116	122	127	132	137	143	148	153	158	183	211
62	104	109	115	120	126	131	136	142	147	153	158	164	191	218
63	107	113	118	124	130	135	141	146	152	158	163	169	197	225
64	110	116	122	128	134	140	145	151	157	163	169	174	204	232
65	114	120	126	132	138	144	150	156	162	168	174	180	210	240
66	118	124	130	136	142	148	153	161	167	173	179	186	216	247
67	121	127	134	140	146	153	159	166	172	178	185	191	223	255
68	125	131	138	144	151	158	164	171	177	184	190	197	230	262
69	128	135	142	149	153	162	169	176	182	189	196	203	236	270
70	132	139	146	153	160	167	174	181	188	195	202	207	243	278
71	136	143	150	157	165	172	179	186	193	200	208	215	250	286
72	140	147	154	162	169	177	184	191	199	206	213	221	258	294
73	144	151	159	166	174	182	189	197	204	212	219	227	265	302
74	148	155	163	171	179	186	194	202	210	218	225	233	272	311
75	152	160	168	176	184	192	200	208	216	224	232	240	279	319
76	156	164	172	180	189	197	205	213	221	230	238	246	287	328

Note: To use this table, find your height in the left-hand column. Move across the row to your weight. The number at the top of the column is the body mass index (BMI) for your height and weight. If your BMI—the ratio of weight to height expressed in units of kilograms per meter squared (kg/m²)—is not on the chart, or if you want to calculate your BMI more precisely, the formula for calculating your exact BMI is relatively easy:

1. Convert your weight in pounds to your weight in kilograms. You do this by dividing your weight in pounds by 2.2.
2. Convert your height in inches to your height in meters. You do this by multiplying your height in inches—not feet—by 0.0254. (For example, if you are 5' tall, your height is 60", or 1.52 meters [m]. If you are 6' tall, your height is 72", or 1.83 m.)
3. Square your height in meters—that is, multiply your height in meters by itself.
4. Divide your weight in kilograms (the number you obtained in item 1) by the number you obtained in item 3.

CHART 9.2
The RealAge Effect of Body Mass Index

	Body Mass Index								
	18.5 or less	18.6– 21.9	22– 24.1	24.2– 26.4	26.5– 28.7	28.8– 31.0	31.1– 33.3	33.4– 35.7	35.7+
Calendar Age	RealAge								
	MEN								
35	35.2	34.7	35	35.4	35.8	36.1	36.1	36.2	36.3
55	55.3	54.3	55	56	57	58.2	58.2	58.5	58.6
70	70.5	69	70	71.4	72.8	74.7	74.7	75.3	75.4
	WOMEN								
35	34.9	34.6	35	35.5	36	36.6	37.1	37.5	37.6
55	54.9	54.4	55	55.8	56.6	57.6	58.6	59.6	60.0
70	69.9	69.2	70	71.0	72.1	73.4	75.0	76.1	76.7

and begin to have fun again as a younger person. Many thousands have e-mailed us, describing their successes and newly regained youth. Once you start, it isn't that difficult to reach most of the RealAge goals that make you 5 to 12 years younger, and it becomes fun as you gain more energy. The alternative, yo-yo dieting, will actually age you. Repeatedly losing and gaining weight stresses your body, accelerates weight gain, decreases your healthy (HDL) cholesterol level, and makes you much older. In fact, yo-yo weight gain and loss is worse than just having the extra weight (see Chart 9.3).

Losing weight without being physically active is difficult. In contrast, it's considerably easier to lose weight slowly if you gradually increase your physical activity until it becomes a regular part of your life. Also, you'll enjoy many benefits that make your RealAge younger:

- A higher caloric burn rate
- Greater muscle mass, which leads to a higher metabolic rate
- Reduced blood pressure and lower levels of bad cholesterol and glucose in the blood
- A lower risk of osteoarthritis of the weight-bearing joints
- Emotional and mental benefits, including increased self-esteem, a greater feeling of self-control, and a reduction in stress levels

CHART 9.3
The RealAge Effect of Frequent Weight Changes

Calendar Age	Percentage of Your Total Weight Lost or Gained in a 5-Year Period		
	Less than 5%	5–10%	More than 10%
	RealAge		
MEN			
35	35	36.6	38.3
55	55	57.8	59.6
70	70	73.4	80.8
WOMEN			
35	35	36.2	38.0
55	55	57.2	59.6
70	70	72.9	79.2

What kind of physical activity is best for someone who is overweight? The easiest and least stressful way to begin is to increase your level of general physical activity slowly and gently, on a daily basis. Be sure to choose activities you enjoy. You could start walking a short distance and gradually work up to a longer distance. For example, park farther away than usual from the grocery store or your workplace. Many of my patients begin by walking one block three times a day.

If you're not able to participate in traditional walking or aerobics programs, swimming or water-walking may be just the prescription for you. Water-walking is relatively strain and stress-free for the joints. If swimming or water walking isn't for you, find something you do like. Sometimes exercise is part of a hobby or task you enjoy, such as gardening, furniture refinishing, room rearranging, lawn mowing, vacuuming, or dancing. You can even exercise in your chair, if your condition keeps you there. Just make sure you like your activity. Whatever you choose, the overall goal is to develop an enjoyable, consistent exercise program that will become a routine part of your life.

Exercise and Your Cardiovascular System

Exercise lowers blood pressure, increases flexibility of the artery walls, helps control stress, and helps prevent blood clots. All of these reduce arterial aging, which, in turn, lessens your risk of heart attack, stroke, memory loss, impo-

REALAGE CAFÉ TIP 9.1

Exercise Away Your Knee Pain

Knee pain? Try exercise. If your knee pain is caused by osteoarthritis, the right kind of exercise may give you relief from pain and disability.

Controlled studies in older persons with osteoarthritis of the knee suggest that low-impact aerobic exercise, as well as resistance (strength) exercise, improves disability, physical performance, and pain. Walking for half an hour at least three times a week will do it. More frequent shorter walks may be easier for some. Exercise performed regularly and at a moderate level appears to present little risk of damage to joints. And remember vitamins C and D and calcium—they help prevent knee pain, too. As a bonus, exercise and those nutrients make your RealAge younger. The hard part is getting started.

tence, and even wrinkling of the skin. Studies show that exercise helps control blood cholesterol levels. When you exercise, the amount of lousy (LDL) cholesterol in your blood decreases, and the amount of healthy (HDL) cholesterol increases.

General Physical Activity: A Good Way to Start

There are three basic types of physical activity that make you younger: (1) stamina-building exercises (also called aerobic or cardiovascular exercises), (2) strength-building exercises (also called weight training or resistance exercise), and (3) the general physical activity of everyday life.

My patients seem to be more successful at keeping up their exercise program if they first start with activities in the general physical activity category (such as walking) and then add strength-building exercises. Finally, they add stamina-building exercises, such as running or fast walking, swimming or walking in a swimming pool, or cycling.

Stamina-Building Exercise

When does general physical activity become aerobic? To qualify as a stamina-building exercise, an activity must cause your heart to reach at least 65 percent of its estimated maximum rate possible, a figure that is calculated based on your calendar age. Chart 9.4 shows the heart rate you should be aiming for when doing stamina-building exercises. The goal is to aim for sixty minutes a week at a heart rate of 65 to 80 percent of your age-adjusted maximum. This heart rate is the level that causes you to sweat in a cool room. Aerobic exercises cause you to sweat in a cool room and are excellent ways to make your arteries and immune system younger.

CHART 9.4

Boosting Your Heart Rate: How Many Heartbeats per Minute Should You Aim For?

Below is the approximate number of heartbeats per minute that different age groups reach when they're exercising at different percentages of their maximum heart rate. To get a good aerobic, stamina-building workout, you should aim for 65–80% of your maximum heart rate.

% of Maximum Heart Rate	Calendar Age (Years)								
	20s	30s	40s	50s	60s	70s	80s	90s	100
100	200	190	180	170	160	150	140	130	120
90	180	171	162	153	144	135	126	117	108
80	160	152	144	136	128	120	112	104	96
70	140	133	126	119	112	105	98	91	84
60	120	114	108	102	96	90	84	78	72
50	100	95	90	85	80	75	70	65	60
40	80	76	73	68	64	60	56	52	48

Note: Reaching 100% of your maximum possible heart rate is very hard to do and impossible to maintain. Also, it may not be a safe thing to do. Only high-level athletes can achieve and maintain a heart rate that is 90% of their maximum. Reaching 80% of your maximum heart rate should be your goal on the days you have a really strenuous workout. If you can get to 70% of your maximum heart rate and maintain it, you will be getting the benefit of a real stamina-building workout. Sixty percent should be your goal when you first start working out. It's a good place to be. Reaching 50% of your maximum heart rate means you're slacking off. If you want to get the benefits of stamina-building exercise, you'll need to boost your heart rate higher than this.

How do you measure your heart rate? When you are well into your workout, stop your exercise for a few seconds. Place the finger of one hand on your opposite wrist and search for the pulse point. It lies on the spot of your wrist just below the base of your thumb. Feel around for it. Make sure to use a finger, not your thumb, to feel for the pulse, since the thumb itself has a pulse point that can distort your reading. Some people advocate feeling your carotid—the artery in your neck. Do not compress both carotid arteries—meaning the left and the right side of your neck—at once, or you may become a candidate for the Darwin award (most physicians recommend that you not take your carotid pulse at all, since there is a small risk of causing a stroke). After you have found a pulse, count the number of heartbeats in 15 sec, subtract 1, and multiply by 4 to get your heart rate for 1 min. Remember, a heartbeat consists of two parts—an "in" and an "out." You should feel both. Count only the out phase. If you find it difficult to get this down, or if you want a more exact measure of your heart rate, buy a heart rate monitor. They are easily found at sporting goods stores, but can be expensive. You can even buy watches that contain a heart rate monitor.

Don't jump into stamina activities immediately. In fact, trying to do stamina-building activities before the other two types is the most common reason most individuals stop their exercise program. They find it too taxing to adopt stamina before general strength-building or resistance exercises. Adopt stamina activities third.

Resistance Exercises

Another reason it might be a good idea to do weight-lifting exercises first is that these kinds of exercises seem to protect the body against damage from free radicals, one of the possible hazards of stamina-building exercises. How does this benefit work?

Free radicals are charged particles that are natural by-products of chemical processes that occur when the body performs such functions as burning fuels or using oxygen. These free radicals can damage cells, promoting illness and aging. Study participants who performed both low- and high-intensity exercises with weights three times a week experienced less free-radical damage after exertion than people who did no weight training. Pumping iron seemed to enhance the body's natural defense system, conditioning the muscles to store more antioxidants for future events requiring stamina. Though we do not know if this storage of more antioxidants is responsible for protecting muscles against damage from free radicals, the protection does occur repeatedly.

Lifting weights or doing resistance exercises for eight of the twelve muscle groups two or three times a week (for as little as ten minutes total each time) just by itself makes you 1.7 years younger. Other age-reducing benefits are a decrease in bad cholesterol levels, an increase in healthy cholesterol levels, and a possible reduction in blood pressure. These benefits are additional to the 1.7 years younger your RealAge becomes from the exercise itself (see Chart 9.5). Of course, if you have ever had irregular heartbeats, severe angina (chest pain), hernias, back or joint pain, or uncontrolled high blood pressure, or are over thirty-five years of age (calendar age), you should discuss your exercise program with your physician first.

CHART 9.5

The RealAge Effect of the Minutes per Week You Spend on Strength-Building Exercises

Calendar Age	None	1–5 min	6–20 min	21–30 min	More than 30 min
			RealAge		
			MEN		
35	36.5	35	34.2	33.8	33.5
55	57.3	55	54.4	53.6	53.3
70	71.8	70	69.2	68.6	68.2
			WOMEN		
35	36.6	35	34.1	33.9	33.6
55	57.1	55	54.3	53.5	53.2
70	72.0	70	69.0	68.4	68.1

Exercise, Your Immune System, and Cancer

Have you noticed that active people seem to experience fewer colds and other illnesses? That's because people who are more physically fit tend to have younger immune systems. Although we don't really know why, we do know that exercise does more for the immune system than simply increase the body's resistance to colds. Exercise may help prevent such cancers as prostate, colon, and breast cancer. The exact relationship is not known, but men who exercise regularly have lower rates of prostate cancer than those who don't exercise regularly. People who are physically active have a 65 percent lower rate of colon cancer. About the same reduction occurs in breast cancer rates in women who exercise regularly, but more studies are required before a definitive statement can be made about the relationship between exercise and breast cancer.

Exercise and Your Bones

Inactivity and a sedentary lifestyle accelerate the aging of your skeletal and muscular systems. The most predictable effect of resistance exercise is that it increases the calcium content in bones, strengthening them and making them more resistant to fracture. Although many people believe that osteoporosis, a disease characterized by weakening of the bones, occurs only in women, it is becoming a growing danger to men as well.

If your exercise program is largely one that builds stamina (if it burns fat but doesn't build muscle), or if your training program is extremely intense, your muscles and bones may not be getting younger and stronger. To strengthen your muscles and bones, you need to perform activities that force your muscles to support weight and overcome resistance. In fact, studies have shown that elite athletes who have extremely low body mass (for example, marathon runners) may actually be at a higher risk of osteoporosis than people who train less intensely. Furthermore, intense stamina training may cause loss of calcium through perspiration. If this sounds like your exercise program, make sure you drink plenty of water while you exercise, and make sure you get approximately 1,600 milligrams of calcium a day, a little more than the usual RealAge optimum.

Exercise and Your Mind

A Great Way to Start the Day

It's tough to get started, but once you get rolling, doesn't exercise feel great? Many of my colleagues and friends work out in the early morning just so they have that feel-good kick for the rest of the day. They tell me that an early morning workout helps them stay positive all day long, laugh more easily, feel less stressed, and remain quick on their feet. Here's a question posed by a user of the RealAge website:

Dr. Mike: I've seen a lot recently in magazines and on TV that says we should do our exercises in the afternoon. For one thing, heart attacks occur more frequently in the morning. Also, one book about the body's time clock says our muscles are stronger and the body is more flexible in the afternoon. I am now uneasy about doing aerobic exercises first thing in the morning. Your opinion?—PS

Dear PS: The best time to exercise is any time you *can*, and anytime you can find time to do so *regularly*. Many people exercise first thing in the morning. As far as your muscles are concerned, a two- to five-minute warm-up walk or warm-up exercise period prior to aerobic exercises works just as well as a full day of "warming up," so it's not more risky to do aerobic exercise in the morning. I do mine in the morning. As soon as I wake up, I take an aspirin and vitamins (with a little fat first), to give me the anti-inflammatory and antioxidant protection those pills provide during and after exercise.—Dr. Mike

---

REALAGE CAFÉ TIP 9.2
Walk Down Memory Lane

Want to improve your memory? Try exercise. Researchers at the University of Illinois found that people who got regular aerobic exercise performed better at short-term memory tasks than people who didn't get such exercise. Subjects who added fifteen minutes to an hour of brisk walking a day to their usual routines improved their mental abilities significantly. Subjects showed better memory recall, quicker reaction times, and a greater ability to juggle complex information.

Emotional Well-Being

Most people experience other important by-products of regular physical activity: an improvement in mood, increased productivity, and a boost in self-esteem and confidence. It's no secret that physical activity improves emotional well-being, decreases stress, and helps ease depression. Researchers believe that the cause may be the release of beta-endorphins and serotonin, naturally occurring substances that help relieve pain and depression.

REALAGE CAFÉ TIP 9.3
Working Out Depression

Researchers have long known that aerobic exercise such as running or cycling can help relieve depression. However, new findings show that even moderate exercise can help brighten your mood. Nonaerobic exercise programs such as weight training or walking can have the same mood-elevating effects as aerobic workouts. Consistency appears to be key in treating depression through exercise: Sticking to a moderate program consistently may be more important than breaking a sweat occasionally.

The Basics of a RealAge Workout Plan

A balanced fitness program helps makes your RealAge 8 or more years younger. For the best results, you need to optimize each of the following three components of what is known as "physical activity":

1 General physical activity
2 Strength-building and flexibility exercises
3 Stamina-building exercises

In the earlier section on exercise and the cardiovascular system, we discussed general definitions and the optimal health order of incorporating these three types of physical activity into your fitness program. We now discuss the specifics of each component.

General Physical Activity

Most people who succeed at maintaining their exercise programs first start by increasing their levels of *general* physical activity—a simple and pleasurable way to make your RealAge as much as 3.4 years younger. Although twenty minutes a day doesn't seem like much, countless health benefits result from even this moderate amount of physical activity. Twenty minutes spent on an evening stroll can reduce your risk of a heart attack or stroke by 15 to 30 per-cent in just twenty weeks. Furthermore, studies suggest that similar health benefits can be attained from two twenty-minute sessions or three smaller sessions—ten or fifteen minutes each—of physical activity scattered through-out the day. The overall goal is to build *slowly* to a level of physical activity in which you are burning 3,500 kilocalories a week. (A kilocalorie is fundamen-tally the same amount of energy as a calorie. The difference is that the term *kilocalorie* is used to describe the expenditure of energy through exercise, and the term *calorie* is used to describe the consumption of energy in food.)

If you have little free time during the day, look for opportunities to be physi-cally active. Many people can take a twenty-minute walk during their lunch break. If you have one-on-one meetings, try a walking meeting. I started this during faculty evaluations—doing forty-five-minute one-on-one walks. My fac-ulty loved this—the meeting was never interrupted by phones or secretaries. And we both benefited by the extra activity. I do at least one of these walking meetings a day. If phone calls are part of your job activity, you can walk while using a cordless phone. If you drive, park a little farther away and walk to your destination.

Also, many everyday chores provide moderate physical exercise. Raking leaves or mowing the lawn with a powered push mower for thirty minutes produces almost half the recommended daily calorie burn. Try gardening or pushing the vacuum cleaner more vigorously and you'll be well on your way to burning the recommended 3,500 kilocalories per week. Chart 9.6 shows the number of

CHART 9.6
Number of Kilocalories Used during Various Activities

Activity	Kilocalories Used per Minute
Walking for pleasure	3.5
Bicycling for pleasure	4
Swimming, slow treading	4
Conditioning exercises, slow stretching	4
Vacuuming the carpet	4
Raking the lawn	4
Walking briskly	4–5
Painting your house	4.5
Mowing the lawn, walking behind power mower	4.5
Racket sports, table tennis, doubles tennis	5
Golf	5.5
General calisthenics	6
Skating (ice skating or roller in-line)	7
Soccer	7
Moving furniture	7
Stair stepper, ski machine	7
Running	8
Basketball	8
Cycling, fast or racing	10
Squash	12
Rowing	12

Source: Modified from B. E. Ainsworth et al., "Compendium of Physical Activities: Classification of Energy Costs of Human Physical Activities," Medicine and Science in Sports and Medicine, 25 (1993): 71–80.

kilocalories you burn in various forms of physical activity, and Chart 9.7 shows the RealAge benefits you receive based on the amount of physical activity you do in a week.

CHART 9.7

The RealAge Effect of the Number of Kilocalories Used in Physical Activity per Week

Calendar Age	Less than 500 kcal	500– 2,000 kcal	2,000– 3,500 kcal	3,500– 6,500 kcal	More than 6,500 kcal
			RealAge		
			MEN		
35	36.7	35	33.1	31.4	32
55	57.7	55	53.3	51.6	52
70	72.9	70	69	66.7	68.2
			WOMEN		
35	36.7	35	34.1	32.4	33
55	57.7	55	54.3	52	53
70	72.8	70	69	67.2	68.2

Strength and Flexibility

The second component of a balanced exercise program is strength-building exercise—the kind of exercise that builds muscle and bone. After the age of thirty, we lose muscle mass at the rate of 5 percent per decade. What's more, regular aerobic exercise won't prevent muscle loss, because it doesn't involve resistance. Even runners lose muscle mass if they don't strength-train, which is why their routines usually contain some form of resistance training, such as pressing or curling weights or running up hills. The key is this: If you can do a particular exercise more than twelve times with excellent form and technique, your strength gains are probably minimal; you're largely building the endurance (stamina) of that muscle. Stretching afterwards (flexibility exercises) helps maintain mobility and lessens the soreness when you start strength exercises. Here are a few important rules when doing strength-building exercises:

- Never sacrifice proper form by using too heavy a weight.
- Always think what muscles you are using when you do an exercise.
- Exercise specific muscles no more frequently than every other day.

Here's another question from the RealAge website:

Dr. Mike: I don't understand why you lump strength and flexibility exercises together. I thought they were two different things.—ST

Dear ST: Although strength and flexibility are very different activities, several studies link these two in determining a quality-of-life difference. Nevertheless, you have to do both in order to make your RealAge as young as it can be.—Dr. Mike

If you are just beginning to integrate strength and flexibility exercises into your workouts, it's important to get some guidance on the correct methods. Lifting weights incorrectly can lead to injury. Follow RealAge Strength Rule Number One:

Never sacrifice proper form for increased weight or increased repetitions.

With a little instruction, you'll be more likely to avoid injury and get the most effective workout possible. A good instructor can show you many possible exercises for strengthening each muscle group, so you can choose resistance exercises you enjoy. Log onto our website (www.RealAge.com) to see choices for each muscle group. We hope you'll enjoy these or find a trainer who will teach you other strength-building exercises you can enjoy.

 REALAGE CAFÉ TIP 9.4
Back Pain Be Gone

A tight tummy can do more than look good—it can actually help ease low back pain. Several studies confirm that stronger abdominal muscles can help minimize and, in some cases, eliminate low back pain. Try this simple exercise to strengthen your stomach.

Lie on your back and cross your arms lightly over your chest. Press the small of your back against the floor. Slowly lift only your head and shoulders off the floor to a height that feels comfortable. Do not do a full sit-up. Hold for a count of three. Repeat eight times. Gradually increase to twenty repetitions (see crunches on the website, www.RealAge.com).

Stamina-Building (Aerobic) Exercise

Would you like to make your heart younger? Go aerobic and increase your stamina. Aerobic exercises are continuous activities that almost always involve the large muscle groups and that last long enough to require the use of oxygen (this is the meaning of "aerobic") to produce energy. Rapid walking, running, cycling, rowing, aerobic dancing, kick-boxing, and swimming are all stamina-building, aerobic exercises. These exercises make your body more efficient at using oxygen to provide energy. Your heart pumps more blood with every stroke, your lungs take in and expel more air with every breath, and your muscles become more adept at extracting oxygen. The overall effect is a stronger, healthier cardiovascular system and a lower risk of cardiovascular disease, including heart disease, stroke, memory loss, impotence, and wrinkling of the skin. This translates to a younger arterial system and a younger RealAge.

Start every workout with a warm-up. Warm up your muscles by walking briskly or jogging slowly for two to five minutes. After your workout, cool down with a few stretches, holding each stretch for twenty seconds. (See our website for my suggestion on stretches. Tracy Hafen, the exercise physiologist for our University of Chicago Program for Executive Health, designed these stretches to be efficient and thorough.)

Build the intensity and duration of your program slowly. If you can walk rapidly for ten minutes at a time this week, try for eleven minutes next week. Don't increase by more than 10 percent per week. Each week your exercise program will seem easier, and you'll soon notice that all of your activities seem easier. You won't get out of breath as quickly, and you won't tire as easily. Then you can bring your exercise program to its former level of difficulty by increasing the intensity of your workouts. Once you have achieved a certain degree of fitness, workouts of shorter duration and higher intensity will provide the same health benefits as moderately intense workouts of longer duration. To assess how hard you're working during aerobic exercise, take the "talk test." If you can talk comfortably and easily while exercising, you could probably work a little harder. But if you're unable to maintain a conversation with your workout buddy, you're doing too much and should decrease your activity level.

Some of my patients use "sweat time" as their guide. They know that if an exercise program makes them sweat for at least twenty minutes three or more times a week, they're probably reaching 70 percent of their maximum heart rate. A regular program of exercise done at this level of intensity can make your RealAge more than 3 years younger (see Chart 9.8). Of course, the sweat

REALAGE CAFÉ TIP 9.5
Step on It

Ever wonder which exercise machine is best at helping you lose weight? A study published in the *Journal of the American Medical Association* compared caloric expenditures on stair-steppers, stationary cycles, rowing machines, combination cycle/rowing machines, cross-country ski machines, and treadmills. The study looked at three levels representing how hard people felt they were exerting themselves—light, medium, and hard. At all three levels, the treadmill came out on top, burning more calories per minute of perceived exertion than the other machines.

has to come from exercise, not environmental factors (a warm room or a hot afternoon) or too-warm clothing.

What is your "maximum heart rate"? Your maximum heart rate is the number of times your heart would beat per minute if it were working at its maximum capacity. To calculate this number, subtract your calendar age from 220. Your goal, during exercise, is to obtain a heart rate that is 65 to 80 percent of this number. For example, if you are fifty years old and have exercised regularly, you

CHART 9.8
The RealAge Effect of Minutes Spent on Stamina-Building Exercises* per Week

Calendar Age	0–5 min	6–15 min	16–35 min	36–60 min	More than 60 min
			RealAge		
			MEN		
35	36.7	35	33.1	32	31.4
55	57.7	55	53.3	52	51.6
70	72.9	70	69	68.2	66.7
			WOMEN		
35	36.7	35	34.1	33	32.4
55	57.7	55	54.3	53	52
70	72.8	70	69.0	68.2	67.2

*At a heart rate that is 65–90% of your age-adjusted maximum.

should aim for a heart rate of 111 to 136 beats a minute for sixty minutes a week (see Chart 9.4). By following these guidelines, you can be sure you're getting all the age-reducing benefits of an aerobic workout. How to determine your heart rate accurately during exercise is also described in Chart 9.4.

REALAGE CAFÉ TIP 9.6
Can Exercise Be Used to Spot-Reduce?

Everyone has one—a body area that just won't get fit. Be it thighs, tummy, or hips, there's a spot that just won't shape up. Can spot reducing make it go away? Unfortunately, no.

Working out a specific area, such as your abdominal or gluteal muscles, will build the muscle beneath the problem area. To reduce the fat on top, however, you have to do whole-body exercise. The body doesn't burn fat in one specific area but, rather, as part of a whole metabolic process. Studies on spot reducing have repeatedly shown that it doesn't work. So, if you want to lose fat from a particular area, focus on increasing your overall caloric expenditure and your muscle strength.

When you get more advanced in your physical activity program, you may need to pay even more attention to the practices that protect you against overuse injuries. Vary the intensity of your program by exercising at a high energy level three days a week and then working out less intensely the other days. You can also decrease your risk of injury by using the proper equipment and shoes for the specific physical activity you undertake. Shoes should provide support for your ankles and feet, particularly if you're involved in sports that stress your legs, knees, and ankles. If you prefer bicycling or skating, wear a helmet that fits. Add knee pads and shin guards to protect you further from injury. Sports equipment may seem expensive, but it's far less costly than medical bills.

Drink Plenty of Water

Dehydration poses perhaps the greatest risk to your health when you exercise, especially when you're exercising outdoors on a hot day. Make sure you're drinking enough water to replace the fluids lost through your exertions.

- Drinking water early and at regular intervals (before, during, and after a workout) is essential to replace all the water lost through sweating. In general, drink as much as you can drink comfortably.
- If adding flavor to your water helps you drink more, go ahead, but adding carbohydrates or salts is not necessary unless you work out heavily for more than an hour.

 REALAGE CAFÉ TIP 9.7
Water and Exercise

Have you ever wondered how much extra water you should drink when you exercise, to remain properly hydrated? The American Dietetic Association recommends drinking one to three extra glasses of water for each hour you exercise. This is in addition to the eight to twelve 8-ounce glasses of water a day that you should be drinking anyway.

When you exercise, drink water before you feel thirsty. According to a report in the *Journal of the American Dietetic Association*, mild dehydration, defined as a 2 percent loss of body weight, makes your athletic performance worse and hurts your health. By the time you begin to feel thirsty, you have already lost 12 percent of your body weight from dehydration.

Cool Down after You Exercise

A cool-down period allows your heart rate and breathing to return to normal slowly, and you will be less likely to experience the dizziness that sometimes results from stopping intense exercise too quickly. Be sure your heart rate decreases significantly *before* you lie down to stretch or bend forward with your shoulders below your waist. These two maneuvers can increase demand on the heart, and your heart is better able to handle this increased demand if it's beating at a slower rate. After exercise, I wait until my heart rate has dropped to 100 beats per minute before I lie down to stretch or bend over too far.

How Do I Get Started?

It's worth putting a little thought into setting up your exercise routine—you're more likely to enjoy your program and stick with it. The ideal physical activity provides just enough challenge to be stimulating and engaging without being frustrating. Furthermore, the fewer injuries you have, the less you feel like you're wasting your time, and the less influenced you are by negative forces around you, the more likely you will be to stick with a program. Here are some general principles for making your exercise program a permanent part of your life.

Set Yourself Up for Success

As Carol did, set goals that are achievable by *you*. She knew she could cross the threshold into a health club three times a week and made the commitment to reward herself if she did. To set yourself up for success, set goals that are well within your physical abilities and your commitment level. For example, it's better to set a goal of doing thirty minutes of exercise twice a week and accomplish that goal than it is to set a goal of thirty minutes three times a week and make it only twice. Although you'd be doing the same amount of physical activity, you'll feel successful when you make the first goal and feel like a failure when you don't make the latter goal. This could discourage you, as *nothing succeeds like success*. So, be like Carol and Janice—set goals that are realistic and achievable for *you*.

Fit Exercise into Your Schedule

When you create a program for exercise, consider what would work best with your schedule. Can you take a quick walk during your lunch break? Is it easier to hit the gym on your way to work? Don't worry if you don't have large stretches of time for exercise. The effects are cumulative, so spending ten minutes jumping rope before work, taking a ten-minute walk during lunch, and following up with a quick jog after work provide almost the same cardiovascular advantages as a thirty-minute aerobics class that expends the same kilocalories. Our website provides a ten-minutes-a-day program (Plan 10) that many of my patients have found doable, plus a sixty-minutes-three-times-a-week program (Plan 60) that other patients have liked. Determine what amount of time you can comfortably plan on, and start your program. You'll feel younger and stronger soon.

Start Gradually

Don't overdo it. Remember, you don't have to engage in strenuous exercise to gain the benefits of exercise. Even a moderate ten-minute walk is a good beginning. If you start with a burst of activity you can't sustain, you're risking exhaustion and injury, which can have a disastrous effect on your motivation.

Keep Building

Each week, do a little more. Whether it's the intensity or the duration of your workout, try to increase your workout by 5 to 10 percent each week. For example, if you lift weights, gradually increase the amount of weight you lift. But remember, never sacrifice proper form for increased weight. If you worked out for ten minutes per session last week, this week shoot for eleven minutes, and next week try to do twelve minutes.

Listen to Your Body

We have all heard the phrase, "No pain, no gain." Forget it. Exercise should not be painful. If it is, you should lower your pace or switch to another activity that uses different muscle groups. Also, your joints should never be painful. If a shoulder, an elbow, or another joint hurts, stop the activity that is causing pain immediately. If the pain recurs, or occurs without exercise, see your physician soon.

You may experience a burning sensation in the muscles that you're working, and, if you're exercising too strenuously, you may feel short of breath. These conditions are perfectly normal—they result when your muscles start to deplete the oxygen stores available to them. However, if you start to feel chest pains, nausea, irregular heartbeats, or lightheadedness and confusion, you should discontinue exercising and consult your doctor immediately.

Add Variety

Just as variety and enjoyment play important roles in your food choices, diversity makes your workouts more fun and more effective. Imagine putting your body through the same routine day after day. How long would the same exercise, with the same frequency, duration, and intensity, continue to be challenging? Not very long. Exercise is most effective when you're *challenging* your heart, lungs, and muscles to become more efficient.

Adding different forms of exercise to your life is easy when you consider the tremendous number of general physical activities, stamina-building activities, and strength- and flexibility-training exercises that are available. Note that all three types are required to gain the most age reduction from exercise.

Choose Enjoyable Activities

I cannot emphasize too much the importance of doing what you enjoy. For some people, exercise is more fun when it involves social interactions—for example, playing golf, or tennis, or tossing a Frisbee at the park. You can also use exercise as a way of spending time with your spouse, a friend, or your dog. If you're uncomfortable exercising in front of others or enjoy quiet solitude, you may prefer walking or running by yourself. Remember—you are far more likely to continue an exercise program if you're doing what you like.

REALAGE CAFÉ TIP 9.8
Workout Tune-up

If you find yourself slowing down toward the end of your workout, you may want to add some upbeat music to your routine. Researchers in England studied the effects of music tempo on exercise. They found that exercisers burned significantly more calories when they listened to fast-paced music.

To help you keep up the pace, add music that matches the tempo of your workout. You can purchase exercise CDs or tapes that allow you to choose the number of beats per minute that best matches your workout rate.

How Can I Stick with It?

Do you find yourself making excuses for not going to the gym? Although we know the benefits of exercise, sometimes it takes more than this to keep us motivated. Boredom with your exercise routine can result in missed sessions, lackadaisical performance, or total abstinence from exercise. Over the years, I've learned a few tricks to help me stick to my program. Simple as they sound, they really work!

Set Goals

If you don't have goals, this may be a big reason why your workouts are more burdensome than pleasurable. Set some short-term and long-term goals.

You can use Chart 9.8 to set your long-term age reduction goals: It shows how young you'll get as you increase the amount of kilocalories expended per week. Whatever your age reduction goals, challenge yourself, and your workouts will

REALAGE CAFÉ TIP 9.9

Dance Your Way to Health

Looking for a fun way to increase your physical activity? Try dancing. People of all ages can enjoy ballroom dancing, also known as dance sport. Whether you swing or samba, dancing fast for just thirty minutes is a terrific way to burn calories (4 to 7 calories per minute) and get a good workout. Also, dancing is a great way to increase your social circle. However, if you have cardiovascular disease or any other health risks, check with your physician before you incorporate dancing into your schedule.

become more meaningful. Post the goals where you'll see them frequently—every morning, for example.

What If It Isn't Fun?

You may need to stick with your exercise for a little longer than you expect before the enjoyment factor kicks in. Most people begin to feel stronger and younger within three months. Some begin to look forward to a workout in three weeks, and some take as long as five months. If you've gone five months and exercise is still not something you look forward to, you may want to try different activities, find a friend you really like to do activities with, or consider a trainer.

Make Exercise a Habit

For many people, once exercise becomes firmly entrenched in their daily routine, it's no longer a question of whether they should or shouldn't go to the gym or the tennis court. One way to make exercise a habit is to construct your daily routine so that exercise is a necessity. For example, leave your hair dryer, make-up, or shaving kit in your gym locker, so that you'll need to go to the gym before you go to work. If you play tennis with a friend, reserve the court for your next game *before* you leave; that way, you'll have a specific appointment with a friend. It's much harder to break an appointment with someone else than with yourself.

Learn Something New

Take up a sport you've never tried before. Learn a new dance style. Add new interest to your activity by hiring a trainer or instructor. An expert can help ensure that you're getting as much from your exercise as possible. He or she may also be able to suggest new elements, like a new dance step or a different exercise for firming your triceps. It's an easy way to pick up the pace of your program. I know many people who are developing a skill when they exercise—whether it's a sports skill or a dance skill.

Anticipate Obstacles

Most people believe they just don't have the time to exercise. You don't have time not to! A long, healthy life is built on physical fitness. Because exercise usually increases your productivity, energy level, and alertness, you're able to accomplish more on a regular basis when you exercise on a regular basis. So, by taking the time to exercise you really gain time—and it's quality time—for the rest of your life. If you are injured, find an alternative activity you can enjoy while the injured part is recovering. Even when traveling, find a hotel with a workout room, or bring resistance tubes or a jump rope with you.

Another common obstacle to exercise is the weather. If you live in a climate where the winter weather becomes harsh or the summers are too hot to exercise outdoors, consider at-home exercises, a health club, or a community center as alternatives to outdoor regimens.

Establish a Support System

Consider having your spouse or a friend join you when you walk or exercise, especially if you're trying to lose weight. One study found that those who participated in a weight-loss program with three friends or family members lost more weight and kept it off more successfully than those who participated by themselves. With a partner, you'll be more likely to show up and more likely to push each other to work harder, and you'll enjoy your workouts more. Even if you prefer to exercise by yourself, try to keep your friends and family involved in your progress. Their encouragement will keep you on track.

Try It for Just Five Minutes

Sometimes the biggest hurdle is just getting started. If it's time to work out and you feel like skipping your session, tell yourself, "I'll try it for *just five minutes.*" Once you get started, you'll feel more motivated, more energetic, and more likely to complete your workout.

Reward Yourself

When you have remained committed to your fitness regimen for a certain amount of time (you decide how long), reward yourself. For every year younger you get, treat yourself to a massage. Or reward yourself for increasing your exercise options by purchasing new gear for those activities. Many of my patients, like Carol, reward themselves with new exercise clothes or a new dress. Even something as simple as buying a new pair of socks and running shoes can inspire you to go for a jog.

Keep Your Perspective

Remember that you're making lifelong changes for a healthier, longer life-time. So, keep your perspective—if, on occasion, you can't do your exercise routine, there's always tomorrow. Just because you've been lax for three days straight—or even three weeks straight—doesn't mean it's all over and your efforts have gone down the drain. Once you've built muscle, even after you begin to lose it, it's just that much easier to get it back. Pick up at the beginning, and you'll be pleasantly surprised to find yourself climbing through the ranks much more quickly than you did the first time. There's always another opportunity—maybe even this afternoon—to make your RealAge younger.

What about the Risks of Exercise?

For most individuals, any risks that exercise might pose are minimal and can be avoided if physical activity is approached with common sense. Just remember not to overwork yourself. Never increase activity by more than 10 percent a week, take precautions to avoid injury, drink plenty of water, and be aware of your environment. Overuse injuries, the most frequent reasons for stopping a physical activity program, almost always occur because a person feels good enough to do much more than usual. Do not fall for that temptation—it may age you. Never, never increase your physical activity by more than 10 percent a week.

Is Exercise for Everyone?

What about Specific Medical Conditions?

Even if you have health problems, you can use exercise to slow the aging process. Whether you have cardiovascular disease or diabetes, or are obese, exercise is for you. But even though everyone can exercise, not every activity is appropriate for every person. If you're over the age of forty-five and have never participated in a program of consistent physical activity before, or if you have cardiovascular disease, asthma, arthritis, diabetes, or another special condition, you should consult a physician before starting your exercise program.

It's Never Too Late to Start

My favorite success stories involve two studies of retired citizens. Visualize a nursing home with people in wheelchairs and walkers. Then visualize these same people being able to abandon their wheelchairs. It's almost like a miracle cure at the hand of a faith-healing preacher. But this study was done by scientists, and the results happened not in one person but in half of all the residents who were dependent on wheelchairs in a nursing home. It happened because they started to do resistance exercises. Pretty amazing, but that's what happened. In this first study (the average age was eighty-three), more than half of the nursing home residents who were in wheelchairs were able to become more functional and independent after just sixteen weeks—only one-third of a year—of strength-training exercises (three forty-five-minute sessions a week).

Now visualize another group of people, who are sitting in a Starbucks. Someone tells half of them that if they start walking while drinking their coffee, they won't lose brain function. That is, they'll not only be able to keep their ability to walk, but they'll also hold onto their memory and intellectual functions. You'd walk, wouldn't you? That's what the scientists found in the second study. Retirees were assigned to groups that either walked while drinking their morning coffee or sat and/or stretched while drinking their morning coffee. When tested after six months, those in the walking groups showed an increase in IQ, whereas members of the sedentary groups showed a loss in IQ. A pretty good reward for such a small change in lifestyle, wouldn't you agree?

And I think there is no better reward than staying more vital and vigorous—living younger longer.

10

Menu Makeovers

The RealAge Plan: Eight Weeks to Better Taste

The RealAge Diet Plan provides two ways for you to shop, cook, and eat the RealAge way. Try Plan 1, Plan 2, or a combination of the two. Either way, it's easy to eat the RealAge way.

Plan 1: An off-the-shelf method of eating that doesn't use recipes but, instead, delicious, age-reducing, ready-to-go foods that you have in your refrigerator or pantry, or can obtain at your local grocery. The emphasis here is on *easy and fast!* We've provided fourteen days of menus to get you started.

Plan 2: Twenty recipes that are world-class delicious, nutrient rich, and calorie poor.

Plan 1: Healthy Eating off the Shelf!

So, you want to eat the RealAge way. You know that healthy eating can make your RealAge younger. But sometimes you just don't have the time to go to the farmers' market, stand in front of the stove peeling tomatoes for that great tomato sauce, or even *think* about food preparation. Also, maybe you don't like to cook. Often it's 6 o'clock and you don't have any ideas about dinner. What can you do? Many people head straight for the nearest place with aging-food—perhaps the one with the golden arches. At these times, if you're like me, you just want to know if there's any kind of delicious, healthful food you can eat that's easy, fast, and ready to go!

The good news is that eating for great flavor that makes you younger with every bite can be as easy as reading the next few pages. They describe a simple, easy-to-follow menu plan that features RealAge foods you can eat every day of the week.

This fast and easy method of healthful eating—Plan 1—has two parts:

- A description of the foods that make your RealAge younger—"RealAge foods"—and how you should eat them. This listing is a general menu guide that shows you how to apply the nutrient-rich, calorie-poor, world-class delicious concepts of earlier chapters. We suggest you eat often— five or even six times a day—so you don't get hungry between meals and eat anything in sight.
- A description of fourteen days' worth of simple, super-fast meals that require very little preparation and either no cooking time or only five or ten minutes of cooking time.

The RealAge Foods

We give the following foods the RealAge "Seal of Approval." They are nutrient rich, calorie poor, and delicious. If possible, purchase these foods fresh and eat them fresh.

Vegetables

Eat vegetables of all kinds, not only for their flavor, but also for their anti-oxidants and beneficial phytochemicals. Especially healthful are *tomatoes, onions, garlic, sweet potatoes, winter squash, kale, asparagus, purslane* (a green used in salads), *mushrooms, avocados,* and *chilies.* Brightly colored vegetables such as squash and asparagus have lots of carotenoids, and leafy greens such as kale and Swiss chard have lots of B vitamins. Almost all vegetables are low in calories and can be eaten in quantity. Eat vegetables raw (tomatoes and avocados), steam or sauté them, or roast them at high temperature. Remember to eat them with a little oil to aid absorption of their great nutrients.

Fruits

Eat them all, but especially *apples, berries, cranberries, grapefruit, grapes, kiwis, oranges,* and *plums.* Berries, apples, and oranges are full of age-reducing flavonoids, and kiwis are a great source of vitamin C. Grapes give us a snack for all ages, plus powerful resveratrol and catechins. Even the skins of citrus contain antioxidants, and just a little scrape of citrus zest gives a lot of flavor. Bake, blend, or eat fresh fruits.

Grains

Eat any and all grains but especially *oats, whole wheat, brown rice, wild rice, quinoa,* and *barley.* The less refined, the better. Packed with fiber, oats consumed in sufficient quantity each day can lower your cholesterol. Quinoa is a wonderful ancient choice and a complete protein to boot. When prepared simply—steamed or in a quick pilaf—grains have relatively few calories yet are filling and satisfying.

Beans

Even though all beans are good—whether black beans, kidney beans, lentils, or peas—*soybeans* and *soy products* have unusually high levels of isoflavones, which may protect against breast cancer and ease the symptoms of menopause. Soybeans also have an excellent omega-3 fatty acid content, which actively lowers (lousy) LDL cholesterol. And, soybeans, like all beans, are packed with lean vegetable protein, which helps fuel the fire of muscle building and age reduction. Luckily, tofu, soy milk, and even soy hot dogs carry these same age-reducing benefits. Cook beans in water (or use canned, drained beans) and then mash them into pâtés and spreads, mix them into casseroles, toss them into salads, or stir them in with rice and chilies.

Fish

All types of fish are good. Many people believe it's the omega-3 fatty acids, particularly prevalent in cold-water saltwater fish, that make fish so age reducing. All we really know, however, is that eating fish makes your RealAge younger. Its protein is lean and high quality and its flavor is, of course, delicious. Fish belongs in the center of your plate. Bake, grill, sauté, or broil fish.

Nuts

All nuts are nutritious, but especially *walnuts, almonds, Brazil nuts,* and *pecans.* Nuts can make you younger, if you're moderate about the portions. Calories are the only issue, so if you are really thin, nuts can be eaten in quantity. Because nuts are high in polyunsaturated fatty acids, when nuts replace saturated, solid-at-room-temperature fat and protein in your diet, they actively prevent heart disease and keep lousy cholesterol from forming plaques in your arteries. Also, nuts are a great source of selenium, a chemical that helps the body fight oxidation. Eat nuts one by one at the start of a meal or mix a few into pancakes and desserts.

Healthy Oils

We recommend olive oil, canola oil, and nut oils. Both olive and canola oils are healthful, but for different reasons. Olive oil has more monounsaturated fat—75 percent—than any other commonly used oil; canola oil is second, with 61 percent. However, canola oil has more omega-3 fats (11 percent) than olive oil (1 percent) and less saturated fat (7 percent) than olive oil (15 percent). Although both olive and canola oils are excellent for cooking, olive oil is especially good for salad dressings. Nut oils, which are also high in polyunsaturated fats, have the extra benefit of imparting an intense, delicious flavor. Remember to use oils sparingly, as all oils contain about 125 calories per tablespoon. Try an oil-mister or drizzle just a little extra-virgin olive oil on a pizza at the very end of the baking process. Also use a little olive oil to dress roasted beets or to finish hummus.

Healthy Sources of Protein

Lean red meat, poultry, and game should be eaten only occasionally. These sources of protein are not for every day, week, or even month. Instead, try fish and other sources of protein. Egg whites are a favorite RealAge food—light as a feather, pure protein, and able to carry flavor easily. Egg whites make great omelets and help lentil and other burgers keep their shape. Skim milk and nonfat and low-fat yogurts are delicious and have just as much calcium as their full-fat counterparts but none of the saturated fat. You can use nonfat milk and yogurts in quick breads, blend them into smoothies, or just snack on them. Low-fat cheeses have great flavor and good calcium and protein content and taste much better than their nonfat counterparts. Low-fat cheeses should be used as garnishes, so that all of their color and flavor is right on top.

Beverages

The beverages we especially recommend are *water, tea, soy milk,* and *red wine.* Water is the best beverage—sparkling, flavored, or just straight from the bottle or tap. Drink lots every day. Tea is another great choice. All natural teas have flavonoids, plant pigments that protect you against upper-digestive-tract cancers, heart disease, and aging. Soy milks are good for everyday cereal and some baking needs, especially rice pudding. Red wine, a glass a day, is also age reducing—maybe due to its resveratrol and catechins, but certainly for its alcohol. Many other beverages—such as coffee, skim milk, and diet soft drinks—do not appear to have a major aging effect one way or the other. If you enjoy these beverages and do not have a specific condition triggered by them, be sure to get extra potassium and calcium, and then enjoy them.

Food Choices to Avoid (Because They Will Cause You to Age Faster)

Some foods will almost invariably make you less vigorous and vital and your RealAge older. We recommend avoiding the following:

- Oils: Beef tallow, butterfat, coconut oil, palm oil, lard, and partially hydrogenated oils
- Animal foods that are not fish, especially fatty red meat, fatty poultry, and game
- Dairy foods that contain saturated fat, especially cream, whipping cream, half-and-half, triple cream cheeses, whole cow's milk, and whole goat's milk

Fourteen Days of Easy Off-the-Shelf Meals

Here are the menus for the fourteen days of the Plan 1 meals. The first day's menu is for the day when you have no time—zero minutes!—to cook. The second day's menu is for the day when you have five minutes to spare for cooking for the whole day. The third day's menu takes about ten minutes. The fourth day is like the first, when you have no time to cook, the fifth like the second, etc. All the menus require less than ten minutes to prepare.

Chart 10.1 shows how the Plan 1 meals and menus stack up against the RealAge optimum values for the factors known to reduce aging. The amazing thing is that each meal tastes great. You can find the ingredients for these meals in most supermarkets, nearly anywhere. Feel free to add beverages from the list above in addition to the ones we've suggested. And, by the way, if you can spare even twenty minutes for cooking, you can always substitute one of the Plan 2 dishes into these Plan 1 menus.

CHART 10.1
The Nutritional Content of the Plan 1 Off-the-Shelf Meals

Here's how the Plan 1 off-the-shelf meals and menus compare with the RealAge Optimum values for the factors that are known to affect aging:

Age-Reducing Factor	Nutritional Content of the Plan 1 Menus	RealAge Optimum Amount
Calories per day (on average)	1,676	
Protein (g/day)	61.6	
Carbohydrates (g/day)	259	
Fat (g/day)	55.9	
% of calories that is fat	26	About 25%
% of fat that is saturated	18.3	Less than 33%
Saturated fat (g/day)	12.0	Less than 20
% of fat that is monounsaturated	35.1	More than 40%
Cholesterol (mg/day)	48.6	Less than 150
Fiber (g/day)	42.8	25 or more
Sodium (mg/day)	2,413	2,400 or less
Potassium (mg/day)	3,716	3,000 or more
Iron (mg/day)	17.1	12–20
Calcium (mg/day)	674	1,200 or more
Folate (mcg/day)	391	700 or more
Vitamin E (IU/day)	10	400 or more
Vitamin C (mg/day)	293	1,200 or more
Fish (ounces/week)	14.0	12 or more
Nuts (ounces/week)	7	5 or more
Lycopene (servings/day)	3	1.5 or more
Flavonoids (mg/day)	31.6	30 or more

Note: These analyses include the nutrients found in the snacks, tea, and desserts in each day's plan. Chapter 5 discusses the supplements we recommend (not included in the nutrient calculations above)

Day One (Required cooking time: None)

Breakfast:	Kashi high-fiber cereal with fresh blueberries and soy milk Orange or grapefruit juice (preferably with extra pulp) Vanilla soy milk and brewed tea
Lunch:	Peanut or soy nut butter and whole-fruit spread or whole-strawberry preserves on whole wheat bread Two plums A glass of soy or skim milk
Dinner:	Six Brazil nuts and six almonds Packaged mixed salad greens, plus chopped scallions, bell peppers, ripe tomatoes, and avocado with chunks of canned tuna packed in water, drizzled with an excellent bottled olive oil-based salad dressing Six whole grain crackers A glass of red wine (optional)
Dessert:	Fresh strawberries dipped in one half ounce of melted dark (not milk) chocolate
Snack:	Whole wheat pretzels with good yellow mustard

Day Two (Required cooking time: Five minutes)

Breakfast:	Purchased cut-up fruit topped with raspberry, blueberry, or strawberry low-fat yogurt Whole wheat English muffin spread with almond butter and apple butter
Lunch:	Six walnuts and six pistachios A microwaved bowl of Progresso tomato or lentil soup Store-bought hummus, spread on whole wheat pita bread Iced tea
Snack:	Frozen-fruit bar or strawberry sorbet
Dinner:	Canned fat-free refried black beans heated with salsa, wrapped in two whole wheat tortillas, with fresh tomato and feta cheese Canned pineapple chunks in their own juice Iced tea
Dessert:	A ripe pear (or canned pear halves) with blue cheese
Snack:	A handful of walnuts and a cup of cut-up fruit

Day Three (Required cooking time: Ten minutes)

Breakfast: Raisin bran with extra raisins or chopped dates
Soy or skim milk
Black tea with soy milk (optional)

Lunch: Sautéed veggie burgers on toasted whole grain English muffin with sliced tomato, red onion, high-quality catsup, and romaine lettuce
Baby carrots with spicy brown mustard
Cranberry juice cocktail

Snack: A small baked sweet potato, with bottled salsa

Dinner: Twelve nuts of any type
Broiled salmon fillet
Whole wheat couscous rehydrated in spicy V8 juice
Microwaved precut broccoli and cauliflower florets, spritzed with lemon juice and toasted diced almonds
Whole grain dinner roll spread with avocado

Dessert: Scoop of frozen chocolate Soy Velvet with fresh raspberries on top

Snack: Low-fat yogurt covered with raisins
An apple

Day Four (Required cooking time: None)

Breakfast: Pineapple-orange smoothie, with silken tofu and low-fat soy milk
Whole toasted whole wheat English muffin spread with peanut butter or apricot preserves or whole fruit spread
Brewed tea

Lunch: Store-bought baba ghanoush (eggplant and tahini dip) on whole wheat pita with salad-bar-purchased chopped fresh tomato, green onions, and jalapeño chiles
Whole baby carrots with yogurt-dill dip or tomato salsa
A glass of low-fat soy or skim milk

Snack: A navel orange
Two soft dried plums stuffed with almonds

Dinner: Progresso or Campbell's Healthy Choice minestrone soup, with added scallions and chopped sundried-tomato bits
Prepared shredded cabbage for coleslaw, tossed with canola oil mayonnaise and Dijon mustard or balsamic vinegar
Seven- or nine-grain crusty bread with a half ounce of feta cheese
A glass of red wine (optional)

Dessert: Frozen strawberries and bananas blended to thicken soy chocolate milk sweetened with chocolate syrup and topped with maraschino cherries

Day Five (Required cooking time: Five minutes)

Breakfast: Hot rolled oats, microwaved with soy milk, and topped with currants, and chunks of mango
Calcium- and vitamin D-enriched, extra-pulp orange, tangerine, or grapefruit juice
Brewed tea

Lunch: Avocado, canned tuna, romaine lettuce, and chipotle chile in adobo sauce or tomato-chipotle salsa, such as Frontera Foods brand, rolled up in corn tortillas
Microwaved corn on the cob
Iced tea

Snack: A handful of toasted honey soy nuts, with a few reserved, to be sprinkled on a toasted whole wheat English muffin topped with peanut butter and honey

Dinner: Whole wheat bulgur simmered for a minute in V8 juice, topped with salad-bar-purchased jalapeño chiles, firm tofu chunks, and spicy black and green olives, or good-quality bottled olives, such as Santa Barbara Olive Company brand
Low-fat vanilla yogurt with red and green grapes and a little granola
A glass of red wine (optional)

Dessert: A banana, split down the center, sprinkled with shaved high-quality dark chocolate or M&M's, and drizzled with no-added-sugar strawberry syrup

Snack: Healthy trail mix (low on saturated or trans fats, high on nuts, dried fruit, and fiber)

Day Six (Required cooking time: Ten minutes)

Breakfast: Cheerios, with fresh apple slices or chopped dried apples, with low-fat soy or skim milk
Sliced honeydew melon
Brewed tea

Lunch: Blended gazpacho soup: fresh tomatoes, cucumbers, onions, sherry vinegar, extra-virgin olive oil and parsley
Feta cheese wedge, with lemon and olives
A bunch of red grapes
Iced tea

Snack: A small handful of toasted walnuts plus nonfat raspberry yogurt

Dinner: Tuna steak brushed with hoisin sauce (or barbecue sauce) and roasted
A sweet potato, microwaved
Microwaved precut broccoli and cauliflower florets, spritzed with lemon juice and toasted sliced almonds
A glass of red wine (optional)

Dessert: Snack-size cans of chocolate pudding, made with good Dutch cocoa, with cinnamon red hots stirred in

Snack: Dried tart cranberries and a ripe pear

Day Seven (Required cooking time: None)

Breakfast: Corn flakes mixed with All-Bran flakes, plus fresh sliced strawberries and low-fat soy milk
Orange or grapefruit juice enriched with calcium and vitamin D and preferably with extra pulp
Brewed tea

Lunch: 1 percent low-fat cottage cheese mixed with fresh tomatoes, chopped green onions, and good salsa
Microwaved broccoli and cauliflower florets, with teriyaki sauce
A glass of low-fat soy milk

Snack: Golden raisins and a banana

Dinner: Takeout grilled portobello mushrooms on a whole wheat burger bun, with arugula, sliced tomato, red onion, and thinly sliced fresh herbed goat cheese
Whole wheat couscous rehydrated in spicy V8 juice
A glass of red wine (optional)

Dessert: Blended frozen mixed berries with a little lime juice and honey, over chocolate nonfat frozen yogurt

Snack: A small handful of toasted sunflower seeds, and sliced jicama sticks

Day Eight (Required cooking time: Five minutes)

Breakfast: Blended smoothie made of fresh cantaloupe, peach yogurt, peach halves, ice, a small amount of honey, and a little silken tofu
Crunchy whole wheat sourdough pretzels, spread with peanut butter
Brewed hot tea

Lunch: Sliced organic skinless rotisserie chicken breast mixed with raisins, olives, and pine nuts, moistened with extra virgin olive oil and tomato sauce
Takeout brown rice
Sliced jicama and fennel, sprinkled with orange juice and ground cumin
Iced tea

Snack: Whole dates and fresh figs or a tangerine

Dinner: Peppered mackerel fillet, such as Ducktrap brand
Canned chickpeas, with fresh tomatoes, sun-dried tomatoes, parsley, lemon juice, and olive oil over packaged mixed salad greens
Whole grain or nutty crackers
A glass of red wine (optional)

Dessert: Slices of orange and grapefruit, splashed with Cointreau (optional), or orange juice concentrate, and toasted sliced almonds

Snack: A small handful of toasted cashews, and thin slices of candied, crystallized ginger

Day Nine (Required cooking time: Ten minutes)

Breakfast: Egg white omelet with whole wheat toast, spread with whole fruit apricot preserves, and sprinkled with sunflower seeds
Toasted whole wheat herb bread
Low-fat soy or skim milk, brewed tea

Lunch: Microwaved zucchini, black olives, and tomatoes over sliced polenta or wild mushroom–flavored polenta from a tube
Takeout grilled shrimp, folded into warm corn tortillas, sprinkled with small amounts of shredded Sonoma garlic-jack cheese and chopped cilantro
Iced tea

Snack: Dried figs and a tangelo

Dinner: Takeout sushi and sashimi, with pickled ginger and wasabi
Salad-bar-purchased salad of baby corn, water chestnuts, watercress, rice-wine vinegar, sunflower seeds
An apple, pear, or apple-pear
A glass of white wine (optional)

Dessert: Pineapple rings caramelized in a hot nonstick skillet, with a few grains of crushed black pepper and a squirt of fresh lime juice, over low-fat vanilla frozen yogurt, such as Häagen-Dazs brand

Snack: A small handful of pecans, and a small piece of very good dark chocolate

Day Ten (Required cooking time: None)

Breakfast: Mixed Corn Chex with Kashi high-fiber flakes, plus slices of banana, a sprinkle of fresh nutmeg, and soy or skim milk
Orange or grapefruit juice enriched with calcium and vitamin D, and preferably with extra pulp
Brewed tea

Lunch: Peanut or soy nut butter and whole strawberry preserves on whole wheat bread
Terra-brand or olive oil vegetable chips
Plums (two)
A glass of low-fat soy or skim milk

Snack: A small handful of dried apricots, and fresh sweet cherries

Dinner: Takeout grape leaves, stuffed with brown rice and tomato
Takeout baba ghanoush (roasted eggplant dip)
Takeout hummus (chickpea dip)
Packaged, washed, mixed salad greens, with an olive oil–based dressing
Toasted whole wheat pita bread
A glass of red wine (optional)

Dessert: Fresh strawberries and candied ginger sticks dipped in melted dark chocolate

Snack: A handful of toasted almonds

Day Eleven (Required cooking time: Five minutes)

Breakfast: A smoothie of peach frozen yogurt, canned peach halves and fresh ginger, blended with low-fat soy milk and silken tofu
Toasted whole wheat English muffin, half spread with almond butter and half with apple butter
Brewed hot tea

Lunch: A microwaved bowl of Progresso or Campbell's Healthy Choice Black Bean Soup
Store-bought tabouli, scooped up with whole grain or nutty crackers, and large sliced red radishes and celery stalks, dressed with lemon and extra-virgin olive oil
Iced tea

Snack: Dried papaya chunks and dried mango slices or fresh whole kiwis, or bananas

Dinner: Frozen salmon burgers, thawed and pan-roasted, on whole wheat buns with canola mayonnaise and minced garlic
Mesclun salad greens, plus canned beets drizzled with walnut oil and balsamic vinegar
A glass of fruity red wine (optional), and iced tea

Dessert: A bowl of mixed whole fresh blueberries, blackberries, strawberries, and raspberries in 1 percent milk, with cinnamon and mini chocolate chips

Snack: A small handful of Brazil nuts, plus some Shredded Wheat Minibites

Day Twelve (Required cooking time: Ten minutes)

Breakfast: Breakfast burrito (sautéed egg whites and one egg yolk with salsa, and cilantro, all wrapped in a large toasted whole wheat tortilla)
Muskmelon or cantaloupe
Low-fat soy or skim milk, tea

Lunch: Microwaved organic white bean soup with added canned diced tomatoes and a sprinkle of curry powder
Rykrisp or other whole grain or nutty crackers
Low-fat whole fruit yogurt, with melon chunks from the salad bar

Snack: Watermelon, with oatmeal cookies

Dinner: Cured, smoked salmon spread with a little horseradish, sprinkled with fresh dill, on toasted nutty whole wheat bagels
Cucumber spears, whole carrots, fennel sticks
Cinnamon applesauce

Dessert: Hot chocolate soy milk, with a little Godiva liqueur (optional) and melted marshmallows

Snack: A small handful of hazelnuts and a few large spiced Sicilian green olives

Day Thirteen (Required cooking time: Five minutes)

Breakfast: Blended smoothie made from frozen raspberries, lemon juice, all-fruit raspberry preserves with sweetener, soy milk, and ice
Toasted whole grain millet bread, such as Natural Ovens brand, with half almond or peanut butter and half pumpkin or apple butter
Brewed hot tea

Lunch:	Focaccia spread with black-olive paste, such as San Remo brand, bottled roasted red peppers, and fresh basil Cherry or grape tomatoes Navel orange
Snack:	A small handful of toasted pine nuts and a few sun-dried tomatoes packed in olive oil, pressed into hearty whole grain millet bread
Dinner:	Sliced, baked five-spice tofu, such as White Wave brand, topped with spicy peach chutney, stuffed into whole wheat pita pockets Cooling mint yogurt, mixed with 1-percent cottage cheese Cucumber and onion salad Iced tea
Dessert:	Lemon sorbet, such as Double Rainbow brand, with strawberries in grappa
Snack:	A small handful of toasted, spiced pecans, and Simon's microwaved popcorn (see RealAge Cafe Tip 4.12)

Day Fourteen (Required cooking time: Ten minutes)

Breakfast:	Old-fashioned rolled oats with plums, prunes, and maple syrup Pineapple-orange juice Low-fat soy or skim milk, roasted green tea
Lunch:	Sliced lean turkey breast, with sliced apple, romaine leaves, and a little fresh goat cheese, layered on a crunchy whole wheat sourdough baguette, slathered with honey mustard Steamed or microwaved whole asparagus, dressed with sesame oil and sesame seeds Store-bought blackberry smoothie, such as Odwalla brand
Snack:	Fresh whole mango, with lime juice and chile powder
Dinner:	Whole wheat couscous, rehydrated in tomatillo salsa and water Whole acorn squash, sliced in eighths, seeded and microwaved, and topped with tomato-garlic sauce and chopped red onion A glass of red wine
Dessert:	Pumpkin pie with toasted almond crust, served warm
Snack:	A small handful of toasted pumpkin seeds, and some Cheerios

Plan 2: Twenty Recipes to Use by Themselves or to Mix and Match with Plan 1 Meals

Plan 2 consists of twenty new and exciting dishes made from nutritious ingredients from all the food groups. These recipes were selected from over two hundred tested and are provided in the next chapter, Chapter 11. To create your own RealAge diet, use the recipes by themselves, or mix and match them with meals from Plan 1. No bland diet foods here. From morning smoothies full of immunity-boosting berries to delightful burrito lunch, to age-defying, day-brightening dinners of Pan-Grilled Citrus Salmon over Asian Slaw, each recipe provides a balance of delicious foods and nutrients and makes you younger.

What criteria did we use when creating our recipes? To be included in this book, each recipe had to meet four requirements:

1 It had to taste "world-class great!"
2 It had to make your RealAge younger.
3 It had to help retrain your palate.
4 It had to be quick to prepare (under thirty minutes).

Over one hundred recipes have now excelled at these four tests, and we hope to have all of these recipes for you before too long. We only have space enough to provide twenty in this book.

"Wow, That Tastes World-Class Great!"

John, who is both a medical doctor and a professional chef, uses RealAge principles to make delicious foods. Most of our recipes were developed in his kitchen. They were then tested at a nutrition center, and then taste-tested in regular homes. For the taste tests, we used a 0 to 10 scale that is specific to this book and in sync with Mike's cut-to-the-chase style. Using the scale, we rated the recipes for taste, color, and texture (Chart 10.2 shows some of the guidelines we used). Only recipes that consistently earned an 8 or higher (order again in a restaurant) from both men and women were included in this book. Food can taste so great there is no need to waste eating on only okay food. Each bit of food you put in your mouth should be "world-class" great.

And you can choose to have only food that tastes that good. Even better, these foods take less than thirty minutes to prepare.

Each Recipe Makes Your RealAge Younger

Each recipe was created to make you younger. Many are loaded with flavonoids, the right vitamins, soluble fiber, excellent antioxidants, and other age-reducing nutrients. Whenever a recipe calls for fat, it's almost always anti-aging monounsaturated and polyunsaturated fats (including omega-3 fatty acids) and not saturated or hydrogenated fats.

To prove that great taste can make you younger, we also calculated how much younger each recipe would make you *if* the dish were eaten twelve times a year ("the RealAge effect").

CHART 10.2

The Rating Scale for the RealAge Recipes

Based on Taste, Color, and Texture:	Rating
I wouldn't feed this to my neighbor's dog—the one that keeps me up all night.	0
I wouldn't send this back at a restaurant, but I wouldn't order it again, either.	6
I'd order this again at a restaurant.	8
This is almost as good as great sex.	10

Each Recipe Helps Retrain Your Palate

When you were born, your palate wasn't particularly fond of foods made with saturated fat—Krispy Kreme doughnuts, Cinnabons, or deep-fried onion "blossoms." The amount of saturated and trans fats in each of these is more than three days' worth of what you really need. In fact, you probably get three days older every time you eat one. If you've become fond of those huge piles of sugar and grease, here's how to retrain your taste buds.

Training the palate to love olive oil or infused, flavored, cold-pressed canola oil, or tuna is just that—training. So, just like an athlete, train gradually. Work up to it a little at a time. If you drink whole milk and decide to switch to skim, it will take about eight weeks before you think that whole milk (or even 2 percent milk) tastes like cream—too rich to drink! After eight weeks of these delicious recipes, either by themselves or combined with the off-the-shelf Plan 1 meals, most "regular food" will taste less healthy, more aging, and not quite right. After eight weeks of retraining your palate, deep-fried tortilla chips will taste greasy and oily, and you'll either not want them at all or only a few.

You'll love the taste of our food. But it will take eight weeks to make the full transition. Give it a try!

Easy-Does-It Recipes

Each RealAge recipe had to be simple to prepare and straightforward to cook. In fact, amateur cooks determined whether the recipe could be prepared—from start to finish—in less than thirty minutes. Brand-name items were suggested only when they were widely available and were particularly suitable for the recipe. If a particular ingredient might be a little difficult for you to find, we suggest possible substitutions.

Here's something else we're working on to make healthy eating a little easier for you. We are trying to make it easier to order your ingredients on the Internet so you can have them delivered to your door! The arrangements for ordering in various cites haven't been completed, but we hope all you'll have to do is go to our website (www.RealAge.com), click on the order button for the week or the recipe, fill in a few blanks, and voilá! The ingredients will be delivered to your door (or even your friend's door, if you want to give a gift of youthful eating).

It Takes Only Eight Weeks of World-Class Eating to Retrain Your Palate

After eight weeks of eating the RealAge way, you will have retrained your palate. You can use one of our twenty recipes as a guide in planning your own meals, or you can create your own. When you're short on time or energy, feel free to repeat your favorites. Creating your own menus allows you to focus on not only your own tastes, but also your own interests in staying young, whether it's reducing your bad cholesterol levels, fighting cancer, or controlling your blood sugar levels. Retraining your palate can be an enjoyable step in making yourself younger.

You can make yourself younger with either plan.

Try Plan 1, Plan 2, or a combination of the two. Following either plan makes your calendar age about 12 to 13 years younger. Once you start, you'll see how much fun it is to continue; the energy and health of more youthful years are the great rewards of consistency.

11

Recipes

Here are twenty recipes that make your RealAge younger. To retrain your palate in eight weeks, mix or match with the off-the-shelf menus in Plan 1.

Coconut-Banana Tapioca Pudding

Preparation time: Two minutes	Four servings (yields about 3 cups pudding)
Cooking time: Twelve minutes	265 calories per serving, 30 percent from fat

RealAge effect if eaten twelve times a year: Can dessert really be good for you? This one can—and it can lower your RealAge by 2.6 days. Thank goodness for the alcohol in rum, and the potassium in bananas (and the flavor in this pudding)!

RealAge effect ingredients: Banana, soy-milk, nuts, alcohol (potassium, alcohol, calcium, healthy protein)

INGREDIENTS

One 14-ounce can light unsweetened coconut milk, such as "A Taste of Thai" brand
¾ cup fat-free or light soy milk
¼ cup quick-cooking tapioca
⅛ teaspoon salt
2 tablespoons packed brown sugar
2 ripe bananas, sliced lengthwise in half and crosswise into ½-inch chunks
¼ cup slivered almonds, toasted
1½ tablespoons dark rum, such as Myers's
2 tablespoons chopped mint leaves (optional)

PREPARATION

In a medium saucepan, combine coconut milk, soy milk, tapioca, and salt. Slowly bring to a simmer over medium heat, stirring constantly. Simmer, stirring constantly until mixture just begins to thicken, about three minutes (mixture will be thin). Remove from heat; stir in sugar until melted. Let stand in saucepan uncovered twelve minutes or until thickened, stirring once. Stir in bananas; transfer to serving cups. Top with almonds and rum. Garnish with mint, if desired.

SUBSTITUTIONS

Fat-free milk may replace the soy milk.

TIPS

Let this pudding sit for a few minutes in your serving cups, after you've made it. It will thicken, while still retaining the mouth-filling warmth you can't wait for.

NUTRITIONAL ANALYSIS

Total Fat (g) 9.0	Sodium (mg) 40	Vitamin A (RE) 10
Fat Calories (kc) 81	Calcium (mg) 57	Beta-carotene (RE) 36
Cholesterol (mg) 4.8	Magnesium (mg) 86	Vitamin C (mg) 8
Saturated Fat (g) 3.2	Zinc (mg) 1.1	Vitamin E (mg) 2.58
Polyunsaturated Fat (g) 1.0	Selenium (mcg) 1	Thiamin B_1 (mg) 0.15
Monounsaturated Fat (g) 2.8	Potassium (mg) 653	Riboflavin B_2 (mg) 0.16

NUTRITIONAL ANALYSIS (*continued*)

Fiber (g) 2.6	Flavonoids (mg) 0	Niacin B_3 (mg) 1.4
Carbohydrates (g) 29.7	Lycopene (mg) 0	Vitamin B_6 (mg) 0.39
Sugar (g) 16.3	Fish (oz) 0	Folic Acid (mcg) 33
Protein (g) 6.1	Nuts (oz) 0.2	Vitamin B_{12} (mcg) 0

Sweet Balsamic-Glazed Oranges and Berries

Preparation time: Ten minutes	Four servings
Cooking time: Three minutes	194 calories per serving, 4 percent from fat

RealAge effect if eaten twelve times a year: 12.1 days younger. This dessert is actually good for your RealAge! It is low in saturated fat, low in calories, and delicious.

RealAge effect ingredients: Oranges, strawberries (vitamin C, fiber, calcium, potassium, folic acid)

INGREDIENTS

4 navel oranges
4 cups hulled strawberries, sliced
¼ cup balsamic vinegar
¼ cup packed light brown sugar
1 tablespoon juniper berries, crushed (optional)
¼ teaspoon nutmeg, preferably freshly grated
Pomegranate seeds (optional)

PREPARATION

Peel oranges and cut crosswise into ¼-inch thick slices. Arrange on four serving plates. Arrange strawberries over the orange slices.

In a small saucepan, combine vinegar, brown sugar, and, if desired, juniper berries. Bring to a boil over medium heat, stirring occasionally. Strain out juniper berries if using. Drizzle mixture over fruit; top with nutmeg. Garnish with pomegranate seeds, if desired.

SUBSTITUTIONS

If you can find them, use blood oranges—their flesh and juice are tomato-red, but orange-sweet.

TIPS

The balsamic glaze thickens as it sits. If you use the juniper berries, be sure to strain them from the glaze before serving. Their aroma lasts just long enough to perfume the sauce, and deepen its flavor. These berries are too strong to eat by themselves. The optional pomegranate seeds provide crunch and visual delight. When they are in season in the fall and winter, make sure to buy a whole pomegranate, just for the wonder of those ruby nuggets of tartness and crunch, and to make this dish exceptional.

NUTRITIONAL ANALYSIS

Total Fat (g) 0.9	Sodium (mg) 11	Vitamin A (RE) 43
Fat Calories (kc) 8.1	Calcium (mg) 111	Beta-carotene (RE) 96
Cholesterol (mg) 0	Magnesium (mg) 38	Vitamin C (mg) 184
Saturated Fat (g) 0.1	Zinc (mg) 0.3	Vitamin E (mg) 1.09
Polyunsaturated Fat (g) 0.3	Selenium (mcg) 2	Thiamin B_1 (mg) 0.19
Monounsaturated Fat (g) 0.1	Potassium (mg) 645	Riboflavin B_2 (mg) 0.17
Fiber (g) 7.9	Flavonoids (mg) 7.4	Niacin B_3 (mg) 0.9
Carbohydrates (g) 48	Lycopene (mg) 0	Vitamin B_6 (mg) 0.17
Sugar (g) 40	Fish (oz) 0	Folic Acid (mcg) 83
Protein (g) 2.7	Nuts (oz) 0	Vitamin B_{12} (mcg) 0

Papaya Fruit Basket with Hint-of-Curry Yogurt Sauce

Preparation time: Eight minutes	Four servings
Cooking time: None	272 calories per serving, 25 percent from fat

RealAge effect if eaten twelve times a year: Lots of potassium and lots of vitamin C combine to make your RealAge 5 days younger.

RealAge effect ingredients: Papayas, grapes, pumpkin seeds (selenium, vitamin C, antioxidants)

INGREDIENTS

2 ripe papayas
2 cups red seedless grapes
1 cup low-fat or fat-free plain yogurt
1 tablespoon honey
¼ teaspoon curry powder
1 tablespoon chopped crystallized ginger
¼ cup pumpkin seeds, toasted

PREPARATION

Cut papayas in half lengthwise; scrape out seeds and arrange papaya halves cut side up in shallow bowls. Fill cavities with grapes. Combine yogurt, honey and curry powder; mix well. Drizzle over fruit; top with ginger and pumpkin seeds.

SUBSTITUTIONS

Brown sugar may replace the honey; cinnamon may replace the curry powder; and toasted cashews, almonds, or mixed nuts may replace the pumpkin seeds. Ground cinnamon is especially sweet here.

TIPS

If you can find it, use ginseng honey. Its sprightly flavor lightens the honey and makes the fruit sparkle.

NUTRITIONAL ANALYSIS

Total Fat (g) 7.7	Sodium (mg) 55	Vitamin A (RE) 75
Fat Calories (kc) 69	Calcium (mg) 181	Beta-carotene (RE) 163
Cholesterol (mg) 3.7	Magnesium (mg) 111	Vitamin C (mg) 128
Saturated Fat (g) 2.0	Zinc (mg) 1.8	Vitamin E (mg) 0.89
Polyunsaturated Fat (g) 3.0	Selenium (mcg) 4.2	Thiamin B_1 (mg) 0.16
Monounsaturated Fat (g) 2.2	Potassium (mg) 992	Riboflavin B_2 (mg) 0.3
Fiber (g) 4.8	Flavonoids (mg) 0	Niacin B_3 (mg) 1.5
Carbohydrates (g) 46.6	Lycopene (mg) 0	Vitamin B_6 (mg) 0.13
Sugar (g) 34.5	Fish (oz) 0	Folic Acid (mcg) 91
Protein (g) 9.6	Nuts (oz) 0	Vitamin B_{12} (mcg) 0.32

Thick Yogurt with Strawberries, Toasted Almonds, and Whole Grain Granola

Preparation time: Six minutes	Four servings
Cooking time: None	530 calories per serving, 25 percent from fat

RealAge effect if eaten twelve times a year: Delicious fiber-rich berries and the B vitamins of whole grains combine to make you 14.3 days younger.

RealAge effect ingredients: Berries, almonds, whole grain granola (fiber, B vitamins, folic acid, healthy fats, calcium)

INGREDIENTS

4 cups fat-free or low-fat strawberry yogurt
4 cups quartered fresh strawberries
2 tablespoons light brown sugar
¾ cup slivered almonds, toasted
1 cup low-fat whole grain granola

PREPARATION

Spoon yogurt into four shallow serving bowls. Combine strawberries and brown sugar; spoon over yogurt. Top with almonds and granola.

SUBSTITUTIONS

Vanilla yogurt may replace the strawberry yogurt and walnuts may replace the almonds. If you use vanilla yogurt, intensify its flavor with a few drops of real vanilla extract or, even better, the inside of a real vanilla bean scraped into the creamy yogurt. Also, soy yogurts are increasingly available, and increasingly delicious. Try one here.

TIPS

Check out the new granolas at your local market. Many are whole grain, lower in fat and sugar, and higher in crunch than just a few years ago. Some like this yogurt sweet, but you may not need the brown sugar—experiment and see.

NUTRITIONAL ANALYSIS

Total Fat (g) 15	Sodium (mg) 193	Vitamin A (RE) 118
Fat Calories (kc) 135	Calcium (mg) 424	Beta-carotene (RE) 26
Cholesterol (mg) 6.7	Magnesium (mg) 112	Vitamin C (mg) 86
Saturated Fat (g) 0.9	Zinc (mg) 3.6	Vitamin E (mg) 6.85
Polyunsaturated Fat (g) 3.1	Selenium (mcg) 19	Thiamin B$_1$ (mg) 0.34
Monounsaturated Fat (g) 8.4	Potassium (mg) 1025	Riboflavin B$_2$ (mg) 0.75
Fiber (g) 7.3	Flavonoids (mg) 4.6	Niacin B$_3$ (mg) 4.9
Carbohydrates (g) 83.9	Lycopene (mg) 0	Vitamin B$_6$ (mg) 0.31
Sugar (g) 61.7	Fish (oz) 0	Folic Acid (mcg) 113
Protein (g) 19.2	Nuts (oz) 0.7	Vitamin B$_{12}$ (mcg) 2.34

Tangy Honey and Lime Fruit Salad

Preparation time: Ten minutes	Four servings
Cooking time: None	76 calories per serving, 4 percent from fat

RealAge effect if eaten twelve times a year: Very little can interfere with the age-reducing quality of fresh fruit. It yields a RealAge effect of 3.8 days younger.

RealAge effect ingredients: Carambola, kiwifruit, grapes, mango or papaya, lime juice (antioxidants, flavonoids, potassium)

INGREDIENTS

1 ripe carambola, also known as star fruit
1 kiwifruit
1 cup whole red seedless grapes
1 cup diced ripe mango or papaya
1½ tablespoons each: honey and fresh lime juice
1 tablespoon chopped fresh mint leaves
Mint sprigs (optional)

PREPARATION

Cut carambola crosswise into thin slices. Partially peel kiwifruit with a vegetable peeler forming strips all around. Cut kiwifruit crosswise into thin slices. Combine the carambola, kiwifruit, grapes, and mango or papaya in a medium bowl. Combine honey and lime juice; add to fruit and toss lightly to coat. Serve immediately or cover and refrigerate up to six hours before serving. Sprinkle with mint and garnish with a mint sprig, if desired.

SUBSTITUTIONS

If fresh mangoes or papayas are not available, look for bottled mango and papaya in the produce section of your supermarket. Seedless green grapes may replace the red grapes, and a sliced banana may be substituted for either the carambola or kiwifruit.

TIPS

Carambola, also called star fruit because of its shape when sliced, is available most of the year. If it is very green, let the fruit ripen in a paper bag at room temperature for a day or two. It will turn a golden-yellow color and the ridges will darken.

Fresh mint is easy to grow in a sunny window. Many supermarkets now sell it in small pots.

To dice a fresh mango, stand it on the blossom end and cut down past the narrow pit on either side, forming two halves. Cut crosswise and lengthwise ½-inch slices (tic-tac-toe fashion) through the mango flesh all the way to the skin, forming ½-inch squares. Hold the scored portion with both hands and bend the peel backwards. Cut cubes away from the skin into a bowl.

NUTRITIONAL ANALYSIS

Total Fat (g) 0.3	Sodium (mg) 3	Vitamin A (RE) 92
Fat Calories (kc) 2.7	Calcium (mg) 19	Beta-carotene (RE) 455
Cholesterol (mg) 0	Magnesium (mg) 14	Vitamin C (mg) 50
Saturated Fat (g) 0	Zinc (mg) 0.1	Vitamin E (mg) 0.50
Polyunsaturated Fat (g) 0	Selenium (mcg) 1	Thiamin B_1 (mg) 0.05
Monounsaturated Fat (g) 0	Potassium (mg) 259	Riboflavin B_2 (mg) 0.05
Fiber (g) 1.7	Flavonoids (mg) 0	Niacin B_3 (mg) 0.5
Carbohydrates (g) 19.6	Lycopene (mg) 0	Vitamin B_6 (mg) 0.09
Sugar (g) 16.6	Fish (oz) 0	Folic Acid (mcg) 25
Protein (g) 0.7	Nuts (oz) 0	Vitamin B_{12} (mcg) 0

Caramelized Banana-Pecan Pancakes

Preparation time: Ten minutes	Four servings, about twelve (4-inch) pancakes
Cooking time: Ten minutes	391 calories per serving, 22 percent from fat

RealAge effect if eaten twelve times a year: The whole grains in these pancakes, plus the isoflavones in the soy milk, combine with the fiber content of the berries to give a RealAge factor of 4 days younger.

RealAge effect ingredients: Whole wheat, cranberries or blueberries, pecans, bananas, soy milk (fiber, isoflavones, antioxidants, flavonoids, nuts, egg whites, healthy fats, potassium)

INGREDIENTS

1 cup whole wheat pancake mix, such as Aunt Jemima brand
1 cup nonfat vanilla soy milk
½ cup dried cranberries or dried blueberries
2 egg whites, slightly beaten
1 tablespoon canola oil
¼ cup chopped pecans, toasted
2 ripe but firm bananas, sliced
¼ cup pure maple syrup

PREPARATION

In a large bowl, combine pancake mix, soy milk, berries, egg whites, and oil, mixing until large lumps disappear. (Do not over mix or pancakes will be tough.) Fold in pecans.

Heat a large nonstick griddle over medium heat until hot. Coat with cooking spray. Drop batter by scant ¼ cupfuls onto hot griddle. Turn when pancakes bubble and bottoms are golden brown; continue to cook until golden brown, about thirty seconds.

Meanwhile, heat a large nonstick skillet over medium heat until very hot. Add bananas; cook until slices are browned, turning once, about thirty seconds per side. Reduce heat to low; add syrup and heat through. Arrange pancakes on four serving plates; top with banana mixture.

SUBSTITUTIONS

Nonfat buttermilk plus ¼ teaspoon vanilla may be substituted for the vanilla soy milk and toasted walnuts may replace the pecans.

TIPS

As they are cooked, the pancakes may be transferred to serving plates and kept warm in a 200°F oven. An electric skillet set at 375°F may be used in place of the griddle. Any extra pancakes may be cooled, placed in plastic freezer bags, and frozen for up to six weeks. Reheat in microwave oven until warm. For a special, fancier look, slice bananas on the bias.

NUTRITIONAL ANALYSIS

Total Fat (g) 9.6	Sodium (mg) 553	Vitamin A (RE) 6
Fat Calories (kc) 86.4	Calcium (mg) 200	Beta-carotene (RE) 39
Cholesterol (mg) 60	Magnesium (mg) 67	Vitamin C (mg) 5
Saturated Fat (g) 0.9	Zinc (mg) 2	Vitamin E (mg) 0.57
Polyunsaturated Fat (g) 3.4	Selenium (mcg) 17	Thiamin B_1 (mg) 0.29
Monounsaturated Fat (g) 8.4	Potassium (mg) 487	Riboflavin B_2 (mg) 0.33
Fiber (g) 4.3	Flavonoids (mg) 3.9	Niacin B_3 (mg) 3.6
Carbohydrates (g) 71	Lycopene (mg) 0	Vitamin B_6 (mg) 0.39
Sugar (g) 44.6	Fish (oz) 0	Folic Acid (mcg) 42
Protein (g) 9	Nuts (oz) 0.3	Vitamin B_{12} (mcg) 0

Hot and Hearty Fig and Apricot Wheatena

Preparation time: Five minutes	Four servings (yields about 5 cups cereal)
Cooking time: Ten minutes	152 per serving, 36 percent from fat

RealAge effect if eaten twelve times a year: The high fiber and nutrients of this cereal and fruit and the monounsaturated fats of almonds make the RealAge factor 5.7 days younger.

RealAge effect ingredients: Whole wheat cereal, figs, apricots, soy milk, almonds (isoflavones, fiber, healthy fats, healthy protein)

INGREDIENTS

1 cup uncooked wheat cereal such as Wheatena brand
2 cups *each:* nonfat or 1 percent vanilla soy milk and water
½ cup *each:* diced dried figs and diced dried apricots
½ teaspoon salt
2 tablespoons honey
Toppings: ¼ cup *each:* nonfat or 1 percent vanilla soy milk and toasted, sliced, unblanched almonds

PREPARATION

Place a medium-size saucepan over medium heat. Add cereal; cook four minutes or until fragrant, stirring occasionally.

Add milk, water, figs, apricots, and salt. Bring to a simmer; cook about five minutes or until thickened, stirring occasionally. Transfer to four warmed serving bowls; let stand one or two minutes (cereal will be very hot). Serve with honey and toppings.

SUBSTITUTIONS

One cup chopped dates or dried mixed fruit bits may be substituted for the figs and apricots. Skim milk plus ½ teaspoon vanilla may be substituted for the vanilla soy milk.

NUTRITIONAL ANALYSIS

Total Fat (g) 6.0	Sodium (mg) 19	Vitamin A (RE) 59
Fat Calories (kc) 54	Calcium (mg) 50	Beta-carotene (RE) 332
Cholesterol (mg) 0	Magnesium (mg) 53	Vitamin C (mg) 2.6
Saturated Fat (g) 0.6	Zinc (mg) 0.7	Vitamin E (mg) 1.91
Polyunsaturated Fat (g) 1.8	Selenium (mcg) 1	Thiamin B_1 (mg) 0.30
Monounsaturated Fat (g) 2.5	Potassium (mg) 377	Riboflavin B_2 (mg) 0.19
Fiber (g) 5.3	Flavonoids (mg) 0	Niacin B_3 (mg) 1.1
Carbohydrates (g) 20.3	Lycopene (mg) 0	Vitamin B_6 (mg) 0.12
Sugar (g) 4.8	Fish (oz) 0	Folic Acid (mcg) 12
Protein (g) 6.5	Nuts (oz) 0.2	Vitamin B_{12} (mcg) 0

Mango Madness

Preparation time: Ten minutes	Makes four (1 cup) servings
Cooking time: None	188 calories per serving, 2 percent from fat

RealAge effect if eaten twelve times a year: Loaded with carotenoids including beta-carotene, with nary a bit of fat, this quick pick-me-upper makes you 1.5 days younger.

RealAge effect ingredients: Mango nectar and mangos, lime juice (flavonoids)

INGREDIENTS

One 11½ ounce can mango nectar, such as Libby's brand
Two ripe mangos, peeled, seeded, cut into chunks (4 cups)
1 cup mango sorbet, such as Häagen-Dazs brand
2 tablespoons fresh lime juice

PREPARATION

Combine nectar and mangos in blender container. Cover and blend until fairly smooth. Add sorbet and lime juice; cover and blend until smooth and thick.

SUBSTITUTIONS

Papaya or guava nectar may replace the mango nectar, and lemon or lime sorbet may replace the mango sorbet. You'll have different flavors, but a delicious, easy balance of sweet and tart.

TIPS

If you like more-liquid shakes, add 2 cups crushed ice to the blender. Use a frosty beer mug to carry Mango Madness from blender to table to your mouth!

NUTRITIONAL ANALYSIS

Total Fat (g) 0.4	Sodium (mg) 4	Vitamin A (RE) 532
Fat Calories (kc) 3.6	Calcium (mg) 16	Beta-carotene (RE) 3075
Cholesterol (mg) 0	Magnesium (mg) 18	Vitamin C (mg) 44
Saturated Fat (g) 0.1	Zinc (mg) 0.1	Vitamin E (mg) 1.16
Polyunsaturated Fat (g) 0.1	Selenium (mcg) 1	Thiamin B_1 (mg) 0.08
Monounsaturated Fat (g) 0.1	Potassium (mg) 223	Riboflavin B_2 (mg) 0.10
Fiber (g) 2.9	Flavonoids (mg) 0	Niacin B_3 (mg) 0.9
Carbohydrates (g) 46.0	Lycopene (mg) 0	Vitamin B_6 (mg) 0.15
Sugar (g) 43	Fish (oz) 0	Folic Acid (mcg) 20
Protein (g) 1.4	Nuts (oz) 0	Vitamin B_{12} (mcg) 0.04

Triple Berry Blender Blaster

Preparation time: Five minutes	Four (8 ounce) servings
Cooking time: None	144 calories per serving, 4 percent from fat

RealAge effect if eaten twelve times a year: 4.6 days younger because it's low in fat and calories.

RealAge effect ingredients: Berries, apple juice, soy protein (antioxidants, potassium, vitamins, healthy proteins)

INGREDIENTS

2 cups mixed frozen berries such as blueberries, raspberries, and strawberries
2 cups unsweetened apple juice or apple cider
1 cup raspberry or strawberry sorbet
¼ cup soy protein powder

PREPARATION

Combine berries and juice in blender container. Cover and blend at high speed thirty seconds. Add sorbet; blend thirty seconds. Add soy powder; blend thirty seconds or until thick and smooth.

SUBSTITUTIONS

Two cups of any one of the frozen berries may replace the mixed berries. Vanilla-flavored soy protein powder may replace the regular soy powder.

TIPS

Frozen berries are a blessing—they add thickness, coolness, and sweetness all in one. They're also less expensive than fresh berries and are perfect for the blender.

NUTRITIONAL ANALYSIS

Total Fat (g) 0.6	Sodium (mg) 32	Vitamin A (RE) 6
Fat Calories (kc) 5.4	Calcium (mg) 20	Beta-carotene (RE) 34
Cholesterol (mg) 0	Magnesium (mg) 22	Vitamin C (mg) 22
Saturated Fat (g) 0.1	Zinc (mg) 0.4	Vitamin E (mg) 0.67
Polyunsaturated Fat (g) 0.2	Selenium (mcg) 9	Thiamin B_1 (mg) 0.05
Monounsaturated Fat (g) 0.1	Potassium (mg) 250	Riboflavin B_2 (mg) 0.06
Fiber (g) 2	Flavonoids (mg) 0.7	Niacin B_3 (mg) 1.7
Carbohydrates (g) 33.2	Lycopene (mg) 0	Vitamin B_6 (mg) 0.13
Sugar (g) 25	Fish (oz) 0	Folic Acid (mcg) 12
Protein (g) 4.2	Nuts (oz) 0	Vitamin B_{12} (mcg) 0

Maple Oatmeal with Prunes and Plums

Preparation time: Ten minutes	Four servings
Cooking time: Eight minutes	478 calories per serving, 10 percent from fat

RealAge effect if eaten twelve times a year: One of nature's best functional foods, whole oats carry the goodness of whole foods and are a complete, unrefined grain. Their soluble fiber, plus the insoluble fiber of the fruit, combine to drop your RealAge by 7.6 days.

RealAge effect ingredients: Oats, apple cider, plums, prunes (fiber, flavonoids, potassium, antioxidants, folic acid)

INGREDIENTS

3 cups fat-free milk
3 cups old-fashioned oats, uncooked
½ cup apple cider or juice
Four small plums, seeded and diced
1 cup dried prunes, diced
3 tablespoons pure maple syrup
¼ teaspoon ground cinnamon

PREPARATION

Bring milk just to a simmer in a medium saucepan; stir in oats and simmer five to eight minutes or until thickened, stirring once or twice. Stir in apple cider, then plums, prunes, and syrup; heat through. Transfer to serving bowls; top with cinnamon.

SUBSTITUTIONS

Four apricots or two nectarines or peaches may replace the plums; dried apricots or mixed fruit bits may replace the prunes. Nutmeg may replace the cinnamon.

TIPS

Here, layered flavors shine through. Prunes are simply dried plums; by adding them with fresh plums, different notes of sweetness blend with the smooth oats. This cooks up well in the microwave, too: Add oats and milk to a 3-quart bowl and cook at HIGH power for seven to eight minutes; then stir in the fruit and syrup and top with cinnamon.

NUTRITIONAL ANALYSIS

Total Fat (g) 5.5	Sodium (mg) 1011	Vitamin A (RE) 216
Fat Calories (kc) 49.5	Calcium (mg) 289	Beta-carotene (RE) 529
Cholesterol (mg) 3.3	Magnesium (mg) 210	Vitamin C (mg) 10
Saturated Fat (g) 0.9	Zinc (mg) 2.8	Vitamin E (mg) 1.22
Polyunsaturated Fat (g) 1.5	Selenium (mcg) 5	Thiamin B_1 (mg) 0.56
Monounsaturated Fat (g) 1.9	Potassium (mg) 1017	Riboflavin B_2 (mg) 0.47
Fiber (g) 9.7	Flavonoids (mg) 0	Niacin B_3 (mg) 1.6
Carbohydrates (g) 95.5	Lycopene (mg) 0	Vitamin B_6 (mg) 0.29
Sugar (g) 42.3	Fish (oz) 0	Folic Acid (mcg) 42
Protein (g) 16.8	Nuts (oz) 0	Vitamin B_{12} (mcg) 0.67

Sun-Dried Tomato and Mushroom Muffuletta Sandwiches

Preparation time: Twenty minutes	Four servings
Cooking time: None	207 calories per serving, 22 percent from fat

RealAge effect if eaten twelve times a year: The lutein in spinach is a powerful antioxidant that slows the aging of the eyes, and reduces cataract formation. The RealAge effect here: 1.5 days younger.

RealAge effect ingredients: Spinach, mushrooms, vegetables, green olives, whole wheat (calcium, healthy fats, antioxidants)

INGREDIENTS

One 8-ounce package sliced button mushrooms
½ cup drained bottled hot or mild pickled vegetables (jardiniere)
¼ cup plus 1 tablespoon coarsely grated Romano cheese
2 tablespoons each: chopped pimiento-stuffed green olives and chopped, drained sun-dried tomatoes in olive oil
2 tablespoons chopped Italian parsley
4 small whole wheat pita bread loaves, such as Sahara brand
1 cup packed spinach or arugula leaves, rinsed well

PREPARATION

In a medium bowl, combine mushrooms, pickled vegetables, ¼ cup cheese, olives, sun-dried tomatoes, and parsley; mix well. Cut pitas in half. Line each pocket with spinach or arugula and fill with mushroom mixture. Sprinkle with remaining 1 tablespoon cheese.

SUBSTITUTIONS

Chopped, pitted kalamata olives or Spanish green olives may be substituted for the pimiento-stuffed olives. Chopped fresh chives may be substituted for the parsley. A mixture of ¼ cup each hot and mild pickled vegetables may replace the ½ cup of just the one.

TIPS

For a pleasant textural contrast, toast the pitas before assembling the sandwiches. These sandwiches are perfect for picnics. Wrap each in plastic wrap and refrigerate up to six hours before serving. Colorful sweet potato chips (such as Terra brand) make a delightful accompaniment.

NUTRITIONAL ANALYSIS

Total Fat (g) 5	Sodium (mg) 677	Vitamin A (RE) 220
Fat Calories (kc) 45	Calcium (mg) 112	Beta-carotene (RE) 1212
Cholesterol (mg) 8.7	Magnesium (mg) 23	Vitamin C (mg) 15
Saturated Fat (g) 1.6	Zinc (mg) 1.1	Vitamin E (mg) 0.65
Polyunsaturated Fat (g) 1.3	Selenium (mcg) 6	Thiamin B_1 (mg) 0.13
Monounsaturated Fat (g) 1.0	Potassium (mg) 370	Riboflavin B_2 (mg) 0.22
Fiber (g) 5.7	Flavonoids (mg) 0.1	Niacin B_3 (mg) 1.9
Carbohydrates (g) 32.3	Lycopene (mg) 0	Vitamin B_6 (mg) 0.13
Sugar (g) 4.2	Fish (oz) 0	Folic Acid (mcg) 29
Protein (g) 10.1	Nuts (oz) 0	Vitamin B_{12} (mcg) 0.20

Sweet Baby Greens in a Light Ranch Dressing with Smoked Trout

Preparation time: Twenty-two minutes	Four servings
Cooking time: None	270 calories per serving, 39 percent from fat

RealAge effect if eaten twelve times a year: Bursting with protective omega-3 fatty acids and full of bright carotenoids, this filling lunch makes your RealAge 9.4 days younger.

RealAge effect ingredients: Garlic, olive oil, soy milk, salad greens, oranges, diced cranberries, trout, soy nuts (healthy protein, healthy fat, calcium, potassium, antioxidants, flavonoids, folic acid)

INGREDIENTS

1 tablespoon each: seasoned rice vinegar, fresh lemon juice, and minced shallot
1 clove garlic, minced
1½ tablespoons olive oil
¼ cup nonfat soy milk
½ teaspoon each: salt and freshly ground black pepper
8 cups packed mesclun salad greens or assorted torn salad greens
2 oranges, peeled, separated into sections, sections halved
⅓ cup dried cranberries
8 ounces smoked rainbow trout, such as Ducktrap brand, skinned, broken into
    chunks
¼ cup toasted soy nuts (optional)

PREPARATION

In a medium bowl, whisk together vinegar, lemon juice, shallot, and garlic. Whisk
in oil, then soy milk, salt, and pepper. In a large bowl, combine salad greens,
oranges, and cranberries. Add dressing; toss to coat well and transfer to four
serving plates. Top with trout and, if desired, soy nuts.

Serve with a crisp flatbread such as Wasa or RyKrisp.

SUBSTITUTIONS

Fat-free milk may replace the soy milk and three tangerines may replace the two
oranges.

TIPS

Using both rice wine vinegar and lemon may seem redundant—they're both acidic
and make your tongue tingle. Together, though, they add smoothness to tastes that
would otherwise be sharp. Also, look for ranch-flavored soy nuts; they would be
perfect here.

NUTRITIONAL ANALYSIS

Total Fat (g) 11.7	Sodium (mg) 996	Vitamin A (RE) 323
Fat Calories (kc) 105	Calcium (mg) 135	Beta-carotene (RE) 1848
Cholesterol (mg) 15.2	Magnesium (mg) 40	Vitamin C (mg) 85
Saturated Fat (g) 2.3	Zinc (mg) 1.4	Vitamin E (mg) 1.48
Polyunsaturated Fat (g) 0.6	Selenium (mcg) 1	Thiamin B_1 (mg) 0.18
Monounsaturated Fat (g) 3.8	Potassium (mg) 574	Riboflavin B_2 (mg) 0.23
Fiber (g) 5.8	Flavonoids (mg) 4.9	Niacin B_3 (mg) 1.1
Carbohydrates (g) 26.9	Lycopene (mg) 0	Vitamin B_6 (mg) 0.44
Sugar (g) 19.8	Fish (oz) 2	Folic Acid (mcg) 167
Protein (g) 17.7	Nuts (oz) 0.4	Vitamin B_{12} (mcg) 1.99

Portuguese Bean Soup

Preparation time: Twelve minutes	Four servings (makes about 7 cups of soup)
Cooking time: Twelve minutes	165 calories per serving, 20 percent from fat

RealAge effect if eaten twelve times a year: Sweet potatoes practically burst with carotenoids—brightly colored antioxidants that protect your arteries, lenses, and joints. The RealAge factor on this baby is 12.5 days younger.

RealAge effect ingredients: Swiss chard, garlic, onions, olive oil, tomatoes, sweet potato, beans (calcium, lycopene, fiber, potassium, carotenoids)

INGREDIENTS

2 teaspoons olive oil
1 cup coarsely chopped white onion
3 cups reduced-sodium chicken broth
1 cup diced (½-inch pieces) unpeeled sweet potato
3 to 4 teaspoons chili garlic sauce or chili puree with garlic, such as Lee Kum Kee brand
1 can (14½ ounces) diced tomatoes, undrained
One 15- or 16-ounce can Great Northern or cannellini beans, undrained
4 cups packed sliced Swiss chard or collard greens
4 teaspoons balsamic vinegar (optional)

PREPARATION

Heat a large saucepan over medium-high heat. Add oil, then onion; cook three minutes, stirring occasionally. Add broth, sweet potato, and chili garlic sauce; bring to a boil over high heat. Reduce heat; simmer uncovered five minutes. Stir in tomatoes and beans; return to a simmer. Stir in Swiss chard or collard greens. Simmer five minutes or until sweet potatoes and chard or greens are tender. Stir in vinegar, if desired, and ladle into four serving bowls.

SUBSTITUTIONS

Diced, peeled butternut or delicata squash may be substituted for the sweet potato. Kale, turnip, or beet greens may replace the Swiss chard or collard greens.

TIPS

Leftover soup may be covered and refrigerated up to three days or frozen up to three months. The soup may be pureed, simmered until thickened, and served as a sauce for cooked whole wheat pasta, underneath a wild-rice pilaf, or on top of a baked potato.

Chili garlic sauce is an Asian condiment found in the ethnic section of your supermarket. It gives a dynamic flavor to this quick-cooking soup.

NUTRITIONAL ANALYSIS

Total Fat (g) 3.7	Sodium (mg) 899	Vitamin A (RE) 569
Fat Calories (kc) 33.3	Calcium (mg) 166	Beta-carotene (RE) 3327
Cholesterol (mg) 2.4	Magnesium (mg) 49	Vitamin C (mg) 39.5
Saturated Fat (g) 0.8	Zinc (mg) 0.4	Vitamin E (mg) 5.07
Polyunsaturated Fat (g) 0.3	Selenium (mcg) 7	Thiamin B_1 (mg) 0.09
Monounsaturated Fat (g) 2.1	Potassium (mg) 801	Riboflavin B_2 (mg) 0.09
Fiber (g) 8.2	Flavonoids (mg) 3.8	Niacin B_3 (mg) 3.3
Carbohydrates (g) 30	Lycopene (mg) 3.3	Vitamin B_6 (mg) 1.06
Sugar (g) 7.3	Fish (oz) 0	Folic Acid (mcg) 214
Protein (g) 9.9	Nuts (oz) 0	Vitamin B_{12} (mcg) 0

Huevos Rancheros Burritos with Chipotle Chili Beans and Corn

Preparation time: Five minutes	Four servings
Cooking time: Ten minutes	446 calories per serving, 23 percent from fat

RealAge effect if eaten twelve times a year: Low in fat and high in fiber, this burrito will get you going—in fact, going 2.7 days younger.

RealAge effect ingredients: Beans, corn, salsa, egg whites (fiber, calcium, healthy protein)

INGREDIENTS

One 15½-ounce can chili beans in spicy sauce, undrained
1 cup frozen whole kernel corn
¼ cup salsa, preferably chipotle, such as Frontera brand
3 large egg whites
2 large eggs
2 tablespoons low-fat sour cream
Cooking spray
4 large (10-inch) flour tortillas
¼ cup chopped cilantro

PREPARATION

In a medium saucepan, combine beans, corn, and salsa. Bring to a boil over high heat; reduce heat; simmer uncovered five minutes.

Beat together egg whites, eggs, and sour cream. Heat a large nonstick skillet over medium-high heat until hot. Coat with cooking spray. Add egg mixture; cook, stirring occasionally until eggs are set. Break into chunks and stir into bean mixture.

Stack tortillas on a clean kitchen towels. Sprinkle a few drops of water on the top of the tortillas. Fold tortillas up in the towel; heat in microwave oven until warm, twenty to thirty seconds. Do not over-warm, or the tortillas will be tough.

Place tortillas on serving plates. Divide egg mixture over tortillas; top with cilantro. Fold sides of tortillas in over filling; roll up, burrito fashion.

SUBSTITUTIONS

Chopped parsley may replace the cilantro, and 2 tablespoons pureed chipotle chilies (smoked, dried jalapenos) in adobo sauce may replace the salsa. When fresh corn is in season, cut the kernels from two ears to replace the cup of frozen corn.

TIPS

For more flavor, brown the corn niblets in the saucepan in a squirt of olive oil over high heat before adding the beans and salsa. Have a little fresh green onion, sliced red radishes, and ½ teaspoon of ground cumin at the ready for extra crunch and spice when garnishing.

NUTRITIONAL ANALYSIS

Total Fat (g) 11.3	Sodium (mg) 928	Vitamin A (RE) 114
Fat Calories (kc) 101.7	Calcium (mg) 170	Beta-carotene (RE) 329
Cholesterol (mg) 113	Magnesium (mg) 32	Vitamin C (mg) 7
Saturated Fat (g) 3.5	Zinc (mg) 2.8	Vitamin E (mg) 1.30
Polyunsaturated Fat (g) 1.3	Selenium (mcg) 30	Thiamin B_1 (mg) 0.12
Monounsaturated Fat (g) 3.8	Potassium (mg) 279	Riboflavin B_2 (mg) 0.48
Fiber (g) 8.6	Flavonoids (mg) 0.2	Niacin B_3 (mg) 3.4
Carbohydrates (g) 68.3	Lycopene (mg) 4.2	Vitamin B_6 (mg) 0.23
Sugar (g) 6.5	Fish (oz) 0	Folic Acid (mcg) 116
Protein (g) 19.1	Nuts (oz) 0	Vitamin B_{12} (mcg) 0.32

Mustard-Crusted Salmon with Sweet Peppers

Preparation time: Ten minutes	Four servings
Cooking time: Twenty minutes	336 calories per serving, 33 percent from fat

RealAge effect if eaten twelve times a year: Red and yellow bell peppers contain an impressive amount of vitamin C—much more than green peppers—and are a good source of fiber. So, when you add the omega-3 fatty acids of salmon, you get 6.4 days younger.

RealAge effect ingredients: Olive oil, onions, bell pepper, salmon, garlic (vitamin C, fiber, healthy fats, flavonoids, potassium)

INGREDIENTS

1 teaspoon olive oil
1 large or 2 medium red or yellow onions, thinly sliced
2 *each:* large red and yellow bell peppers, cut into long, thin strips
6 cloves garlic, thinly sliced
¼ cup plus 1 tablespoon honey
¼ cup cider vinegar
½ teaspoon salt, or to taste
⅛ teaspoon ground white pepper (optional)
1½ teaspoons Dijon mustard
4 (4- to 5-ounce) salmon fillets with skin
½ teaspoon paprika
2 tablespoons chopped fresh tarragon or chives (optional)

PREPARATION

Heat a large deep skillet over medium heat. Add oil, then onion; cook over medium heat three minutes, stirring occasionally. Add bell peppers and garlic; cover and cook five minutes or until vegetables are softened. Add ¼ cup honey, cider vinegar, salt, and, if desired, white pepper; mix well. Cook uncovered over medium-high heat five to eight minutes or until sauce is slightly thickened and vegetables are tender, stirring occasionally.

Meanwhile, combine remaining 1 tablespoon honey with mustard; mix well. Place salmon, skin side down, on rack of broiler pan. Brush honey mixture over salmon; sprinkle with paprika. Broil four to five inches from heat for six to eight minutes or until salmon is opaque and firm to the touch. Transfer vegetable mixture to four warmed serving plates; top with salmon. Sprinkle with tarragon or chives, if desired.

SUBSTITUTIONS

Halibut or sea bass fillets may be substituted for the salmon, and pommery or horseradish mustard may be substituted for the Dijon mustard.

NUTRITIONAL ANALYSIS

Total Fat (g) 14	Sodium (mg) 411	Vitamin A (RE) 906
Fat Calories (kc) 126	Calcium (mg) 48	Beta-carotene (RE) 4828
Cholesterol (mg) 67	Magnesium (mg) 63	Vitamin C (mg) 283
Saturated Fat (g) 2.7	Zinc (mg) 1.4	Vitamin E (mg) 3.58
Polyunsaturated Fat (g) 4.8	Selenium (mcg) 42	Thiamin B_1 (mg) 0.24
Monounsaturated Fat (g) 5.3	Potassium (mg) 811	Riboflavin B_2 (mg) 0.33
Fiber (g) 3.8	Flavonoids (mg) 0	Niacin B_3 (mg) 9.5
Carbohydrates (g) 37.9	Lycopene (mg) 1.5	Vitamin B_6 (mg) 0.40
Sugar (g) 27.8	Fish (oz) 4.5	Folic Acid (mcg) 66
Protein (g) 24.9	Nuts (oz) 0	Vitamin B_{12} (mcg) 3.83

Warm Spinach Salad with Chicken, Apples, and Toasted Almonds

Preparation time: Ten minutes	Four servings
Cooking time: Five minutes	290 calories per serving, 28 percent from fat

RealAge effect if eaten twelve times a year: Nuts are a terrific source of healthy protein, unsaturated fats, and, of course, great flavor. These plus the B vitamins in dark leafy spinach combine to make you 8.5 days younger.

RealAge effect ingredients: Spinach, apple juice, olive oil, onions, almonds, apples (B vitamins, healthy fats, potassium, flavonoids, calcium)

INGREDIENTS

¼ cup sliced almonds
1 cup plus 3 tablespoons apple juice, preferably unfiltered
12 ounces shredded or chopped cooked skinless chicken breast (about 3 cups)
1 teaspoon canola or olive oil
⅓ cup sliced shallots or chopped sweet onion
1 tablespoon brown sugar
¼ teaspoon cinnamon
¼ teaspoon salt
6 cups (10 ounces) packed torn spinach leaves
1 apple, preferably Fuji or Gala, unpeeled and cut into ½-inch cubes
Ground black pepper, if desired

PREPARATION

Place almonds on a baking sheet and bake in a 350°F oven until lightly browned and fragrant, six to eight minutes; set aside.

In a very large bowl, combine 3 tablespoons apple juice and chicken; toss well and set aside. Heat a large skillet over medium heat. Add oil, then shallots or onions; sauté five minutes. Add remaining 1 cup apple juice, brown sugar, cinnamon, and salt. Simmer five minutes, stirring occasionally. Add spinach, apple, and almonds to chicken mixture. Add hot shallot mixture; toss well and transfer to four serving plates. Serve with freshly ground black pepper, if desired.

SUBSTITUTIONS

Fuji and Gala are crisp, sweet eating apples, which are usually available all year long. You may, however, substitute any red eating apple (not cooking apples). You may substitute walnuts, pecans, or toasted pumpkin seeds for the almonds.

TIPS

Toast extra almonds to eat as a snack or to add to cereal for breakfast. Toasting doubles the flavor, enabling you to use just half what you would use otherwise. Using thinly sliced almonds (instead of whole ones or slivered ones) is another way to get more flavor out of the same nut: Thinner slices go further and carry more flavor.

NUTRITIONAL ANALYSIS

Total Fat (g) 8.9	Sodium (mg) 270	Vitamin A (RE) 499
Fat Calories (kc) 80.1	Calcium (mg) 121	Beta-carotene (RE) 2927
Cholesterol (mg) 72.0	Magnesium (mg) 114	Vitamin C (mg) 27
Saturated Fat (g) 1.3	Zinc (mg) 1.6	Vitamin E (mg) 3.9
Polyunsaturated Fat (g) 2.1	Selenium (mcg) 26	Thiamin B_1 (mg) 0.15
Monounsaturated Fat (g) 4.5	Potassium (mg) 843	Riboflavin B_2 (mg) 0.34
Fiber (g) 3.8	Flavonoids (mg) 2.2	Niacin B_3 (mg) 12.6
Carbohydrates (g) 22.6	Lycopene (mg) 0	Vitamin B_6 (mg) 0.73
Sugar (g) 15.9	Fish (oz) 0	Folic Acid (mcg) 150
Protein (g) 29.7	Nuts (oz) 0.2	Vitamin B_{12} (mcg) 0.28

Pan-Grilled Citrus Salmon over Asian Slaw

Preparation time: Twelve minutes	Four servings
Cooking time: Eight minutes	240 calories per serving, 38 percent from fat

RealAge effect if eaten twelve times a year: 5.6 days younger

RealAge effect ingredients: Grapefruit, salmon, pea pods, cabbage, radishes (fiber, lycopene, vitamins, healthy fat, healthy protein)

INGREDIENTS

½ large (or 1 small) pink or red grapefruit

2 tablespoons hoisin sauce, such as KAME brand

2 teaspoons dark sesame oil

Four 4-ounce skinless salmon fillets

¾ teaspoon salt

2 cups (6 ounces) pea pods, cut lengthwise into thin strips

1 cup sliced Napa cabbage

½ cup sliced radishes

2 teaspoons sesame seeds, toasted (optional)

PREPARATION

Peel and coarsely chop grapefruit, saving juices. Measure juice; if necessary, squeeze more juice from chopped grapefruit to yield 2 tablespoons.

Combine the 2 tablespoons grapefruit juice, hoisin sauce, and sesame oil. Transfer 2 tablespoons of the mixture to a large bowl. Brush remaining mixture over salmon fillets; sprinkle with ½ teaspoon salt. Heat a ridged grill pan° over

°If a ridged pan is not available, broil the salmon 4 to 5 inches away from heat for three to four minutes per side.

medium heat until hot. Add salmon; cook three to four minutes per side or until salmon is opaque and firm to the touch.

Meanwhile, add pea pods, cabbage, radishes, reserved chopped grapefruit, and remaining ¼ teaspoon of salt to bowl with reserved hoisin sauce mixture; toss well. Arrange on four serving plates; top with salmon and sprinkle with sesame seeds, if desired.

SUBSTITUTIONS

Daikon (Japanese radish) may replace the red radishes, and 1 cup thinly sliced red cabbage may replace Napa cabbage. One tablespoon molasses plus 1 tablespoon soy sauce may replace the 2 tablespoons hoisin sauce.

TIPS

The grapefruit makes the marinade, because the acidity of its juice delicately penetrates the flesh of the salmon, allowing more flavor to seep in before you grill.

NUTRITIONAL ANALYSIS

Total Fat (g) 10	Sodium (mg) 628	Vitamin A (RE) 28
Fat Calories (kc) 90	Calcium (mg) 52	Beta-carotene (RE) 94
Cholesterol (mg) 64	Magnesium (mg) 50	Vitamin C (mg) 47
Saturated Fat (g) 0.5	Zinc (mg) 0.9	Vitamin E (mg) 1.73
Polyunsaturated Fat (g) 3.2	Selenium (mcg) 43	Thiamin B_1 (mg) 0.30
Monounsaturated Fat (g) 3.4	Potassium (mg) 818	Riboflavin B_2 (mg) 0.5
Fiber (g) 3.4	Flavonoids (mg) 1.0	Niacin B_3 (mg) 7.8
Carbohydrates (g) 9.9	Lycopene (mg) 0.5	Vitamin B_6 (mg) 0.56
Sugar (g) 3.9	Fish (oz) 4	Folic Acid (mcg) 54
Protein (g) 26.1	Nuts (oz) 0	Vitamin B_{12} (mcg) 3.06

Tuna with Garlic and Olives over Pasta with Fresh Basil

Preparation time: Fifteen minutes	Four servings
Cooking time: Fifteen minutes	572 calories per serving, 24 percent from fat

RealAge effect if eaten twelve times a year: With a full day's omega-3 in one dish, plus vitamin C and calcium to burn, this dish will make your RealAge 4 days younger.

RealAge effect ingredients: Tuna, garlic, olives, herbs (lycopene, flavonoids, healthy fats)

INGREDIENTS

12 ounces (5 cups) whole wheat rotini pasta, uncooked
2 tablespoons extra virgin olive oil, divided
½ cup chopped red onion
1 red bell pepper, diced

2 tablespoons minced garlic
½ cup dry red wine (optional)
4 cups bottled spaghetti sauce, such as Classico brand
Two 6-ounce cans white tuna in water, drained, broken into chunks
12 kalamata olives, quartered
¼ cup sliced or chopped fresh basil leaves

PREPARATION

Cook pasta according to package directions. Meanwhile, heat a large saucepan over medium-high heat. Add 1 tablespoon oil, then onion. Cook four minutes, stirring frequently. Add bell pepper. Cook four to five minutes or until vegetables are tender, stirring occasionally. Stir in garlic; cook thirty seconds. If desired, add wine; cook, stirring constantly, until liquid evaporates. Reduce heat; stir in spaghetti sauce. Bring to a simmer, stirring constantly. Stir in tuna and olives; heat through. Drain pasta; transfer to serving plates; top with sauce and basil. Drizzle remaining 1 tablespoon oil over all.

SUBSTITUTIONS

Flat-leaf Italian parsley may replace the basil, yellow bell pepper may replace the red pepper, and whole wheat shell pasta may replace the rotini.

TIPS

Although red wine is optional, it adds a little richer, deeper color and extra zing to the meal—try it and see. Any dry red wine will work, though we like California zinfandel for its fruitiness and flavor.

NUTRITIONAL ANALYSIS

Total Fat (g) 15.5	Sodium (mg) 1292	Vitamin A (RE) 249
Fat Calories (kc) 139.5	Calcium (mg) 67	Beta-carotene (RE) 1327
Cholesterol (mg) 36	Magnesium (mg) 97	Vitamin C (mg) 82
Saturated Fat (g) 2.2	Zinc (mg) 1.5	Vitamin E (mg) 1.50
Polyunsaturated Fat (g) 2.4	Selenium (mcg) 107	Thiamin B_1 (mg) 0.37
Monounsaturated Fat (g) 8.1	Potassium (mg) 433	Riboflavin B_2 (mg) 0.39
Fiber (g) 10.9	Flavonoids (mg) 7.9	Niacin B_3 (mg) 15.2
Carbohydrates (g) 78	Lycopene (mg) 67.9	Vitamin B_6 (mg) 1.32
Sugar (g) 14.3	Fish (oz) 3	Folic Acid (mcg) 27
Protein (g) 35.0	Nuts (oz) 0	Vitamin B_{12} (mcg) 1.99

Black Bean and Fresh Cheese Enchiladas with Warm Tomatillo Salsa

Preparation time: Fifteen minutes	Four servings
Cooking time: Six minutes	424 calories per serving, 13 percent from fat

RealAge effect if eaten twelve times a year: 4.2 days younger

RealAge effect ingredients: Beans, onions, tomatoes, salsa (fiber, antioxidants, flavonoids, lycopene)

INGREDIENTS

One 15-ounce can low-fat or fat-free refried black beans, such as Bearitos brand
1 large tomato, seeded and diced°
¾ cup sliced green onions
2 teaspoons ground coriander
1¾ cups tomatillo salsa or salsa verde, such as Frontera or Arriba brands
Eight small (6-inch) flour tortillas
1 cup (4 ounces) crumbled queso añejo or farmer's cheese

PREPARATION

Preheat broiler. In a microwave-safe bowl, combine beans, tomato, green onions, coriander, and ½ cup of the salsa; mix well. Cook in microwave oven until heated through, one to two minutes. Spoon ¼ cup of the salsa on the bottom of a 13 × 9-inch baking pan or ovenproof dish.

Spoon about ⅓ cup hot bean mixture down center of each tortilla; roll up and place seam side down in prepared pan. Spread remaining 1 cup salsa evenly over tortillas; top with cheese. Broil 5 to 6 inches from heat until enchiladas are heated through and cheese melts, five to six minutes. Transfer to warmed serving plates; garnish as desired.

SUBSTITUTIONS

Ground cumin may replace the ground coriander for a rounder, softer flavor. Low-fat or fat-free refried pinto beans may replace the black beans—the taste will be smoother and less distinct.

TIP

°To quickly seed a tomato, cut it in half crosswise and scoop out the seeds with your finger while gently squeezing each half. Serve the dish with your favorite garnishes: chopped cilantro, sliced radishes, diced ripe avocado, sliced romaine lettuce, pickled jalapeño, fat-free or light sour cream, and additional salsa.

NUTRITIONAL ANALYSIS

Total Fat (g) 6.2	Sodium (mg) 964	Vitamin A (RE) 35
Fat Calories (kc) 55.8	Calcium (mg) 105	Beta-carotene (RE) 208
Cholesterol (mg) 0	Magnesium (mg) 9	Vitamin C (mg) 39
Saturated Fat (g) 0	Zinc (mg) 0.1	Vitamin E (mg) 1.33
Polyunsaturated Fat (g) 1.9	Selenium (mcg) 0.3	Thiamin B_1 (mg) 0.42
Monounsaturated Fat (g) 0.1	Potassium (mg) 290	Riboflavin B_2 (mg) 0.14
Fiber (g) 6.7	Flavonoids (mg) 4.0	Niacin B_3 (mg) 1.9
Carbohydrates (g) 82	Lycopene (mg) 31.7	Vitamin B_6 (mg) 0.05
Sugar (g) 18.4	Fish (oz) 0	Folic Acid (mcg) 18.8
Protein (g) 11.5	Nuts (oz) 0	Vitamin B_{12} (mcg) 0.48

Warm Teriyaki Beef with Pea Shoots

Preparation time: Ten minutes	Four servings
Cooking time: Six minutes; standing time: five minutes	313 calories per serving, 38 percent from fat

RealAge effect if eaten twelve times a year: Our special Asian Beef provides a whopping 136 mcg of folate, making your RealAge 2.8 days younger.

RealAge effect ingredients: Salad greens, pea shoots, baby corn (calcium, potassium, folic acid, healthy protein, healthy fats)

INGREDIENTS

⅓ cup light teriyaki sauce, such as Kikkoman brand

2 teaspoons dark sesame oil

1 pound well-trimmed boneless beef top sirloin steak, cut 1 inch thick

1 tablespoon rice wine or cider vinegar

6 cups packed mesclun salad mix or torn salad greens

1 cup pea shoots

One 8¾-ounce can whole baby corn, such as Dynasty brand, drained

½ cup corn nuts

PREPARATION

Combine teriyaki sauce and sesame oil. Spoon 2 tablespoons of the mixture over both sides of steak; let stand five minutes.

Combine remaining teriyaki mixture and vinegar; set aside. Prepare a charcoal or gas grill, or heat a ridged grill pan over medium-high heat until hot. Add steak; grill or pan sear two to three minutes per side for rare steak or longer to desired doneness. Transfer to a carving board; let stand five minutes.

Toss mesclun with 3 tablespoons of the reserved teriyaki mixture; transfer to serving plates and top with pea shoots. Cut steak crosswise into ⅛-inch thick slices; arrange over salad. Arrange four baby corncobs around edges of salad, forming a "box." Sprinkle corn nuts over beef and drizzle remaining reserved teriyaki mixture over all.

SUBSTITUTIONS

Sunflower seed sprouts or mung bean sprouts may replace the pea shoots—you will get a more intense bean flavor. Salted, roasted soy nuts may replace the corn nuts. In the summer, look for fresh whole baby corn in your supermarket produce section to replace the canned corn.

TIPS

Using a marinade to serve more than one purpose—meat tenderizer, flavor enhancer, and salad dressing—is an easy way to make your work go further. Look for ways to do this in other dishes as well.

NUTRITIONAL ANALYSIS

Total Fat (g) 13.3	Sodium (mg) 587	Vitamin A (RE) 228
Fat Calories (kc) 120	Calcium (mg) 61	Beta-carotene (RE) 1354
Cholesterol (mg) 76	Magnesium (mg) 68	Vitamin C (mg) 15
Saturated Fat (g) 4.1	Zinc (mg) 6.0	Vitamin E (mg) 1.0
Polyunsaturated Fat (g) 1.9	Selenium (mcg) 30	Thiamin B_1 (mg) 0.2
Monounsaturated Fat (g) 5.6	Potassium (mg) 816	Riboflavin B_2 (mg) 0.5
Fiber (g) 3.8	Flavonoids (mg) 1.2	Niacin B_3 (mg) 4.3
Carbohydrates (g) 19.1	Lycopene (mg) 0	Vitamin B_6 (mg) 0.72
Sugar (g) 4.7	Fish (oz) 0	Folic Acid (mcg) 136
Protein (g) 30	Nuts (oz) 1.0	Vitamin B_{12} (mcg) 3.24

Key References

Aging

Fraser, G. E., Lindsted, K. D., and Beeson, W. L. "Effect of Risk Factor Values on Lifetime Risk of and Age at First Coronary Event. The Adventist Health Study." *American Journal of Epidemiology* 142 (1995):746–58.

Gaziano, J. M. "When Should Heart Disease Prevention Begin?" *New England Journal of Medicine* 338 (1998):1690–92.

Kant, A. K., Schatzkin, A., Graubard, B. I., and Schairer, C. "A Prospective Study of Diet Quality and Mortality in Women." *Journal of the American Medical Association* 283 (2000):2109–15.

Lee, C. K., Klopp, R. G., Weindruch, R., and Prolla, T. A. "Gene Expression Profile of Aging and Its Retardation by Caloric Restriction." *Science* 285 (1999):1390–93.

Stampfer, M. J., Hu, F. B., Manson, J. E., Rimm, E. B., and Willett, W. C. "Primary Prevention of Coronary Heart Disease in Women through Diet and Lifestyle." *New England Journal of Medicine* 343 (2000):16–22.

Vaupel, J. W., Carey, J. R., Christensen, K., Johnson, T. E., Yashin, A. I., Holm, N. V., Iachine, I. A., Kannisto, V., Khazaeli, A. A., Liedo, P., Longo, V. D., Zeng, Y., Manton, K. G., and Curtsinger, J. W. "Biodemographic Trajectories of Longevity." *Science* 280 (1998):855–60.

Vita, A. J., Terry, R. B., Hubert, H. B., and Fries, J. F. "Aging, Health Risks, and Cumulative Disability." *New England Journal of Medicine* 338 (1998):1035–41.

Wright, J. C., and Weinstein, M. C. "Gains in Life Expectancy from Medical Interventions—Standardizing Data on Outcomes." *New England Journal of Medicine* 339 (1998):380–86.

Alcohol

Bobak, M., Skodova, Z., and Marmot, M. "Effect of Beer Drinking on Risk of Myocardial Infarction: Population Based Case-Control Study." *British Medical Journal* 320 (2000):1378–79.

Fuchs, C. S., Stampfer, M. J., Colditz, G. A., Giovannucci, E. L., Manson, J. E., Kawachi, I., Hunter, D. J., Hankinson, S. E., Hennekens, C. H., and Rosner, B. "Alcohol Consumption and Mortality among Women." *New England Journal of Medicine* 332 (1995):1245–50.

Solomon, C. G., Hu, F. B., Stampfer, M. J., Colditz, G. A., Speizer, F. E., Rimm, E. B., Willett, W. C., and Manson, J. E. "Moderate Alcohol Consumption and Risk of Coronary Heart Disease among Women with Type 2 Diabetes Mellitus." *Circulation* 102 (2000):494–99.

Body Mass Index

Lindsted, K., Tonstad, S., and Kusma, J. W. "Body Mass Index and Patterns of Mortality among Seventh-Day Adventist Men." *International Journal of Obesity* 15 (1991):397–406.

Breakfast

Kaplan, G. A., Seeman, T. E., Cohen, R. D., Knudson, L. P., and Guralnik, J. "Mortality among the Elderly in the Alameda County Study: Behavioral and Demographic Risk Factors." *American Journal of Public Health* 77 (1987):307–12.

Diet and Diseases

Campbell, L. V., Marmot, P. E., Dyer, J. A., Borkman, M., and Storlien, L. H. "The High-Monounsaturated Fat Diet as a Practical Alternative for NIDDM." *Diabetes Care* 17 (1994):177–82.

Graves, P. L., Thomas, C. B., and Mead, L. A. "Familial and Psychological Predictors of Cancer." *Cancer Detection and Prevention* 15 (1991):59–64.

Haffner, S. M., Lehto, S., Ronnemaa, T., Pyorala, K., and Laakso, M. "Mortality from Coronary Heart Disease in Subjects with Type 2 Diabetes and in Nondiabetic Subjects with and without Prior Myocardial Infarction." *New England Journal of Medicine* 339 (1998):229–34.

Hu, F. B., Stampfer, M. J., Manson, J. E., Grodstein, F., Colditz, G. A., Speizer, F. E., and Willett, W. C. "Trends in the Incidence of Coronary Heart Disease and Changes in Diet and Lifestyle in Women." *New England Journal of Medicine* 343 (2000):530–37.

Janne, P. A., and Mayer, R. J. "Chemoprevention of Colorectal Cancer." *New England Journal of Medicine* 342 (2000):1960–68.

Lichtenstein, P., Holm, N. V., Verkasalo, P. K., Iliadou, A., Kaprio, J., Koskenvuo, M., Pukkala, E., Skytthe, A., and Hemminki, K. "Environmental and Heritable Factors in the Causation of Cancer—Analyses of Cohorts of Twins from Sweden, Denmark, and Finland." *New England Journal of Medicine* 343 (2000):78–85.

Lynch, J. W., Kaplan, G. A., and Shema, S. J. "Cumulative Impact of Sustained Economic Hardship on Physical, Cognitive, Psychological, and Social Functioning." *New England Journal of Medicine* 337 (1997):1889–95.

Parillo, M., Rivellese, A. A., Ciardullo, A. V., Capaldo, B., Giacco, A., Genovese, S., and Riccardi, G. "A High-Monounsaturated-Fat/Low-Carbohydrate Diet Improves Peripheral Insulin Sensitivity in Non-Insulin-Dependent Diabetic Patients." *Metabolism* 41 (1992):1373–78.

Saito, I., Folsom, A. R., Brancati, F. L., Duncan, B. B., Chambless, L. E., and McGovern, P. G. "Nontraditional Risk Factors for Coronary Heart Disease Incidence among Persons with Diabetes: The Atherosclerosis Risk in Communities (ARIC) Study." *Annals of Internal Medicine* 133 (2000):81–91.

Simopoulos, A. P. "Essential Fatty Acids in Health and Chronic Disease." *American Journal of Clinical Nutrition* 70 suppl (1999):560S–69S.

Steinmetz, K. A., and Potter, J. D. "Vegetables, Fruit, and Cancer. II. Mechanisms." *Cancer Causes and Control* 2 (1991):427–42.

Diet Diversity

Kant, A. K., Schatzkin, A., and Ziegler, R. G. "Dietary Diversity and Subsequent Cause-Specific Mortality in the NHANES I Epidemiologic Follow-Up Study." *Journal of the American College of Nutrition* 14 (1995):233–38.

Fat in the Diet

Carroll, K. K., and Khor, H. T. "Dietary Fat in Relation to Tumorigenesis." *Progress in Biochemical Pharmacology* 10 (1975):308–53.

Hoerger, T. J., Bala, M. V., Bray, J. W., Wilcosky, T. C., and LaRosa, J. "Treatment Patterns and Distribution of Low-Density Lipoprotein Cholesterol Levels in Treatment-Eligible United States Adults." *American Journal of Cardiology* 82 (1998):61–65.

Hu, F. B., Stampfer, M. J., Manson, J. E., Rimm, E., Colditz, G. A., Rosner, B. A., Hennekens, C. H., and Willett, W. C. "Dietary Fat Intake and the Rise of Coronary Heart Disease in Women." *New England Journal of Medicine* 337 (1997):1491–99.

Hu, F. B., Stampfer, M. J., Rimm, E. B., Manson, J. E., Ascherio, A., Colditz, G. A., Rosner, B. A., Spiegelman, D., Speizer, F. E., Sacks, F. M., Hennekens, C. H., and Willett, W. C. "A Prospective Study of Egg Consumption and Risk of Cardiovascular Disease in Men and Women." *Journal of the American Medical Association* 281(1999):1387–94.

Hunt, J. N., Smith, J. L., and Jiang, C. L. "Effect of Meal Volume and Energy Density on the Gastric Emptying of Carbohydrates." *Gastroenterology* 89 (1985):1326–30.

Moore, J. G., Christian, P. E., and Coleman, R. E. "Gastric Emptying of Varying Meal Weight and Composition in Man. Evaluation by Dual Liquid- and Solid-Phase Isotopic Method." *Digestive Diseases and Sciences* 26 (1981):16–22.

Shekelle, R. B., Shryock, A. M., Paul, O., Lepper, M., Stamler, J., Liu, S., and Raynor, W. J. Jr. "Diet, Serum Cholesterol, and Death from Coronary Heart Disease. The Western Electric Study." *New England Journal of Medicine* 304 (1981):65–70.

Stamler, J., and Shekelle, R. "Dietary Cholesterol and Human Coronary Heart Disease. The Epidemiologic Evidence." *Archives of Pathology and Laboratory Medicine* 112 (1988):1032–40.

Wardle, J., Rogers, P., Judd, P., Taylor, M. A., Rapoport, L., Green, M., and Nicholson Perry, K. "Randomized Trial of the Effects of Cholesterol-Lowering Dietary Treatment on Psychological Function." *American Journal of Medicine* 108 (2000):547–53.

Fiber and Grain

Ascherio, A., Rimm, E. B., Giovannucci, E. L., Spiegelman, D., Stampfer, M., and Willett, W. C. "Dietary Fat and Risk of Coronary Heart Disease in Men: Cohort Follow Up Study in the United States." *British Medical Journal* 313 (1996):84–90.

Jacobs, D. R. Jr., Meyer, K. A., Kushi, L. H., and Folsom, A. R. "Is Whole Grain Intake Associated with Reduced Total and Cause-Specific Death Rates in Older Women? The Iowa Women's Health Study." *American Journal of Public Health* 89 (1999):322–29.

Key, T. J., Thorogood, M., Appleby, P. N., and Burr, M. L. "Dietary Habits and Mortality in 11,000 Vegetarians and Health Conscious People: Results of a 17 Year Follow Up." *British Medical Journal* 313 (1996):775–79.

Khaw, K. T., and Barrett-Connor, E. "Dietary Fiber and Reduced Ischemic Heart Disease Mortality Rates in Men and Women: A 12-Year Prospective Study." *American Journal of Epidemiology* 126 (1987):1093–102.

Pietinen, P., Ascherio, A., Korhonen, P., Hartman, A. M., Willett, W. C., Albanes, D., and Virtamo, J. "Intake of Fatty Acids and Risk of Coronary Heart Disease in a Cohort of Finnish Men. The Alpha-Tocopherol, Beta-Carotene Cancer Prevention Study." *American Journal of Epidemiology* 145 (1997):876–87.

Thun, M. J., Calle, E. E., Namboodiri, M. M., Flanders, W. D., Coates, R. J., Byers, T., Boffetta, P., Garfinkel, L., and Heath, C. W. Jr. "Risk Factors for Fatal Colon Cancer in a Large Prospective Study." *Journal of the National Cancer Institute* 84 (1992):1491–500.

Todd, S., Woodward, M., Tunstall-Pedoe, H., and Bolton-Smith, C. "Dietary Antioxidant Vitamins and Fiber in the Etiology of Cardiovascular Disease and All-Causes Mortality: Results from the Scottish Heart Health Study." *American Journal of Epidemiology* 150 (1999):1073–80.

Willett, W. C., Stampfer, M. J., Manson, J. E., Colditz, G. A., Speizer, F. E., Rosner, B. A., Sampson, L. A., and Hennekens, C. H. "Intake of Trans Fatty Acids and Risk of Coronary Heart Disease among Women." *Lancet* 341 (1993):581–85.

Wolk, A., Manson, J. E., Stampfer, M. J., Colditz, G. A., Hu, F. B., Speizer, F. E., Hennekens, C. H., and Willett, W. C. "Long-Term Intake of Dietary Fiber and Decreased Risk of Coronary Heart Disease among Women." *Journal of the American Medical Association* 281 (1999):1998–2004.

Fish

Daviglus, M. L., Stamler, J., Orencia, A. J., Dyer, A. R., Liu, K., Greenland, P., Walsh, M. K., Morris, D., and Shekelle, R. B. "Fish Consumption and the 30-Year Risk of Fatal Myocardial Infarction." *New England Journal of Medicine* 336 (1997):1046–53.

von Schacky, C., Angerer, P., Kothny, W., Theisen, K., and Mudra, H. "The Effect of Dietary Omega-3 Fatty Acids on Coronary Atherosclerosis. A Randomized, Double-Blind, Placebo-Controlled Trial." *Annals of Internal Medicine* 130 (1999):554–62.

Zhang, J., Sasaki, S., Amano, K., and Kesteloot, H. "Fish Consumption and Mortality from All Causes, Ischemic Heart Disease, and Stroke: An Ecological Study." *Preventative Medicine* 28 (1999):520–29.

Flavonoids

Hertog, M. G., Feskens, E. J., Hollman, P. C., Katan, M. B., and Kromhout, D. "Dietary Antioxidant Flavonoids and Risk of Coronary Heart Disease: The Zutphen Elderly Study." *Lancet* 342 (1993):1007–11.

Knekt, P., Jarvinen, R., Reunanen, A., and Maatela, J. "Flavonoid Intake and Coronary Mortality in Finland: A Cohort Study." *British Medical Journal* 312 (1996):478–81.

Yochum, L., Kushi, L. H., Meyer, K., and Folsom, A. R. "Dietary Flavonoid Intake and Risk of Cardiovascular Disease in Postmenopausal Women." *American Journal of Epidemiology* 149 (1999):943–49.

Folate

Pancharuniti, N., Lewis, C. A., Sauberlich, H. E., Perkins, L. L., Go, R. C., Alvarez, J. O., Macaluso, M., Acton, R. T., Copeland, R. B., Cousins, A. L., et al. "Plasma Homocyst(e)ine, Folate, and Vitamin B-12 Concentrations and Risk for Early-Onset Coronary Artery Disease." *American Journal of Clinical Nutrition* 59 (1994):940–48.

Selhub, J., Jacques, P. F., Bostom, A. G., D'Agostino, R. B., Wilson, P. W., Belanger, A. J., O'Leary, D. H., Wolf, P. A., Schaefer, E. J., and Rosenberg, I. H. "Association between

Plasma Homocysteine Concentrations and Extracranial Carotid-Artery Stenosis." *New England Journal of Medicine* 332 (1995):286–91.

Fruits and Vegetables

Joshipura, K. J., Ascherio, A., Manson, J. E., Stampfer, M. J., Rimm, E. B., Speizer, F. E., Hennekens, C. H., Spiegelman, D., and Willett, W. C. "Fruit and Vegetable Intake in Relation to Risk of Ischemic Stroke." *Journal of the American Medical Association* 282 (1999):1233–39.

Patterson, B. H., Block, G., Rosenberger, W. F., Pee, D., and Kahle, L. L. "Fruits and Vegetables in the American Diet: Data from the NHANES II Survey." *American Journal of Public Health* 80 (1990):1443–49.

Rimm, E. B., Ascherio, A., Giovannucci, E., Spiegelman, D., Stampfer, M. J., and Willett, W. C. "Vegetable, Fruit, and Cereal Fiber Intake and Risk of Coronary Heart Disease among Men." *Journal of the American Medical Association* 275 (1996):447–51.

Steinmetz, K. A., Kushi, L. H., Bostick, R. M., Folsom, A. R., and Potter, J. D. "Vegetables, Fruit, and Colon Cancer in the Iowa Women's Health Study." *American Journal of Epidemiology* 139 (1994):1–15.

Ziegler, R. G. "Vegetables, Fruits, and Carotenoids and the Risk of Cancer." *American Journal of Clinical Nutrition* 53 suppl (1991):251S–59S.

Lycopene

Giovannucci, E. "Tomatoes, Tomato-Based Products, Lycopene, and Cancer: Review of the Epidemiologic Literature." *Journal of the National Cancer Institute* 91 (1999):317–31.

Kohlmeier, L., Kark, J. D., Gomez-Garcia, E., Martin, B. C., Steck, S. E., Kardinaal, A. F., Ringstad, J., Thamm, M., Masaev, V., Riemersma, R., Martin-Moreno, J. M., Huttunen, J. K., and Kok, F. J. "Lycopene and Myocardial Infarction Risk in the EURAMIC Study." *American Journal of Epidemiology* 146 (1997):618–26.

Meat

Thorogood, M., Mann, J., Appleby, P., and McPherson, K. "Risk of Death from Cancer and Ischaemic Heart Disease in Meat and Non-Meat Eaters." *British Medical Journal* 308 (1994):1667–70.

Minerals

He, J., Odgen, L. G., Vupputuri, S., Bazzano, L. A., Loria, C., and Whelton, P. K. "Dietary Sodium Intake and Subsequent Risk of Cardiovascular Disease in Overweight Adults." *Journal of the American Medical Association* 282 (1999):2027–34.

Khaw, K. T., and Barrett-Connor, E. "Dietary Potassium and Stroke-Associated Mortality: A 12-Year Prospective Population Study." *New England Journal of Medicine* 316 (1987):235–40.

Nuts

Fraser, G. E., and Shavlik, D. J. "Risk Factors for All-Cause and Coronary Heart Disease Mortality in the Oldest-Old. The Adventist Health Study." *Archives of Internal Medicine* 157 (1997):2249–58.

Hu, F. B., Stampfer, M. J., Manson, J. E., Rimm, E. B., Colditz, G. A., Rosner, B. A., Speizer, F. E., Hennekens, C. H., and Willett, W. C. "Frequent Nut Consumption and Risk of Coronary Heart Disease in Women: Prospective Cohort Study." *British Medical Journal* 317 (1998):1341–45.

Physical Activity

Blair, S. N., Kohl, H. W. III, Paffenbarger, R. S. Jr., Clark, D. G., Cooper, K. H., and Gibbons, L. W. "Physical Fitness and All-Cause Mortality. A Prospective Study of Healthy Men and Women." *Journal of the American Medical Association* 262 (1989):2395–401.

Kujala, U. M., Kaprio, J., Sarna, S., and Koskenvuo, M. "Relationship of Leisure-Time Physical Activity and Mortality. The Finnish Twin Cohort." *Journal of the American Medical Association* 279 (1998):440–44.

Paffenbarger, R. S. Jr., Hyde, R. T., Wing, A. L., Lee, I. M., Jung, D. L., and Kampert, J. B. "The Association of Changes in Physical-Activity Level and Other Lifestyle Characteristics with Mortality among Men." *New England Journal of Medicine* 328 (1993):538–45.

Paffenbarger, R. S. Jr., Kampert, J. B., Lee, I. M., Hyde, R. T., Leung, R. W., and Wing, A. L. "Changes in Physical Activity and Other Lifeway Patterns Influence Longevity." *Medicine and Science in Sports and Exercise* 26 (1994):857–65.

Sherman, S. E., D'Agostino, R. B., Silbershatz, H., and Kannel, W. B. "Comparison of Past Versus Recent Physical Activity in the Prevention of Premature Death and Coronary Artery Disease." *American Heart Journal* 138 (1999):900–7.

Stamina-Building Exercises

Blair, S. N, Kohl, H. W. III, Barlow, C. E., Paffenbarger, R. S. Jr., Gibbons, L. W., and Macera, C. A. "Changes in Physical Fitness and All-Cause Mortality. A Prospective Study of Healthy and Unhealthy Men." *Journal of the American Medical Association* 273 (1995):1093–98.

Strength-Building Exercises

Kushi, L. H., Fee, R. M., Folsom, A. R., Mink, P. J., Anderson, K. E., and Sellers, T. A. "Physical Activity and Mortality in Postmenopausal Women." *Journal of the American Medical Association* 277 (1997):1287–92.

Province, M. A., Hadley, E. C., Hornbrook, M. C., Lipsitz, L. A., Miller, J. P., Mulrow, C. D., Ory, M. G., Sattin, R. W., Tinetti, M. E., and Wolf, S. L. "The Effect of Exercise on Falls in Elderly Patients. A Preplanned Meta-Analysis of the FICSIT Trials. Frailty and Injuries: Cooperative Studies of Intervention Techniques." *Journal of the American Medical Association* 273 (1995):1341–47.

Tinetti, M. E., and Williams, C. S. "Falls, Injuries Due to Falls, and the Risk of Admission to a Nursing Home." *New England Journal of Medicine* 337 (1997):1279–84.

Protein

Hu, F. B., Stampfer, M. J., Manson, J. E., Rimm, E., Colditz, G. A., Speizer, F. E., Hennekens, C. H., and Willett, W. C. "Dietary Protein and Risk of Ischemic Heart Disease in Women." *American Journal of Clinical Nutrition* 70 (1999):221–27.

Vitamins (Diet)

Bronstrup, A., Hages, M., Prinz-Langenohl, R., and Pietrzik, K. "Effects of Folic Acid and Combinations of Folic Acid and Vitamin B-12 on Plasma Homocysteine Concentrations in Healthy, Young Women." *American Journal of Clinical Nutrition* 68 (1998):1104–10.

Giles, W. H., Kittner, S. J., Croft, J. B., Anda, R. F., Casper, M. L., and Ford, E. S. "Serum Folate and Risk for Coronary Heart Disease: Results from a Cohort of US Adults." *Annals of Epidemiology* 8 (1998):490–96.

Gloth, F. M. III, Gundberg, C. M., Hollis, B. W., Haddad, J. G. Jr., and Tobin, J. D. "Vitamin D Deficiency in Homebound Elderly Persons." *Journal of the American Medical Association* 274 (1995):1683–86.

Roodenburg, A. J., Leenen, R., van het Hof, K. H., Westrate, J. A., and Tijburg, L. B. "Amount of Fat in the Diet Affects Bioavailability of Lutein Esters But Not Alpha-Carotene, Beta-Carotene, and Vitamin E in Humans." *American Journal of Clinical Nutrition* 71 (2000):1187–93.

Yong, L. C., Brown, C. C., Schatzkin, A., Dresser, C. M., Slesinski, M. J., Cox, C. S., and Taylor, P. R. "Intake of Vitamins E, C, and A and Risk of Lung Cancer. The NHANES I Epidemiologic Followup Study. First National Health and Nutrition Examination Survey." *American Journal of Epidemiology* 146 (1997):231–43.

Vitamins (Supplements)

Enstrom, J. E., Kanim, L. E., and Klein, M. A. "Vitamin C Intake and Mortality among a Sample of the United States Population." *Epidemiology* 3 (1992):194–202.

Folsom, A. R., Nieto, F. J., McGovern, P. G., Tsai, M. Y., Malinow, M. R., Eckfeldt, J. H., Hess, D. L., and Davis, C. E. "Prospective Study of Coronary Heart Disease Incidence in Relation to Fasting Total Homocysteine, Related Genetic Polymorphisms, and B Vitamins: The Atherosclerosis Risk in Communities (ARIC) Study." *Circulation* 98 (1998):204–10.

Giovannucci, E., Stampfer, M. J., Colditz, G. A., Hunter, D. J., Fuchs, C., Rosner, B. A., Speizer, F. E., and Willett, W. C. "Multivitamin Use, Folate, and Colon Cancer in Women in the Nurses' Health Study." *Annals of Internal Medicine* 129 (1998):517–24.

Hodis, H. N., Mack, W. J., LaBree, L., Cashin-Hemphill, L., Sevanian, A., Johnson, R., and Azen, S. P. "Serial Coronary Angiographic Evidence That Antioxidant Vitamin Intake Reduces Progression of Coronary Artery Atherosclerosis." *Journal of the American Medical Association* 273 (1995):1849–54.

"NIH Consensus Conference. Optional Calcium Intake. NIH Consensus Development Panel on Optimal Calcium Intake." *Journal of the American Medical Association* 272 (1994):1942–48.

Rimm, E. B., Willett, W. C., Hu, F. B., Simpson, L., Colditz, G. A., Manson, J. E., Hennekens, C., and Stampfer, M. J. "Folate and Vitamin B6 from Diet and Supplements in

Relation to Risk of Coronary Heart Disease among Women." *Journal of the American Medical Association* 279 (1998):359–64.

Sahyoun, N. R., Jacques, P. F., and Russell, R. M. "Carotenoids, Vitamins C and E, and Mortality in an Elderly Population." *American Journal of Epidemiology* 144 (1996):501–11.

Stampfer, M. J., Hennekens, C. H., Manson, J. E., Colditz, G. A., Rosner, B., and Willett, W. C. "Vitamin E Consumption and the Risk of Coronary Disease in Women." *New England Journal of Medicine* 328 (1993):1444–49.

Watson, K. E., Abrolat, M. L., Malone, L. L., Hoeg, J. M., Doherty, T., Detrano, R., and Demer, L. L. "Active Serum Vitamin D Levels Are Inversely Correlated with Coronary Calcification." *Circulation* 96 (1997):1755–60.

Water and Beverages

Curhan, G. C., Willett, W. C., Speizer, F. E., and Stampfer, M. J. "Beverage Use and Risk for Kidney Stones in Women." *Annals of Internal Medicine* 128 (1998):534–40.

Lane, J. D., Phillips-Bute, B. G., and Pieper, C. F. "Caffeine Raises Blood Pressure at Work." *Psychosomatic Medicine* 60 (1998):327–30.

Michaud, D. S., Spiegelman, D., Clinton, S. K., Rimm, E. B., Curhan, G. C., Willett, W. C., and Giovannucci, E. L. "Fluid Intake and the Risk of Bladder Cancer in Men." *New England Journal of Medicine* 340 (1999):1390–97.

Ross, G. W., Abbott, R. D., Petrovich, H., Morens, D. M., Grandinetti, A., Tung, K. H., Tanner, C. M., Masaki, K. H., Blanchette, P. L., Curb, J. D., Popper, J. S., and White, L. R. "Association of Coffee and Caffeine Intake with the Risk of Parkinson Disease." *Journal of the American Medical Association* 283 (2000):2674–79.

Weight Management

Olson, M. B., Kelsey, S. F., Bittner, V., Reis, S. E., Reichek, N., Handberg, E. M., and Merz, C. N. "Weight Cycling and High-Density Lipoprotein Cholesterol in Women: Evidence of an Adverse Effect: A Report from the NHLBI-Sponsored WISE Study. Women's Ischemia Syndrome Evaluation Study Group." *Journal of the American College of Cardiology* 36 (2000):1565–71.

Ross, R., Dagnone, D., Jones, P. J., Smith, H., Paddags, A., Hudson, R., and Janssen, I. "Reduction in Obesity and Related Comorbid Conditions after Diet-Induced Weight Loss or Exercise-Induced Weight Loss in Men. A Randomized, Controlled Trial." *Annals of Internal Medicine* 133 (2000):92–103.

Yang, M. U., and Van Itallie, T. B. "Composition of Weight Lost during Short-Term Weight Reduction: Metabolic Responses of Obese Subjects to Starvation and Low-Calorie Ketogenic and Nonketogenic Diets." *Journal of Clinical Investigation* 58 (1976):722–30.

Index

About the Authors

Michael F. Roizen, M.D.

Michael F. Roizen, M.D., the creator of the RealAge concept, is a professor of medicine and chair of the Department of Anesthesia and Critical Care at the University of Chicago's Pritzker School of Medicine, one of the top ten departments of anesthesia in the United States. He is a fifty-five-year-old internist and anesthesiologist who lives his RealAge Reduction Plan and has a RealAge of 38.

Dr. Roizen is a Phi Beta Kappa and magna cum laude graduate of Williams College and an Alpha Omega Alpha graduate of the University of California Medical School in San Francisco. He performed his residency in internal medicine at Harvard's Beth Israel Hospital in Boston and completed a tour of duty in the Public Health Service at the National Institutes of Health in the laboratory of Irv Kopin and Nobel Prize winner Julius Axelrod.

Dr. Roizen has been a chair of a Food and Drug Administration advisory committee, an editor or associate editor of six medical journals, and an editor of the University of Chicago's *Better Health Newsletter*. He has published more than 140 peer-reviewed scientific papers, 100 textbook chapters, 30 editorials, and 3 medical books. He is a past president of the Society of Cardiovascular Anesthesiologists.

Both Dr. Roizen and Dr. Nancy Roizen, his wife, are named in the Woodward-White list of the Best Physicians in the United States.

Dr. Michael Roizen continues to practice internal medicine and uses the RealAge measurement routinely to motivate patients to healthier behaviors. He has provided medical care to numerous CEOs, seven Nobel Prize winners, and hundreds of other individuals. He is the medical director of the University of Chicago's Program for Executive Health.

His first book for readers who are not doctors was *RealAge: Are You as Young as You Can Be?*, published by Cliff Street Books, HarperCollins, in 1999. It has been translated into twenty-two languages and was number one on the *New York Times* bestseller list. Dr. Roizen has been featured on the television shows

Oprah, 20/20, Good Morning America, CBN Breakfast Club, Today, Donny and Marie, and seventy-four other national shows. His work has been featured in *Newsweek,* the *Los Angeles Times,* the *Chicago Tribune,* the *Chicago Sun Times,* the *Wall Street Journal,* the *New York Post, USA Today, Reader's Digest, Health, Men's Health, Cosmopolitan, Ladies Home Journal, Prevention, McCall's, Time, Veja, Mademoiselle, O,* and more than twenty other national magazines. More than 7 million people have learned their RealAges at the RealAge website, and 1.5 million subscribe to the RealAge "Tip of the Day" by e-mail. The RealAge health column is syndicated to forty newspapers.

John La Puma, M.D.

A board-certified internist and professionally trained chef, Dr. La Puma practices preventive internal medicine and teaches medical cooking in Chicago. He is medical director of the CHEF (Cooking, Healthy Eating, and Fitness) Clinic in Elk Grove Village, Illinois (www.CHEFClinic.com), and a professor of nutrition at Kendall College and School of the Culinary Arts in Evanston, Illinois. His calendar age is forty-four, and his RealAge is 31.

Dr. La Puma is a Phi Beta Kappa graduate of the University of California, Santa Barbara, and a graduate of Baylor College of Medicine in Houston. He performed his residency in internal medicine at the University of California at Los Angeles and the West Los Angeles Veterans Administration Medical Center. He completed the first postgraduate fellowship in the United States in clinical ethics and internal medicine at the University of Chicago's Pritzker School of Medicine. He also completed the professional cooking curriculum of the Cooking and Hospitality Institute of Chicago. For almost four years, Dr. La Puma cooked at Rick Bayless's Frontera Grill/Topolobampo once a week.

Formerly a clinical associate professor of medicine at the University of Chicago, Dr. La Puma has testified about his patients' concerns before the U.S. Senate. His work has been published in the *New England Journal of Medicine,* the *Journal of the American Medical Association,* the *New York Times,* the *Encyclopedia Britannica,* and the *Wall Street Journal.* He has authored or co-authored more than two hundred articles and book chapters and three medical books and has edited three medical books. He is a fellow of the American College of Physicians, founded and edits *Alternative Medicine Alert* (the leading newsletter in its field), and serves on the boards of *Nutrition in Clinical Care,* the *Journal of Clinical Ethics,* and *Managed Care Magazine.* He has been written about in *USA Today, Prevention,* and *Newsweek* and has appeared on PBS and NBC in Chicago. His recipes are online at www.CHEFClinic.com.

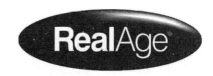